Make the Connection!

Welcome to your first leap into the study of medical language. You may be curious about the title of this book and why it is so important to "get connected." In this socially networked world, where we can organize the meaningful aspects of our lives and link them with others, it is clear that successful experiences involve making connections. Medical terminology is no different. Let us illustrate.

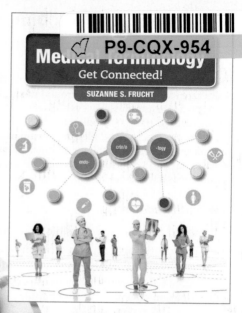

Medical Terminology is about connecting...

with peers and classmates to help you study

word parts to form medical terms

dermat/o

-logy

organs and structures that comprise body systems

with colleagues and patients for accurate medical communication

This text will give you the ability to build and interpret medical terms with accuracy and confidence. It will demonstrate the interconnectedness of body structures and systems. It will provide you with activities and online resources that will foster peer-to-peer study opportunities. And finally, it will help you acquire the tools necessary to communicate effectively in a professional healthcare environment.

So let's get connected with the features of this book.

What Makes This Book Different

You will quickly notice that this book is not arranged like most other medical terminology texts. Others present medical terms within the framework of basic human anatomy and physiology, creating a mini-A&P course. Rather, this book organizes and presents terms by medical specialty. This gives you an immediate window into how the health care world is organized—around medical specialties, and not by organ systems.

This is a true introductory-level "essentials" text focusing solely on medical terminology, and on teaching how to construct and translate medical terms. Designed to be fun, accessible, and eye-catching, it guides readers step-by-step toward mastery of relevant word parts, understanding word roots, and assembling terms. To help you learn meanings, correct spelling, pronunciation, and other components of each term, the book contains numerous exercises, tips, and colorful figures for learning and practice. It is flexible enough to be used either in support of lectures, or as a workbook to support independent study.

New for this edition

- Increased anatomy and physiology content for the organs presented in the Building Terms section.
- An augmented art program more fully illustrates the organs being described and provides visual information to correlate with the textual content.
- Reorganized Learning Objectives provide students with an up-front, quick preview of the information covered in each chapter.
- All terms and definitions have been reviewed and updated.
- Revised design uses color schemes that are more accessible to students with visual difficulties.
- Case Study and Practice Exercises have been reviewed and updated to better reinforce the Learning Objectives of each chapter.

Here is a summary of the key objectives of the book.

Describe each of the medical specialties

Each chapter in Section Two begins with a brief description of its particular medical specialty, along with some examples of healthcare workers in this specialty and some conditions that they treat.

Define relevant combining forms, suffixes, and prefixes

This section in each chapter introduces the word parts that build the terms most common to each medical specialty. Color-coded word parts (**red combining forms**, **blue suffixes**, and **green prefixes**) allow for quick recognition throughout the book.

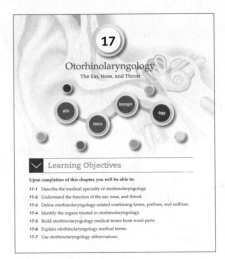

Second Edition

Medical Terminology

Get Connected!

Suzanne S. Frucht, PhD

Associate Professor Emeritus
Northwest Missouri State University
Maryville, MO

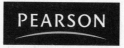

Boston   Columbus   Indianapolis   New York   San Francisco
Amsterdam   Cape Town   Dubai   London   Madrid   Milan   Munich   Paris   Montreal   Toronto
Delhi   Mexico City   São Paulo   Sydney   Hong Kong   Seoul   Singapore   Taipei   Tokyo

Publisher: Julie Levin Alexander
Publisher's Assistant: Sarah Henrich
Executive Editor: John Goucher
Program Manager: Nicole Ragonese
Editorial Assistant: Amanda Losonsky
Development Editor: Danielle Doller
Director of Marketing: David Gesell
Marketing Manager: Brittany Hammond
Marketing Specialist: Michael Sirinides
Project Management Lead: Cynthia Zonneveld
Project Manager: Patricia Gutierrez
Operations Specialist: MaryAnn Gloriande

Art Director: Andrea Nix
Text Designer: Maria Guglielmo-Walsh
Cover Designer: Wee Design Group
Cover Image 1: Soulsisz/Fotolia
Cover Image 2: Rawpixel/Shutterstock
Media Director: Amy Peltier
Lead Media Project Manager: Lorena Cerisano
Full-Service Project Management: Michelle Gardner
Composition: SPi-Global
Printer/Binder: R.R. DONNELLEY
Cover Printer: Phoenix Color/Hagerstown
Text Font: Palatino LT Pro 8.5/10.5

Credits and acknowledgments for content borrowed from other sources and reproduced, with permission, in this textbook appear on appropriate page within text.

Notice: The author and the publisher of this book have taken care to make certain that the information given is correct and compatible with the standards generally accepted at the time of publication. Nevertheless, as new information becomes available, changes in treatment and in the use of equipment and procedures become necessary. The reader is advised to carefully consult the instruction and information material included in each piece of equipment or device before administration. Students are warned that the use of any techniques must be authorized by their medical advisor, where appropriate, in accordance with local laws and regulations. The publisher disclaims any liability, loss, injury, or damage incurred as a consequence, directly or indirectly, of the use and application of any of the contents of this book.

Many of the designations by manufacturers and sellers to distinguish their products are claimed as trademarks. Where those designations appear in this book, and the publisher was aware of a trademark claim, the designations have been printed in initial caps or all caps.

Library of Congress Cataloging-in-Publication Data

Names: Frucht, Suzanne S., author.
Title: Medical terminology: get connected! / Suzanne S. Frucht.
Description: 2nd edition. | Boston: Pearson, 2016. | Includes index.
Identifiers: LCCN 2015038254 | ISBN 9780134318134
Subjects: LCSH: Medicine—Terminology.
Classification: LCC R123 .F78 2016 | DDC 610.1/4—dc23
LC record available at http://lccn.loc.gov/2015038254

10 9 8 7 6 5 4 3 2 1

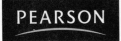

www.pearsonhighered.com

ISBN-13: 978-0-13-431813-4
ISBN-10: 0-13-431813-7

DEDICATION

*For Rikki, the classiest
and bravest woman in my life.*

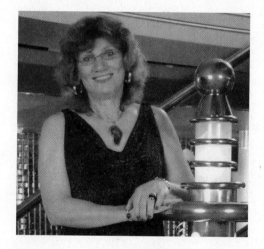

Identify organs treated by the medical specialty

Each medical specialty chapter presents a quick visual summary of the appropriate organs. To reinforce the combining forms introduced in the preceding section, this art is labeled with both the names and combining forms (**in red**) of each organ.

Build medical terms from word parts

Perhaps the heart of each chapter, this is where you will apply your knowledge. Each word part is explained and then followed by a list of phrases followed by a color-coded blank line divided by slash marks. These marks indicate how many word parts are necessary to build the term. You complete this activity by filling in the blanks as you work through this section. NEW for the second edition, more anatomy and physiology content has been provided for the organs presented in this section. This information gives more detail of the structure of each organ, how it accomplishes its functions, and how it interacts with other organs in the system.

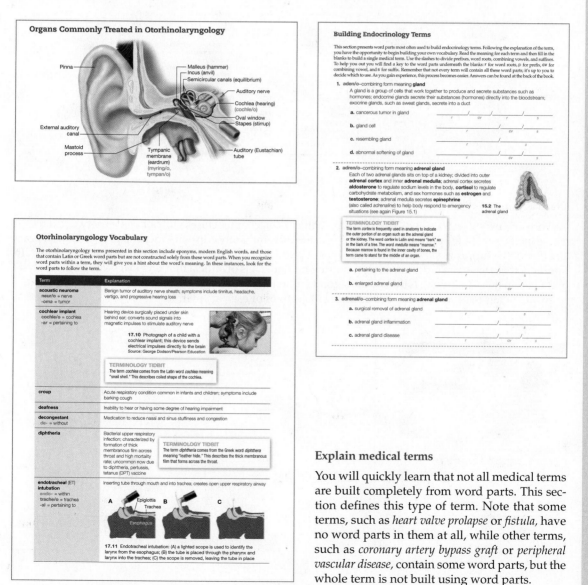

Explain medical terms

You will quickly learn that not all medical terms are built completely from word parts. This section defines this type of term. Note that some terms, such as *heart valve prolapse* or *fistula*, have no word parts in them at all, while other terms, such as *coronary artery bypass graft* or *peripheral vascular disease*, contain some word parts, but the whole term is not built using word parts.

Use abbreviations

Abbreviations are an essential part of the medical language because they save time. However, only approved abbreviations may be used in order to prevent misunderstandings. This section of each chapter presents the most commonly used abbreviations for that medical specialty.

Cardiology Abbreviations

The following list presents common cardiology abbreviations.

ACG	angiocardiography	HTN	hypertension
AF	atrial fibrillation	ICD	implantable
AS	arteriosclerosis		cardioverter defibrillator
ASCVD	arteriosclerotic cardiovascular disease	ICU	intensive care unit
		IV	intravenous
ASD	atrial septal defect	LDH	lactate dehydrogenase
ASHD	arteriosclerotic heart disease	LVH	left ventricular hypertrophy
AV, A-V	atrioventricular	MI	myocardial infarction
BP	blood pressure	mmHg	millimeters of mercury
bpm	beats per minute	MS	mitral stenosis
CABG	coronary artery bypass graft	MVP	mitral valve prolapse
CAD	coronary artery disease	NSR	normal sinus rhythm
cath	catheterization	P	pulse
CC	cardiac catheterization	PTCA	percutaneous transluminal coronary angioplasty
CCU	coronary care unit		
CHD	congestive heart disease	PVC	premature ventricular contraction
CHF	congestive heart failure	PVD	peripheral vascular disease
CK	creatine kinase	SA, S-A	sinoatrial
CP	chest pain	SGOT	serum glutamic oxaloacetic transaminase
CPR	cardiopulmonary resuscitation		
CSD	congenital septal defect	SK	streptokinase
CV	cardiovascular	SOB	shortness of breath
DVT	deep vein thrombosis	TEE	transesophageal echocardiogram
ECG	electrocardiogram	tPA	tissue plasminogen activator
ECHO	echocardiogram	V Fib	ventricular fibrillation
EKG	electrocardiogram	VSD	ventricular septal defect
GOT	glutamic oxaloacetic transaminase	VT, V-tach	ventricular tachycardia
HR	heart rate		

Practice using medical terms

As with any newly learned skill, practice is essential. Each chapter closes with a large variety of exercises. These include real-life application exercises (Case Study and Transcription Practice), pronunciation practice (Sound It Out), as well as more typical types of recall exercises (labeling, fill-in-the-blank, matching). In addition, this section includes exercises requiring higher levels of critical thinking (Medical Term Analysis and Photomatch Challenge). NEW for the second edition, these activities have been reviewed and updated to ensure better reinforcement of the Learning Objectives of each chapter.

The Total Teaching and Learning Package

We are committed to providing students and instructors with exactly the tools they need to be successful in the classroom and beyond. To this end, *Medical Terminology: Get Connected!, Second Edition* is supported by the most complete and dynamic set of resources available today.

The ultimate personalized learning tool is available at **www.mymedicalterminologylab.com.** This online course correlates with the textbook and is available for purchase separately or for a discount when packaged with the book. **MyMedicalTerminologyLab** is an immersive study experience.

MyMedicalTerminologyLab saves instructors time by providing quality feedback, ongoing individualized assessments for students, and instructor resources all in one place. It offers instructors the flexibility to make technology an integral part of their course, or a supplementary resource for students.

Visit **www.mymedicalterminologylab.com** to log in to the course or purchase access. Instructors may contact their Pearson sales representative for a demonstration or for information on discount bundle options.

Help each student learn through personalized Dynamic Study Modules

Help students study effectively on their own by continuously assessing their activity and performance in real time. Here's how it works: students complete a set of questions with a unique answer format that also asks them to indicate their confidence level. Questions repeat until the student can answer them all correctly and confidently. Once completed, Dynamic Study Modules explain the concept using materials from the text. These are available as graded assignments prior to class, and accessible on smartphones, tablets, and computers. Available for select titles.

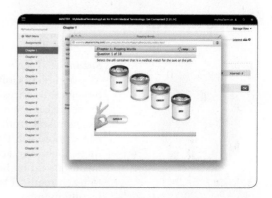

Comprehensive Instructional Package

Perhaps the most gratifying part of an educator's work is the "aha" learning moment when the light bulb goes off and a student truly understands a concept — when a connection is made. Along these lines, Pearson is pleased to help instructors foster more of these educational connections by providing a complete battery of resources to support teaching and learning. Qualified adopters are eligible to receive a wealth of materials, including a comprehensive test bank, PowerPoint lecture notes, an image library, guided lectures that can be used in class or for student self-study — all designed to help instructors prepare, present, and assess. For more information, please contact your Pearson sales representative or visit **www.pearsonhighered. com/educator**.

About the Author

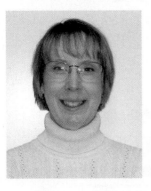

Suzanne S. Frucht was an Associate Professor of Physiology at Northwest Missouri State University (NWMSU). She holds baccalaureate degrees in biological sciences and physical therapy from Indiana University, an MS in biological sciences at NWMSU, and a PhD in molecular biology and biochemistry from the University of Missouri–Kansas City. For 14 years she worked full time as a physical therapist in various health care settings, including acute care hospitals, extended care facilities, and home health. Based on her educational and clinical experience she was invited to teach medical terminology part time in 1988 and became a full-time faculty member three years later as she discovered her love for the challenge of teaching. Before retiring in 2008, she taught a variety of courses including medical terminology, human anatomy, human physiology, and animal anatomy and physiology. She received the Governor's Award for Excellence in Teaching in 2003.

About the Illustrators

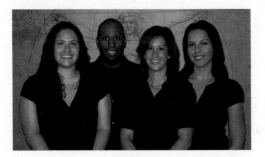

Marcelo Oliver is president and founder of Body Scientific International, LLC. He holds a master's degree in Medical and Biological Illustration from the University of Michigan. For the past 15 years, his passion has been to condense complex anatomical information into visual education tools for students, patients, and medical professionals. Body Scientific's contributing medical artists in this publication were **Carol Gudanowski, Liana Bauman**, and **Dawn Scheuerman**. Their contribution in the publication was key in the creation and editing of artwork throughout. Body Scientific invites you to visit their website at **www.bodyscientific.com**.

Acknowledgments

No textbook can ever reach the hands of students without the extraordinary contributions of numerous talented and dedicated professionals. *Medical Terminology: Get Connected!, Second Edition* is certainly no exception and I would like to take this opportunity to acknowledge their contributions.

Foremost, I would like to acknowledge Pearson Education, particularly John Goucher, Executive Editor, for his continued support. This project has benefitted from an unparalleled team, especially Nicole Ragonese, Program Manager, and I believe this second edition fulfills everyone's high expectations.

Many, many thanks go to Danielle Doller, Development Editor. Her professionalism, expertise, sound ideas, and friendship always keep me on track. I know any project I undertake is more successful because of her.

Marcello Oliver and his team of illustrators at Body Scientific International, LLC, provided the outstanding art that enhances the text. Their skills are clear everywhere in the book.

And last, but certainly not least, my utmost appreciation goes to Garnet Tomich, Quality Assurance Editor, and the myriad reviewers whose comments and suggestions at each turn helped make this second edition even better.

Without the hard work and dedication of each of these individuals, plus everyone else who has had a hand in this project, there might be a book, but certainly not this one. Words can never express my thanks.

-Suzanne Frucht

Editorial Development Team

The content and format of *Medical Terminology: Get Connected!, Second Edition* are the result of an incredible collaboration of expert educators from all around. This book represents the collective insights, experience, and thousands of hours of work performed by members of this development team. Their influence will continue to have an impact for decades to come. Let us introduce the members of our team.

Reviewers of the Second Edition

Dean Chiarelli, MA, RDN, HFS, CHES, REHS
Arizona State University
Phoenix, Arizona

Colleen Croxall, PhD
Eastern Michigan University
Ypsilanti, Michigan

Julie Hall, MPH, RT(R)(CT)(ARRT)
Roane State Community College
Oak Ridge, Tennessee

Stephen M. Johnson, MS, MT (ASCP)
Saint Vincent Hospital, School of Medical Technology
Erie, Pennsylvania

Allison Kaczmarek, MPH
University of Tampa
Tampa, Florida

Jane K. Walker, BBA, PhD, RN, CPN, CNE
Walters State Community College
Morristown, Tennessee

Amy Way, PhD
Lock Haven University
Clearfield, Pennsylvania

Barbara Worley, DPM, BS, RMA (AMT)
King's College
Charlotte, North Carolina

First Edition Reviewers

Steven G. Bassett, PhD
Seton Hill University
Greensburg, Pennsylvania

Karen Boriack, RN, BSN, MA Ed
Porterville College
Porterville, California

Ranelle Brew, EdD
Grand Valley State University
Grand Rapids, Michigan

Amanda J. Davis
Meridian Community College
Meridian, Mississippi

Dianne Davis, MS
West Virginia University
at Parkersburg
Parkersburg, West Virginia

Duane A. Dreyer, PhD
Miller-Motte College
Cary, North Carolina

Marie A. Fenske, EdD, RRT
GateWay Community College
Phoenix, Arizona

Melissa Mapp Francisco, BA, MAOM
Suwanee Hamilton Technical Center
Live Oak, Florida

Elaine Garcia, RHIT
Spokane Community College
Spokane, Washington

Krista L. Hoekstra, RN, MA
Hennepin Technical College
Brooklyn Park, Minnesota

Traci Hotard, RHFA
Louisiana Technical College
Morgan City, Louisiana

Donna M. Kubesh, BS, MA, PhD
Luther College
Decorah, Iowa

Anita Lane, MEd, OTR
Navarro College
Corsicana, Texas

Molly Lee, PhD
Harrisburg Area Community College
Harrisburg, Pennsylvania

Tricia Leggett, MSEd, RT(R)(QM)
Zane State College
Zanesville, Ohio

Sue Moe, RN
Northwest Technical College
East Grand Forks, Minnesota

Cynthia K. Moore, PhD, RD
University of Arkansas — Fayetteville
Fayetteville, Arkansas

Paulette Nitkiewicz, BSN, RN, CMA
Westmoreland County Community College
Youngwood, Pennsylvania

Tonya Oakley, BS, RT(R)
Forsyth Technical Community College
Winston-Salem, North Carolina

Michelle Parolise, MBA, OTR/L
Santa Ana College
Santa Ana, California

Karen Plawecki, PhD, RD, LDN
University of Illinois
Urbana, Illinois

Martha L. Rew, MS, RD, LD
Texas Woman's University
Denton, Texas

Michael Sells, RN, Certified Surgical Tech
Kirkwood Community College
Cedar Rapids, Iowa

Don Steinert, MA, RRT, MT, CLS
University of the District of Columbia
Washington, D.C.

Halcyon Watkins, BS, DVM
Prairie View A&M University
Prairie View, Texas

Amy Way, PhD
Lock Haven University
Clearfield, Pennsylvania

Sherry B. Wilson, RN, MSN
Durham Technical Community College
Durham, North Carolina

Medical Terminology Advisory Board

Jeff Anderson, MA, RRT
Boise State University
Boise, Idaho

Beverly Bartholomew, MEd, CPC
Wake Tech Community College
Raleigh, North Carolina

Amy Bolinger Snow, MS
Greenville Technical College
Greenville, South Carolina

Richard Brown, MS, CPhT/RPT
Program Chair, MAA/MOBS
Ultimate Medical Academy
Clearwater, Florida

Kerry Cirillo, MS, BS
Mildred Elley
New York, New York

Rosana Darang, MD, Dept. Chair
Bay State College
Boston, Massachusetts

Robert Fanger, MSEd
Del Mar College
Corpus Christi, Texas

Gerry Gordon, BA CPC, CPB
Daytona College
Ormond Beach, Florida

Timothy J. Jones, BA, MA (English), MA (Classics)
Oklahoma City Community College
Oklahoma City, Oklahoma
The University of Oklahoma
Norman, Oklahoma

Tammie Petersen, RNC, BSN
Austin Community College
Austin, Texas

Focus Group Members

Edward W. Kolk, DPM
Suffolk Community College
Brentwood, New York

Glenn Ross
The College of Westchester
White Plains, New York

Denise Vill'neuve, MA, RT(R)(CT)(M)
County College of Morris
Randolph, New Jersey

A Commitment to Accuracy

As a learner embarking on a career in health care, you probably already know how critically important it is to be precise in your work. Patients and co-workers will be counting on you to avoid errors on a daily basis. Likewise, we owe it to you—the reader—to ensure accuracy in this book. We have gone to great lengths to verify that the information provided in *Medical Terminology: Get Connected!, Second Edition* is complete and correct. To this end, here are the steps we have taken:

1. Editorial review—We have assembled a large team of developmental consultants to critique every word and every image in this book. In addition, some members of our developmental team were specifically assigned to focus on the precision of each illustration that appears in the book.

2. Medical Illustrations—A team of medically trained illustrators was hired to prepare each piece of art that graces the pages of this book. These illustrators have a higher level of scientific education than the artists for most textbooks, and they worked directly with the author and members of our development team to make sure that their work was clear, correct, and consistent with what is described in the text.

3. Accurate Ancillaries—The teaching and learning ancillaries are often as important to instruction as the textbook itself. Therefore we took steps to ensure accuracy and consistency of these components by reviewing every ancillary component.

While our intent and actions have been directed at creating an error-free text, we have established a process for correcting any mistakes that may have slipped past our editors. Pearson takes this issue seriously and therefore welcomes any and all feedback that you can provide along the lines of helping us enhance the accuracy of this text. If you identify any errors that need to be corrected in a subsequent printing, please send them to:

Pearson Education
Medical Terminology Corrections/Health Science
221 River Street, Hoboken NJ 07030

Thank you for helping Pearson reach its goal of providing the most accurate medical terminology textbooks available.

CONTENTS

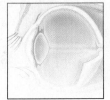
*Glossary can be found online at www.mymedicalterminologylab.com

1

Introduction to Medical Terminology

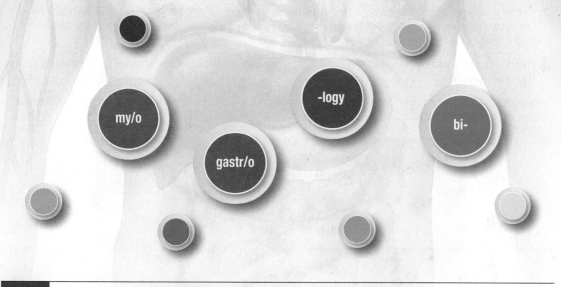

Learning Objectives

Upon completion of this chapter, you will be able to:

1-1 Identify the three types of medical terms.

1-2 Explain the differences between prefixes, suffixes, word roots, and combining vowels.

1-3 Form combining forms.

1-4 Explain how to analyze (build and interpret) medical terms.

1-5 Describe how to pluralize medical terms.

1-6 Understand how to pronounce medical terms.

A Brief Introduction to Medical Terminology

In our daily lives, each of us is surrounded by medical terminology. Of course, health care professionals use it to communicate with each other (Figure 1.1), but every person is exposed to these terms whether in the doctor's office, talking with friends, reading the newspaper, or watching television. Using medical terminology is an efficient method of conveying very specific and important information. Because each term has a precise meaning, detailed information can be quickly shared using only a few words. Therefore, everyone has something to gain from learning how to understand and use medical terminology whether in your professional or personal life.

There are three common types of medical terms:

1. Terms built from **Latin** and **Greek** word parts; examples are *cardiology* and *tonsillectomy*.

2. Terms based on a person's name, called **eponyms**; examples are Alzheimer disease and Parkinson disease. The current trend in writing eponyms is away from using the possessive form of the person's name; this text will follow that practice.

3. Terms utilizing **modern English** words; examples are *magnetic resonance imaging* and *irritable bowel syndrome.*

Without doubt, the majority of medical terms are based on Latin and Greek word parts. The remainder of this chapter teaches you how to build and analyze this type of medical term.

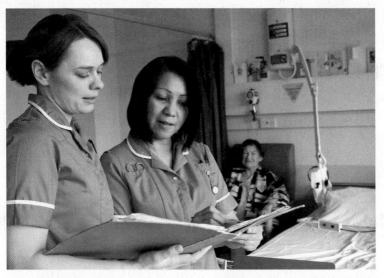

1.1 A nurse and medical assistant review a patient's chart and plan her daily care
Source: Life in View/Science Source

Elements of Latin- and Greek-Based Medical Terms

Learning medical terminology is similar to learning a foreign language because the basis for the majority of medical terms is Latin or Greek. In mastering this "language of medicine" you will:

- Begin by memorizing individual word parts
- Learn to analyze and build terms from word parts
- Gain skill and confidence through repetitious use of terms
- Make these terms a permanent part of your professional vocabulary.

Latin- and Greek-based medical terms are constructed using word parts from four different categories: **word roots**, **suffixes**, **prefixes**, and **combining vowels**.

Word Roots

The word root is the foundation of most medical terms and gives the essential meaning of the term. It frequently but not always refers to a body structure, organ, or system. See examples in Table 1.1.

Table 1.1 Examples of Word Roots

Word Root	Meaning
arthr	joint
carcin	cancer
cardi	heart
cephal	head
electr	electricity
gastr	stomach
hepat	liver
my	muscle
oste	bone
rhin	nose

Suffixes

A suffix is found at the end of a medical term. The type of information it provides includes conditions, diseases, surgical procedures, and diagnostic procedures involving the word root. See examples in Table 1.2. To help you recognize **suffixes** in this text, they are color-coded in blue. *Note that when a suffix is written by itself, a hyphen is placed at the front.*

Table 1.2 Examples of Suffixes

Suffix	Meaning	Used in Medical Term	Meaning of Medical Term
-ectomy	surgical removal	gastrectomy	surgical removal of stomach
-gram	record or picture	electrocardiogram	record of heart's electrical (activity)
-itis	inflammation	arthritis	joint inflammation
-logy	study of	cardiology	study of the heart
-megaly	enlarged	hepatomegaly	enlarged liver
-pathy	disease	myopathy	muscle disease

Prefixes

A prefix is found at the beginning of a medical term. It often indicates information such as abnormal conditions, numbers, positions, or times. See examples in Table 1.3. Many medical terms do not have a prefix. To help you recognize **prefixes** in this text, they are color-coded in green. *Note that when a prefix is written by itself, a hyphen is placed at the end.*

Table 1.3 Examples of Prefixes

Prefix	Meaning	Used in Medical Term	Meaning of Medical Term
a-	without	apnea	without breathing
bi-	two	bilateral	two sides
dys-	abnormal, difficult, painful	dysuria	painful or difficult urination
inter-	between	intervertebral	between vertebrae
post-	after	postsurgical	after surgery
sub-	under, beneath	subcutaneous	underneath the skin

Combining Vowels

Combining vowels are used for two reasons: to connect word parts and to make medical terms easier to spell and pronounce. Combining vowels are placed either between a word root and suffix or between two word roots. They are not used between a prefix and word root. See Table 1.4 for examples. *Note that the slashes (/) are used to divide the term into its word parts.*

Table 1.4 Examples of the Use of Combining Vowels

Term with Combining Vowels	Meaning
electr/o/cardi/o/gram	record of heart's electrical (activity)
hepat/o/megaly	enlarged liver
oste/o/arthr/itis	bone and joint inflammation
rhin/o/plasty	surgical repair of the nose

However, combining vowels are *not* always necessary.

- To decide whether one is needed between a word root and suffix, you must look at the first letter of the suffix. Do *not* use a combining vowel between a word root and suffix if the suffix begins in a vowel. For example, the correct way to combine the word root **arthr** and the suffix **-itis** is *arthr/itis*, not *arthr/o/itis*.
- Place a combining vowel between two word roots, even if the second word root begins with a vowel. The term *gastr/o/enter/o/logy* is correct, while *gastr/enter/o/logy* is incorrect.

Combining Forms

Combining forms consist of a word root and its combining vowel. Throughout this text, combining forms will be written with a slash (/) between the two word parts. For example, **electr/o** is the combining form meaning electricity. See Figure 1.2 for more examples of combining forms in the body. To help you recognize **combining forms** in this text, they are color-coded in red.

A combining form is not another category of word part because it consists of two other word parts. However, word roots are normally presented as combining forms; these are easier to pronounce and therefore, to remember. Word roots will be given as combining forms throughout this text.

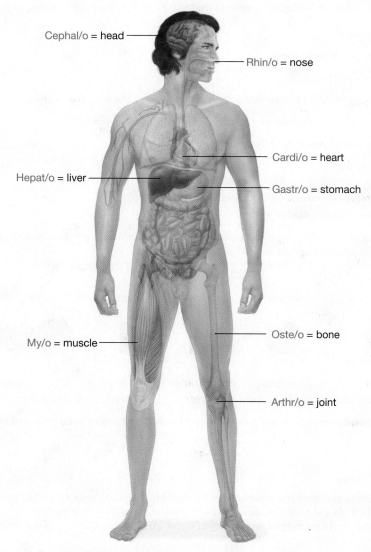

Cephal/o = head

Rhin/o = nose

Cardi/o = heart

Hepat/o = liver

Gastr/o = stomach

Oste/o = bone

My/o = muscle

Arthr/o = joint

1.2 Common combining forms for body organs

Strategies for Analyzing Medical Terms

Using medical terms is a two-way street; you will need to learn both how to define medical terms used by other people and how to build medical terms for yourself. There are some specific strategies that will help you learn both.

Defining Medical Terms

When you first encounter an unfamiliar medical term, don't panic! Remember that the meaning of the individual word parts will give you the information needed to understand at least the basic meaning of the word.

Follow these simple steps:

1. Divide the term into its word parts.

2. Define each word part.

3. Put the meaning of the word parts together in order to see what the term is describing.

For example, follow the steps to define the term *dysmenorrhea*.

1. Divide the term into its word parts: dys / men / o / rrhea

2. Define each word part
   - **dys-** → prefix meaning abnormal, difficult, painful
   - **men/o** → combining form meaning menses, menstruation
   - **-rrhea** → suffix meaning discharge, flow

3. Put the meaning of individual word parts together: abnormal, difficult, or painful menstrual flow. See Figure 1.3 for an overview of this process.

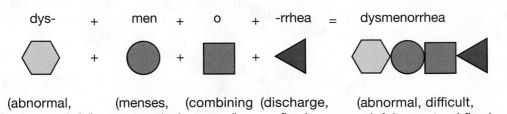

1.3 You can figure out the meaning of a medical term by dividing it into its word parts and then defining each part

Building Medical Terms

Building medical terms is almost the reverse of defining them. Begin by selecting word parts that convey the meaning needed. Then place the word parts in the correct order to build a complete term.

For example, build a term for the phrase *fibrous skin tumor*. First, choose word parts that represent each portion of the phrase.

- combining form, *fibr/o*, means *fibrous*
- combining form, *dermat/o*, means *skin*
- suffix, *-oma*, means *tumor, mass*

Then place these word parts in the correct order to complete the whole term: *dermatofibroma*.

It is important to realize that not all possible combinations of word parts will build actual medical terms used by medical professionals. When first learning to build medical terms, this is very frustrating, but do not give up! After working with medical terms for only a short period of time, you will find making correct choices gets easier and easier.

Rules for Building Plurals

Latin- and Greek-style medical terms do not follow the same pluralization rules used in English. Refer to the rules presented in Table 1.5 when deciding how to pluralize medical terms.

Table 1.5   Rules for Pluralizing Medical Terms

If the Word Ends In	Singular	Plural
–a, keep –a and add –e	vertebra	vertebrae
–ax, drop –x and add –ces	thorax	thoraces
–ex, drop –ex and add –ices	apex	apices
–is, drop –is and add –es	metastasis	metastases
–ix, drop –x and add –ces	appendix	appendices
–ma, keep –ma and add –ta	sarcoma	sarcomata
–on, drop –on and add –a	spermatozoon	spermatozoa
–us, drop –us and add –i	alveolus	alveoli
–um, drop –um and add –a	ovum	ova
–x, drop –x and add –ges	phalanx	phalanges
–y, drop –y and add –ies	biopsy	biopsies

Pronouncing Medical Terms

Often medical terms are difficult to pronounce because the word parts are unfamiliar to us, or they contain letter combinations that do not occur in English words. Refer to Table 1.6 for hints to pronounce these letter combinations. Refer to the audio glossary at www.mymedicalterminologylab.com for a phonetic pronunciation of each term presented in this text. Any syllable that should be stressed is written in uppercase.

Table 1.6 Hints for Pronouncing Medical Terms

Hint	Examples
-ae or -oe, pronounce only second letter	bursae (BER-see) coelom (SEE-loam)
c and g have soft sound if followed by e, i, or y	cerebrum (ser-REE-brum) gingivitis (jin-jih-VIGH-tis)
c and g have hard sound if followed by other letters	cardiac (CAR-dee-ak) gastric (GAS-trik)
ch- at beginning of word has hard k sound	cholesterol (koh-LES-ter-all) chemical (KEM-ih-call)
-e or -es at end of word pronounced as separate syllable	syncope (SIN-koh-pee) nares (NAIR-eez)
-i at end of word pronounced "eye"	bronchi (BRONG-keye) nuclei (NOO-clee-eye)
pn- at beginning of word, pronounce only n	pneumonia (noo-MOH-nee-ah) pneumogram (NOO-moe-gram)
pn in middle of word, pronounce hard p and hard n	tachypnea (tak-ip-NEE-ah) hypopnea (high-POP-nee-ah)
ps- at beginning of word, pronounce only s	psychiatry (sigh-KIGH-ah-tree) psychology (sigh-KOL-oh-jee)

PRACTICE

Recognizing Types of Medical Terms

Indicate whether each of the medical terms below is a Latin/Greek term, eponym, or modern English term.

1. hepatitis _____

2. ball and socket _____

3. Bell palsy _____

4. arthrogram _____

5. cardiomegaly _____

6. Addison disease _____

7. activities of daily living _____

8. Hodgkin disease _____

9. pacemaker _____

10. gastritis _____

Forming Plurals

Fill in the following blanks with the missing singular or plural form of the term.

Singular	Plural
1. bursa	_____
2. diverticulum	_____
3. _____	adenomata
4. ganglion	_____
5. index	_____
6. _____	diagnoses
7. _____	alveoli

Practice Defining Medical Terms

These medical terms have already been subdivided into their word parts. Each word part has been defined for you. First, label each word part as a prefix, word root, suffix, or combining vowel. Then put together the meanings of all the word parts to define the term.

1. encephal/o/malacia
   * **encephal** is a _____ meaning brain
   * **o** is a _____
   * **-malacia** is a _____ meaning abnormal softening
   * *encephalomalacia* means _____

2. sub/cutane/ous
   * **sub-** is a _____ meaning beneath, under
   * **cutane** is a _____ meaning skin
   * **-ous** is a _____ meaning pertaining to
   * *subcutaneous* means _____

3. hyster/o/pexy
   * **hyster** is a _____ meaning uterus
   * **o** is a _____
   * **-pexy** is a _____ meaning surgical fixation
   * *hysteropexy* means _____

4. pan/sinus/itis
   - **pan-** is a _____ meaning all
   - **sinus** is a _____ meaning sinus
   - **-itis** is a _____ meaning inflammation
   - *pansinusitis* means _____

5. angi/o/rrhaphy
   - **angi** is a _____ meaning vessel
   - **o** is a _____
   - **-rrhaphy** is a _____ meaning to suture
   - *angiorrhaphy* means _____

6. inter/ventricul/ar
   - **inter-** is a _____ meaning between
   - **ventricul** is a _____ meaning ventricle
   - **-ar** is a _____ meaning pertaining to
   - *interventricular* means _____

Practice Building Medical Terms

Use the following list of word parts to build a medical term for each definition. The blanks following each definition provide an outline of the term showing the placement of prefixes, word roots, combining vowels, and suffixes.

Term	Category	Meaning
-ar	suffix	pertaining to
arthr	word root	joint
intra-	prefix	within
-logy	suffix	study of
laryng	word root	voice box
muscul	word root	muscle
neur	word root	nerve
o	combining vowel	
-oma	suffix	tumor, mass
ophthalm	word root	eye
-plasty	suffix	surgical repair
scapul	word root	shoulder blade
-scope	suffix	instrument for viewing
sub-	prefix	beneath, under

1. surgical repair of the voice box _____/_____/_____

2. instrument for viewing a joint _____/_____/_____

3. pertaining to under the shoulder blade _____/_____/_____

4. study of the eye _____/_____/_____

5. nerve tumor _____/_____

6. pertaining to within a muscle _____/_____/_____

MyMedicalTerminologyLab™

MyMedicalTerminologyLab is a premium online homework management system that includes a host of features to help you study. Registered users will find:

- A multitude of activities and assignments built within the MyLab platform
- Powerful tools that track and analyze your results—allowing you to create a personalized learning experience
- Videos and audio pronunciations to help enrich your progress
- Streaming lesson presentations and self-paced learning modules
- A space where you and your instructors can view and manage your assignments

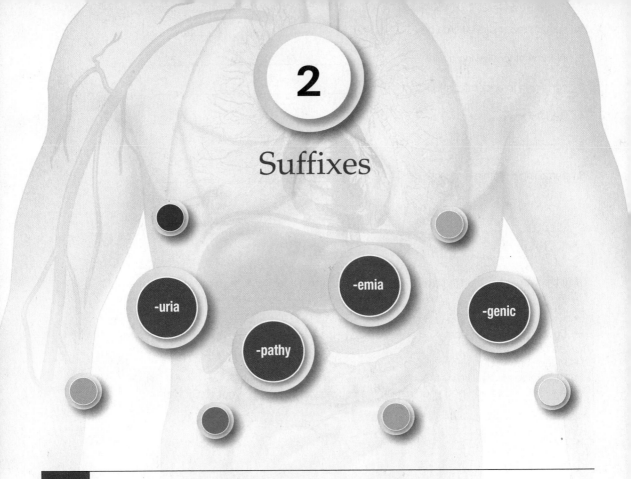

2

Suffixes

-uria

-emia

-pathy

-genic

⌄ Learning Objectives

Upon completion of this chapter, you will be able to:

2-1 Explain the role of suffixes in building medical terms.

2-2 Use suffixes to indicate diseases or abnormal conditions.

2-3 Use suffixes to indicate surgical procedures.

2-4 Use suffixes to indicate diagnostic procedures.

2-5 Use general suffixes to build additional medical terms.

2-6 Use suffixes to indicate medical specialties or personnel.

2-7 Use suffixes to convert word roots into adjectives.

A Brief Introduction to Suffixes

A suffix on the end of a medical term adds specific meaning to the term. All medical terms built from Latin or Greek word parts must have a suffix. Changing the suffix added to a term changes the meaning of the entire term. This can be illustrated with the combining form for heart, *cardi/o*.

- **cardi/o** + **-logy** = *cardiology* meaning *study of heart*
- **cardi/o** + **-dynia** = *cardiodynia* meaning *heart pain*
- **cardi/o** + **-megaly** = *cardiomegaly* meaning *enlarged heart*

Most suffixes are not associated with only one medical specialty or body system. Therefore, you will use many of the same suffixes with each new set of combining forms introduced in each chapter of this text. Suffixes can be placed into one of several categories. The following list makes learning them easier by subdividing them into smaller groups:

- Suffixes indicating diseases or abnormal conditions
- Suffixes indicating a surgical procedure
- Suffixes indicating a diagnostic procedure
- General suffixes
- Suffixes indicating medical specialties or personnel
- Suffixes that convert word roots into adjectives

Suffixes Indicating Diseases or Abnormal Conditions

Added to a word root, the following suffixes are used to indicate a diseased state or body abnormality.

Suffix	Meaning	Example (Translation)
-algia	pain	gastralgia (stomach pain)
-asthenia	weakness	myasthenia (muscle weakness)

> **TERMINOLOGY TIDBIT**
> The suffix *-asthenia* comes from combining the prefix *a-* meaning "without" and the Greek word *sthenos* meaning "strength."

Suffix	Meaning	Example (Translation)
-cele	protrusion	cystocele (protrusion of urinary bladder)
-dynia	pain	cardiodynia (heart pain)
-cytosis	abnormal cell condition (too many)	erythrocytosis (too many red cells)
-ectasis	dilated	bronchiectasis (dilated bronchi)
-edema	swelling	lymphedema (lymphatic swelling)
-emesis	vomiting	hematemesis (vomiting blood)
-emia	blood condition	leukemia (white [cell] blood condition)
-ia	state, condition	pneumonia (lung condition)
-iasis	abnormal condition	lithiasis (abnormal condition of stones)

Suffix	Meaning	Example (Translation)
-ism	state of	hypothyroidism (state of insufficient thyroid [hormones])
-itis	inflammation	dermatitis (skin inflammation)
-lith	stone	cystolith (bladder stone)
-lysis	to destroy	osteolysis (to destroy bone)
-lytic	destruction	thrombolytic (clot destruction)
-malacia	abnormal softening	chondromalacia (abnormal cartilage softening)
-megaly	enlarged	cardiomegaly (enlarged heart)
-oma	tumor, mass	carcinoma (cancerous tumor)
-osis	abnormal condition	cyanosis (abnormal condition of blue [skin])
-pathy	disease	myopathy (muscle disease)
-penia	too few	cytopenia (too few cells)

> **TERMINOLOGY TIDBIT**
> The suffix -penia comes from the Greek word penia meaning "poverty."

Suffix	Meaning	Example (Translation)
-phobia	fear	photophobia (fear of [sensitivity to] light)
-plegia	paralysis	paraplegia (paralysis of both lower extremities)
-ptosis	drooping	proctoptosis (drooping rectum)
-rrhage	excessive, abnormal flow	hemorrhage (excessive bleeding)
-rrhagia	abnormal flow condition	menorrhagia (abnormal menstrual flow condition)
-rrhea	discharge, flow	rhinorrhea (discharge from nose)

> **TERMINOLOGY TIDBIT**
> The suffixes -rrhea and -rrhagia are very similar but come from different Greek words. -rrhea comes from rhoia meaning "to flow"; -rrhagia comes from rhegnymi meaning "to burst forth" and now means excessive flow.

Suffix	Meaning	Example (Translation)
-rrhexis	rupture	hysterorrhexis (rupture of uterus)
-sclerosis	hardening	arteriosclerosis (hardening of artery)
-spasm	involuntary muscle contraction	bronchospasm (involuntary contraction of bronchi muscles)
-stasis	stopping	hemostasis (stopping blood flow)
-stenosis	narrowing	angiostenosis (narrowing of a vessel)
-toxic	poison	cytotoxic (poisonous to cells)
-uria	urine condition	hematuria (blood in urine condition)

Suffixes Indicating Surgical Procedures

The following suffixes are used to indicate surgical procedures. The word root paired with the surgical suffix indicates what area of the body is being operated on.

Suffix	Meaning	Example (Translation)
-clasia	surgical breaking	osteoclasia (surgical breaking of bone)
-desis	surgical fusing	arthrodesis (surgical fusing of joint)
-ectomy	surgical removal	gastrectomy (surgical removal of stomach)
-ostomy	surgically create an opening	colostomy (surgically create opening for colon [through abdominal wall])
-otomy	cutting into	thoracotomy (cutting into chest)

> **TERMINOLOGY TIDBIT**
> The suffixes -ectomy and -otomy have very specific meanings that relate back to the original Greek words. -ectomy comes from *ektome* meaning "to cut out" while -otomy comes from *tomia* meaning "to cut into."

Suffix	Meaning	Example (Translation)
-pexy	surgical fixation	nephropexy (surgical fixation of kidney)
-plasty	surgical repair	dermatoplasty (surgical repair of skin)
-rrhaphy	suture	myorrhaphy (suture together muscle)
-tome	instrument to cut	dermatome (instrument to cut skin)
-tripsy	surgical crushing	lithotripsy (surgical crushing of stone)

Suffixes Indicating Diagnostic Procedures

The following suffixes indicate common diagnostic procedures.

Suffix	Meaning	Example (Translation)
-centesis	puncture to withdraw fluid	arthrocentesis (puncture to withdraw fluid from joint)

> **TERMINOLOGY TIDBIT**
> The suffix -centesis comes from the Greek word *kentesis* meaning "to prick or pierce."

Suffix	Meaning	Example (Translation)
-gram	record or picture	electrocardiogram (record of heart's electrical [activity])
-graph	instrument for recording	myograph (instrument for recording muscle)
-graphy	process of recording	electrocardiography (process of recording heart's electrical [activity])
-manometer	instrument for measuring pressure	sphygmomanometer (instrument for measuring pulse [blood] pressure)

Suffix	Meaning	Example (Translation)
-meter	instrument for measuring	audiometer (instrument to measure hearing)
-metry	process of measuring	audiometry (process of measuring hearing)
-scope	instrument for viewing	gastroscope (instrument to view stomach)
-scopy	process of visually examining	gastroscopy (process of visually examining stomach)

General Suffixes

These suffixes belong to a group not specifically referring to a medical condition or procedure. However, they add meaning to the term.

Suffix	Meaning	Example (Translation)
-cle	small	vesicle (small sac [blister])
-cyesis	pregnancy	salpingocyesis (uterine tube pregnancy)
-cyte	cell	leukocyte (white [blood] cell)
-derma	skin condition	leukoderma (white skin condition)
-dipsia	thirst	polydipsia (much [frequent] thirst)
-esthesia	feeling, sensation	anesthesia (without sensation)
-gen	that which produces	mutagen (that which produces mutations)
-genesis	produces, generates	osteogenesis (produces bone)
-genic	producing	carcinogenic (producing cancer)

> **TERMINOLOGY TIDBIT**
> The suffixes -genesis, -genic, and -gen all come from the Greek word gignesthai meaning "to be born."

Suffix	Meaning	Example (Translation)
-globin	protein	hemoglobin (blood protein)
-globulin	protein	immunoglobulin (protective protein)
-gravida	pregnancy	multigravida (many pregnancies)
-kinesia	movement	bradykinesia (slow movement)
-oid	resembling	lipoid (resembling fat)
-ole	small	arteriole (small artery)
-opia	vision	diplopia (double vision)
-opsy	view of	biopsy (view of life)
-osmia	sense of smell	anosmia (no sense of smell)
-oxia	oxygen	anoxia (without oxygen)

Suffix	Meaning	Example (Translation)
-para	to bear (offspring)	nullipara (to bear no children)
-partum	childbirth	postpartum (after childbirth)
-pepsia	digestion	bradypepsia (slow digestion)
-phagia	eating, swallowing	dysphagia (difficulty swallowing)
-phasia	speech	aphasia (lack of speech)
-phil	attracted to	eosinophil (attracted to rosy [dye])
-phonia	voice	aphonia (without voice)
-plasia	formation of cells	hyperplasia (excessive formation of cells)
-plasm	formation	neoplasm (new formation [of tissue])
-pnea	breathing	apnea (lack of breathing)
-poiesis	formation	hematopoiesis (blood formation)
-porosis	porous	osteoporosis (porous bone)
-ptysis	spitting up, coughing up	hemoptysis (spitting or coughing up blood)
-therapy	treatment	chemotherapy (treatment with chemicals)
-thorax	chest	hemothorax (blood in the chest)
-trophic	development	amyotrophic (without muscle development)
-trophy	development	hypertrophy (excessive development)
-ule	small	venule (small vein)

Suffixes Indicating Medical Specialties or Personnel

The word root placed with these suffixes indicates the area of medicine in which the specialist works.

Suffix	Meaning	Example (Translation)
-er	one who	radiographer (one who takes X-rays)
-iatric	medical specialty	psychiatric (medical specialty of the mind)
-iatrist	physician	psychiatrist (physician specializing in the mind)
-iatry	treatment, medicine	podiatry (treatment of the foot)
-ician	specialist	pediatrician (specialist for children)
-ist	specialist	pharmacist (drug specialist)
-logist	one who studies	cardiologist (one who studies the heart)
-logy	study of	cardiology (study of the heart)

Suffixes Used to Convert Word Roots into Adjectives

The following suffixes are used to convert word roots into adjectives. Often a term such as *ulcer* will need to be paired with a second term to indicate location. For example, *-ic* combined with **gastr/o** forms the term *gastric* to give the adjective form for stomach. *Gastric* is then paired with *ulcer* to indicate that the ulcer is located in the stomach. The accepted meaning for these adjective suffixes is *pertaining to* or *relating to*.

Suffix	Meaning	Example (Translation)
-ac	pertaining to	cardiac (pertaining to heart)
-al	pertaining to	duodenal (pertaining to duodenum)
-an	pertaining to	ovarian (pertaining to ovary)
-ar	pertaining to	ventricular (pertaining to ventricle)
-ary	pertaining to	pulmonary (pertaining to lungs)
-atic	pertaining to	lymphatic (pertaining to lymph)
-eal	pertaining to	esophageal (pertaining to esophagus)
-ic	pertaining to	gastric (pertaining to stomach)
-ine	pertaining to	uterine (pertaining to uterus)
-ior	pertaining to	superior (pertaining to above)
-nic	pertaining to	embryonic (pertaining to embryo)
-ory	pertaining to	auditory (pertaining to hearing)
-ose	pertaining to	adipose (pertaining to fat)
-ous	pertaining to	venous (pertaining to vein)
-tic	pertaining to	hepatic (pertaining to liver)

PRACTICE

Recognizing Categories of Suffixes

On each of the following blanks, indicate the category to which each suffix belongs and its translation. The suffix categories included in this exercise are disease/abnormal condition, surgical, diagnostic, and general.

Suffix	Category	Translation
1. -plegia	_____	_____
2. -metry	_____	_____
3. -cyte	_____	_____
4. -otomy	_____	_____

Suffix	Category	Translation
5. -lith	_____	_____
6. -scope	_____	_____
7. -thorax	_____	_____
8. -graphy	_____	_____
9. -emesis	_____	_____
10. -clasia	_____	_____
11. -lysis	_____	_____
12. -ectomy	_____	_____

Matching

Match each suffix to its definition.

_____	1. -pepsia	A.	cell
_____	2. -pnea	B.	formation
_____	3. -phasia	C.	movement
_____	4. -cyesis	D.	producing
_____	5. -kinesia	E.	digestion
_____	6. -genic	F.	speech
_____	7. -dipsia	G.	treatment
_____	8. -cyte	H.	pregnancy
_____	9. -porosis	I.	thirst
_____	10. -therapy	J.	vision
_____	11. -plasm	K.	porous
_____	12. -opia	L.	breathing

Choosing the Correct Adjective Form

One of the most difficult things to master in learning medical terminology is correct use of adjective forms. There are several ways to technically construct a word, but only one of them is an actual medical term. The rest simply aren't used. Unfortunately, there is no rule to help; you can learn this only by becoming familiar with which adjective form is correct. After a short while, a term will just "sound" correct and you won't forget it again.

The following exercise is a start to this process. Read the translation, sound out each choice, and circle the one that "sounds" correct to you.

1. **pertaining to the heart**

   cardiac   cardial   cardior   carditic

2. **pertaining to the ovary**

   ovarous   ovariac   ovarian   ovarial

3. **pertaining to the duodenum**

   duodenar   duodenal   duodeniac   duodentic

4. **pertaining to a ventricle**

   ventricultic   ventriculous   ventricular   ventriculac

5. **pertaining to the lungs**

   pulmonal   pulmontic   pulmonous   pulmonary

6. **pertaining to the esophagus**

   esophageal   esophagic   esophagous   esophagar

7. **pertaining to the stomach**

   gastran   gastric   gastral   gastreal

8. **pertaining to the uterus**

   uterior   uterary   uterotic   uterine

9. **pertaining to a vein**

   venous   ventic   venary   veniac

10. **pertaining to the liver**

    hepatar   hepatary   hepatic   hepatac

Build Medical Terms

Now you are ready to start building actual medical terms. The following format will be used for this exercise and word building throughout the rest of this text:

- Translation phrase for the medical term
- Blanks are subdivided into prefix (if needed), word root, combining vowel (if needed), and suffix

Examples

- Instrument to view the stomach   gastr / o / scope
- Enlarged liver   hepat / o / megaly
- Pertaining to the kidney   ren / al
- Inflammation of skin   dermat / itis

Remember that whether or not to use a combining vowel depends on the first letter of the suffix. If it begins in a consonant, use a combining vowel (first two examples). If the suffix begins with a vowel, a combining vowel is not necessary (last two examples). Refer back to Chapter 1 if you need more help with this rule.

Finally, you will need a short list of combining forms to use with the suffixes you learned in this chapter. The following list contains several common combining forms for use in these exercises.

Combining Form	Meaning	Combining Form	Meaning
angi/o	vessel	hepat/o	liver
arteri/o	artery	my/o	muscle
arthr/o	joint	nephr/o	kidney
bronch/o	bronchus	neur/o	nerve
col/o	colon	rhin/o	nose
cyst/o	urinary bladder, sac	thorac/o	chest
dermat/o	skin	trache/o	trachea
gastr/o	stomach		

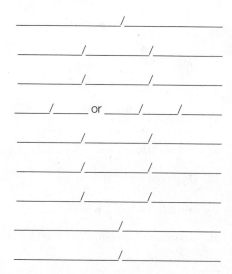

1. Surgical removal of the stomach _____/_____

2. Instrument for viewing inside the stomach _____/_____/_____

3. Process of visually examining the stomach _____/_____/_____

4. Stomach pain _____/_____ or _____/_____/_____

5. Bladder stone _____/_____/_____

6. Instrument for viewing inside the bladder _____/_____/_____

7. Process of visually examining the bladder _____/_____/_____

8. Surgically create an opening in the bladder _____/_____

9. Pertaining to the bladder _____/_____

10. Surgical repair of a vessel   _____ / _____ / _____

11. Vessel tumor   _____ / _____

12. Process of recording a vessel   _____ / _____ / _____

13. Picture of a vessel   _____ / _____ / _____

14. Narrowing of a vessel   _____ / _____ / _____

15. Hardening of an artery   _____ / _____ / _____

16. Involuntary muscle contraction in an artery   _____ / _____ / _____

17. Ruptured artery   _____ / _____ / _____

18. Small artery   _____ / _____

19. Inflamed joint   _____ / _____

20. Instrument for viewing inside a joint   _____ / _____ / _____

21. Process of visually examining a joint   _____ / _____ / _____

22. Surgical repair of a joint   _____ / _____ / _____

23. Puncture to withdraw fluid from a joint   _____ / _____ / _____

24. Study of the skin   _____ / _____ / _____

25. One who studies the skin   _____ / _____ / _____

26. Inflamed skin   _____ / _____

27. Abnormal condition of the skin   _____ / _____

28. Inflamed liver   _____ / _____

29. Liver tumor   _____ / _____

30. Enlarged liver   _____ / _____ / _____

31. Liver cell   _____ / _____ / _____

32. Pertaining to the liver   _____ / _____

33. Discharge from the nose   _____ / _____ / _____

34. Surgical repair of the nose   _____ / _____ / _____

35. Condition of abnormal flow from the nose   _____ / _____ / _____

36. Inflamed bronchus   _____/_____

37. Instrument for viewing inside the bronchus   _____/_____/_____

38. Process of visually examining the bronchus   _____/_____/_____

39. Surgically create an opening into the trachea   _____/_____

40. Cut into the trachea   _____/_____

41. Protrusion of the trachea   _____/_____/_____

42. Abnormal softening of the trachea   _____/_____/_____

43. Pertaining to the trachea   _____/_____

44. Surgically create an opening into the colon   _____/_____

45. Surgical removal of the colon   _____/_____

46. Surgical fixation of the colon   _____/_____/_____

47. Study of the kidney   _____/_____/_____

48. One who studies the kidney   _____/_____/_____

49. Abnormal softening of the kidney   _____/_____/_____

50. Abnormal condition of the kidney   _____/_____

51. Kidney disease   _____/_____/_____

52. Surgical fixation of the kidney   _____/_____/_____

53. Cut into the chest   _____/_____

54. Puncture to withdraw fluid from the chest   _____/_____/_____

55. Chest pain   _____/_____/_____ or _____/_____

56. Study of the nerves   _____/_____/_____

57. One who studies the nerves   _____/_____/_____

58. Surgical repair of a nerve   _____/_____/_____

59. Crushing a nerve   _____/_____/_____

60. Nerve pain   _____/_____ or _____/_____/_____

61. Suture a muscle   _____/_____/_____

62. Muscle disease   _____ / _____ / _____

63. Muscle pain   _____ / _____ or _____ / _____ / _____

64. Instrument to cut muscle   _____ / _____ / _____

65. Instrument for recording a muscle   _____ / _____ / _____

66. Record of a muscle   _____ / _____ / _____

67. Process of recording a muscle   _____ / _____ / _____

MyMedicalTerminologyLab™

MyMedicalTerminologyLab is a premium online homework management system that includes a host of features to help you study. Registered users will find:

- A multitude of activities and assignments built within the MyLab platform
- Powerful tools that track and analyze your results—allowing you to create a personalized learning experience
- Videos and audio pronunciations to help enrich your progress
- Streaming lesson presentations and self-paced learning modules
- A space where you and your instructors can view and manage your assignments

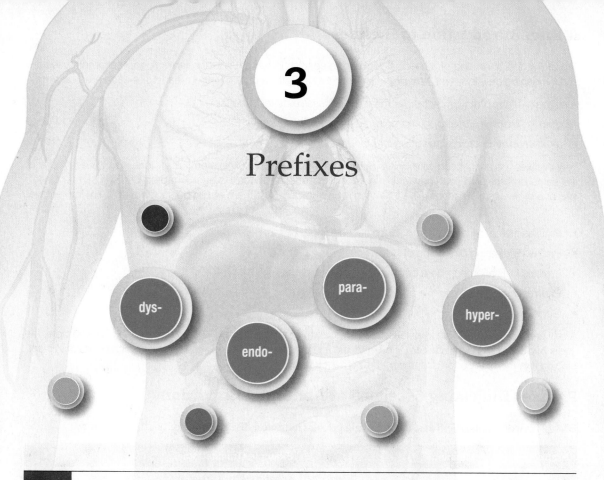

3

Prefixes

Learning Objectives

Upon completion of this chapter, you will be able to:

3-1 Explain the role of prefixes in building medical terms.

3-2 Use prefixes to indicate diseases or abnormal conditions.

3-3 Use prefixes to indicate directions or body positions.

3-4 Use prefixes to indicate numbers or quantity measurements.

3-5 Use prefixes to indicate time.

3-6 Use prefixes to build additional medical terms.

A Brief Introduction to Prefixes

A prefix at the beginning of a medical term adds specific information to the term. A good example uses the suffix meaning development, *-trophy*. Using different prefixes changes the meaning of each medical term.

- *hyper-* + *-trophy* = *hypertrophy* meaning *excessive development*
- *dys-* + *-trophy* = *dystrophy* meaning *abnormal development*
- *a-* + *-trophy* = *atrophy* meaning *lack of development*

Few prefixes are associated with only one medical specialty or body system. Therefore, you will use many of the same prefixes with each new set of combining forms introduced in each chapter. Prefixes can be placed into one of several categories. The following list makes learning them easier by subdividing them into smaller groups:

- Prefixes indicating diseases or abnormal conditions
- Prefixes indicating directions or body positions
- Prefixes indicating numbers or quantity measurements
- Prefixes indicating time
- General prefixes

A few prefixes have multiple translations. Therefore, they appear in more than one category. For example, the prefix *hypo-* can be translated as *below,* placing it in the direction or body position category, or as *insufficient,* placing it in the number or quantity measurement category.

Prefixes Indicating Diseases or Abnormal Conditions

Used with word roots or suffixes, the following prefixes indicate a diseased state or body abnormality.

Prefix	Meaning	Example (Translation)
a-	without	aphasia (without speech)
an-	without	anoxia (without oxygen)
anti-	against	antibiotic (against life)
brady-	slow	bradycardia (slow heartbeat)
de-	without	dehydration (without water)
dys-	painful, difficult, abnormal	dyspnea (painful breathing)
		TERMINOLOGY TIDBIT The prefix *dys-* comes from the Greek word *dus,* which has a general negative meaning. It can be translated several ways such as "bad, difficult, abnormal, incorrect," and "painful."
pachy-	thick	pachyderma (thick skin)
tachy-	fast	tachycardia (fast heartbeat)

Prefixes Indicating Directions or Body Positions

Used with word roots or suffixes, the following prefixes indicate directions or body positions.

Prefix	Meaning	Example (Translation)
ante-	before, in front of	anteorbital (in front of eye socket)
endo-	within, inner	endoscope (instrument for viewing within)
epi-	above	epigastric (above stomach)
ex-	outward	exophthalmos (eyes [bulging] outward)
extra-	outside of	extraocular (outside of eye)
hypo-	below	hypogastric (below stomach)
infra-	below	infraorbital (below eye socket)
inter-	between	intervertebral (between vertebrae)
intra-	within	intravenous (inside vein)
para-	beside; two like parts of a pair	paranasal (beside the nose); paraplegia (paralysis of two like parts of a pair [the legs])
peri-	around	periodontal (around tooth)
retro-	behind	retroperitoneal (behind the peritoneum)
sub-	beneath, under	subcutaneous (under skin)
supra-	above	suprapubic (above pubic bone)
trans-	across	transurethral (across urethra)

> **TERMINOLOGY TIDBIT**
> The prefixes *intra-* and *inter-* are commonly confused. Both come from Latin words, *intra* meaning "within" and *inter* meaning "between."

Prefixes Indicating Time

Used with word roots or suffixes, the following prefixes indicate time periods.

Prefix	Meaning	Example (Translation)
ante-	before	antepartum (before birth)
neo-	new	neonate (newborn)
post-	after	postpartum (after birth)
pre-	before	premenstrual (before menstruation)

Prefixes Indicating Numbers or Quantity Measurements

Used with word roots or suffixes, the following prefixes indicate the number of items or quantity measurement.

Prefix	Meaning	Example (Translation)
bi-	two	bilateral (two sides)
di-	two	diplegic (paralysis of two extremities)
hemi-	half	hemiplegia (paralysis of one side [half] of body)
hyper-	excessive	hyperemesis (excessive vomiting)
hypo-	insufficient	hypocalcemia (insufficient calcium in blood)
micro-	small	microscope (instrument for viewing small things)
mono-	one	monoplegia (paralysis of one extremity)
multi-	many	multigravida (more than one pregnancy)
nulli-	none	nulligravida (no pregnancies)
pan-	all	pansinusitis (inflammation of all sinuses)
poly-	many	polyarteritis (many inflamed arteries)
primi-	first	primigravida (first pregnancy)
quadri-	four	quadriplegia (paralysis of all four extremities)
tri-	three	triplegia (paralysis of three extremities)
ultra-	excess	ultrasound (excess [high] sound wave frequency)
uni-	one	unilateral (one side)

> **TERMINOLOGY TIDBIT**
> The prefix *hypo-* is used several different ways. It comes from the Greek word *hupo* meaning "under" and is used to indicate a smaller than normal amount. It is also used to indicate a position underneath another structure.

General Prefixes

These prefixes belong to a group not specifically referring to a disease, abnormal condition, direction, body position, number, or time. However, they add meaning to the term.

Prefix	Meaning	Example (Translation)
auto-	self	autograft (graft from one's own body)
eu-	normal, good	eupnea (normal breathing)
hetero-	different	heterograft (graft from a different species)
homo-	same	homograft (graft from same species)
per-	through	percutaneous (through skin)

> **TERMINOLOGY TIDBIT**
> The prefix *eu-* comes from the Greek word *eu* and has a general positive meaning. It can be translated as "good, normal," or "well." It is the opposite of *dys-*.

PRACTICE

Recognizing Categories of Prefixes

On each of the following blanks, indicate the category to which each prefix belongs and its translation. The categories included in this exercise are disease/abnormality prefixes, direction/body position prefixes, number prefixes, and time prefixes.

Prefix	Category	Translation
1. dys-		
2. hypo-		
3. nulli-		
4. brady-		
5. an-		
6. neo-		
7. inter-		
8. post-		
9. micro-		
10. peri-		
11. epi-		
12. anti-		

Matching

Match each prefix to its definition.

_____	**1.** auto-	**A.** same
_____	**2.** poly-	**B.** four
_____	**3.** per-	**C.** fast
_____	**4.** homo-	**D.** many
_____	**5.** eu-	**E.** first
_____	**6.** pan-	**F.** within
_____	**7.** primi-	**G.** self
_____	**8.** quadri-	**H.** different
_____	**9.** intra-	**I.** excessive
_____	**10.** hetero-	**J.** normal, good
_____	**11.** hyper-	**K.** all
_____	**12.** tachy-	**L.** through

Build Medical Terms

Now you are ready to practice using prefixes to build medical terms. The following format will be used for this exercise:

- Translation phrase for the medical term
- Blanks are subdivided into prefix and word root/suffix

You will need additional word parts for this practice exercise. The following list contains word roots that have already been joined with a suffix, making them ready to combine with a prefix.

Word Root + Suffix	Meaning	Word Root + Suffix	Meaning
-cardia	heart	-pepsia	digestion
-carditis	heart inflammation	-phagia	eating
-cellular	pertaining to cells	-plegia	paralysis
-dermal	pertaining to skin	-pnea	breathing
-graft	skin graft	-scapular	pertaining to the scapula
-lateral	pertaining to the side	-trophy	development
-operative	operation	-uria	condition of the urine
-para	woman who has given birth		

1. Fast heart _____/_____

2. Slow heart _____/_____

3. Inflammation within the heart _____/_____

4. Inflammation around the heart _____/_____

5. Inflammation of the entire heart _____/_____

6. Pertaining to within the cell _____/_____

7. Pertaining to outside the cell _____/_____

8. Pertaining to many cells _____/_____

9. Pertaining to one cell _____/_____

10. Pertaining to within the skin _____/_____

11. Pertaining to beneath the skin _____/_____

12. Pertaining to above the skin _____/_____

13. Graft from same source _____/_____

14. Graft from other source _____/_____

15. Graft from self _____/_____

16. Pertaining to two sides _____/_____

17. Pertaining to one side _____/_____

18. Before an operation _____/_____

19. After an operation _____/_____

20. Within an operation _____/_____

21. First birth _____/_____

22. No births _____/_____

23. Many births _____/_____

24. No eating _____/_____

25. Abnormal eating _____/_____

26. Eating too much (many) _____/_____

27. Without digestion _____/_____

28. Abnormal digestion   _____/_____

29. Slow digestion   _____/_____

30. Without development   _____/_____

31. Abnormal development   _____/_____

32. Half paralysis   _____/_____

33. Four paralysis   _____/_____

34. One paralysis   _____/_____

35. No breathing   _____/_____

36. Normal breathing   _____/_____

37. Fast breathing   _____/_____

38. Slow breathing   _____/_____

39. Excessive breathing   _____/_____

40. Insufficient breathing   _____/_____

41. Pertaining to below the scapula   _____/_____

42. Pertaining to above the scapula   _____/_____

43. Pertaining to beneath the scapula   _____/_____

44. Condition of no urine   _____/_____

45. Condition of too much (many) urine   _____/_____

46. Condition of abnormal urine   _____/_____

MyMedicalTerminologyLab™

MyMedicalTerminologyLab is a premium online homework management system that includes a host of features to help you study. Registered users will find:

- A multitude of activities and assignments built within the MyLab platform
- Powerful tools that track and analyze your results—allowing you to create a personalized learning experience
- Videos and audio pronunciations to help enrich your progress
- Streaming lesson presentations and self-paced learning modules
- A space where you and your instructors can view and manage your assignments

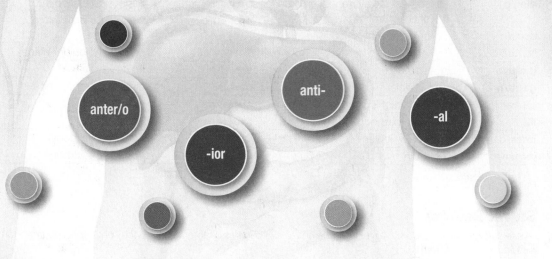

4

Anatomical Terminology

anter/o

anti-

-ior

-al

Upon completion of this chapter, you will be able to:

4-1 Visualize patients in the anatomical position.

4-2 Identify the planes and sections of the body.

4-3 Use correct directional terms.

4-4 Use anatomical terms to refer to body surface structures.

4-5 Place internal organs into the correct body cavity.

4-6 Use either anatomical divisions or clinical divisions to describe the abdominopelvic cavity.

Anatomical Combining Forms

abdomin/o	abdomen		**later/o**	side
anter/o	front (side of body)		**lumb/o**	low back
brachi/o	arm		**medi/o**	middle
caud/o	tail		**nas/o**	nose
cephal/o	head		**or/o**	mouth
cervic/o	neck		**orbit/o**	eye socket
chondr/o	cartilage		**ot/o**	ear
crani/o	skull		**patell/o**	patella (kneecap)
cubit/o	elbow		**pelv/o**	pelvis
dist/o	farthest (away from beginning of structure)		**poster/o**	back (side of body)
			proxim/o	nearest (to beginning of structure)
dors/o	back (side of body)		**scapul/o**	scapula (shoulder blade)
femor/o	femur (thigh bone)			
gastr/o	stomach		**spin/o**	spine
genit/o	genitals		**stern/o**	sternum (breast bone)
glute/o	buttocks		**super/o**	above, upper
ili/o	ilium (part of pelvis)		**thorac/o**	chest
infer/o	below, lower		**ventr/o**	belly (side of body)
inguin/o	groin		**vertebr/o**	vertebra (backbone)

Suffix Review

These suffixes introduced in Chapter 2 are being reviewed in this chapter because they are especially important for building anatomical terms.

-ac	pertaining to		**-iac**	pertaining to
-al	pertaining to		**-ic**	pertaining to
-ar	pertaining to		**-ior**	pertaining to

Prefix Review

These prefixes introduced in Chapter 3 are being reviewed here because they are especially important for building anatomical terms.

ante-	before, in front of		**hypo-**	below, insufficient
epi-	above		**retro-**	behind

Anatomical Position

When describing body positions or using directional terms, health professionals visualize the patient in the **anatomical position** (see Figure 4.1).

> **TERMINOLOGY TIDBIT**
> The term *anatomy* comes from combining two Greek words: *ana* meaning "apart" and *tome* meaning "to cut." It was necessary to cut apart the body in order to study its internal structure.

Therefore, it is not necessary to describe the patient's actual position. It does not matter whether the patient is lying down or sitting up or whether the health professional is on the patient's right or left side. Unless stated otherwise, it is assumed that the patient is:

- Standing upright
- Legs together
- Feet pointing forward
- Arms down at sides
- Palms facing forward
- Eyes looking straight ahead

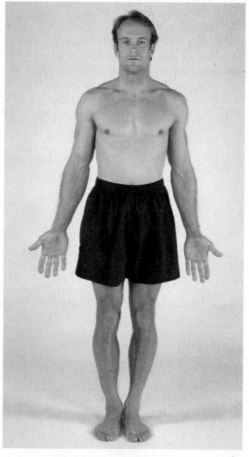

4.1 The anatomical position: Standing upright, gazing straight ahead, arms down at sides, palms facing forward, fingers extended, legs together, and toes pointing forward
Source: Pearson Education

Planes and Sections

The human body is three-dimensional. Therefore, it can be divided into sections along three different planes: frontal (coronal), sagittal, and transverse (see Figure 4.2). A two-dimensional image of the body, for example an X-ray, taken along one of the planes is called a *section*. Each plane yields a different section.

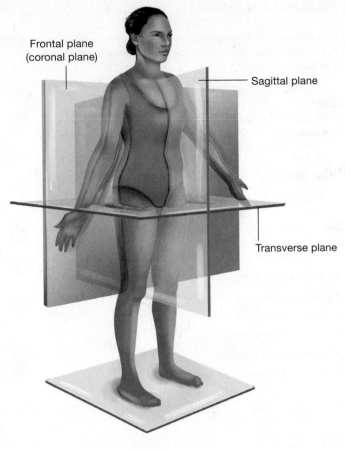

Frontal plane
(coronal plane)

Sagittal plane

Transverse plane

4.2 The planes of the body; sagittal plane is vertical from front to back, the frontal plane is vertical from left to right, and the transverse plane is horizontal

1. **Frontal (or coronal) plane:** A vertical plane that runs from side to side; it slices the body into anterior and posterior portions; a cut along the frontal plane produces a **frontal** or **coronal section** (see Figure 4.3A)

2. **Sagittal plane:** Also a vertical plane but runs from front to back; it slices the body into left and right portions; a cut along the sagittal plane produces a **sagittal section** (see Figure 4.3B); a line down the center of the body dividing it into equal left and right halves is called the **midsagittal line**

3. **Transverse plane:** Only horizontal plane; slices the body into upper and lower portions; a cut along the transverse plane produces a **transverse section** (see Figure 4.3C)

The terms **longitudinal section** and **cross-section** are often used to describe internal views of the body. A lengthwise slice along the long axis of a structure produces a longitudinal section. A cut down the length of the arm is an example of a longitudinal section. A cross-section is produced by a slice perpendicular to the long axis of a structure. A cut across the upper arm yields a cross-section view.

TERMINOLOGY TIDBIT

Imagine slicing down the length of a banana; that is a longitudinal section. Slicing across the banana, like you would to put it on your cereal, is a cross-section.

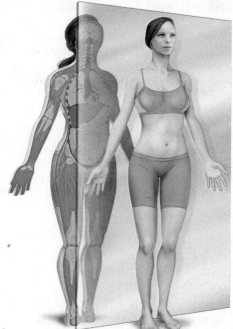

A

4.3 Figures illustrating how the different body sections are formed. (A) Frontal or coronal section, (B) sagittal section, (C) transverse section

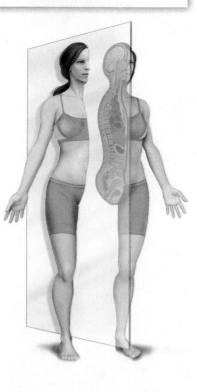

B

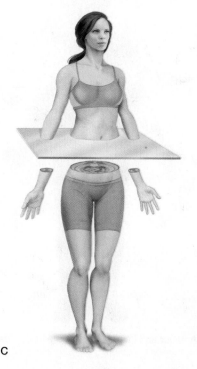

C

Directional Terminology

Directional terms indicate the position of a structure *in relation* to another structure. For example, the heart is above the stomach. The position of these two organs relative to each other can be expressed as either the heart is superior to the stomach or the stomach is inferior to the heart. This example also demonstrates another characteristic of directional terms: They come in opposite pairs; for each directional term there is a second term that means the opposite (see Figure 4.4).

Building Directional Terms

Most directional terms are Latin-style terms and therefore can be built from word parts. They consist of a word root and an adjective suffix, usually –ic, –ior, or –al.

For each of the following word roots and suffixes, build the corresponding directional term. Terms not built from word parts are simply presented with their definition.

1. **anter/o + -ior**

   a. pertaining to front (side of body) _____/_____

2. **caud/o + -al**

   a. pertaining to the tail _____/_____

3. **cephal/o + -ic**

   a. pertaining to the head _____/_____

4.4 Anterior and lateral views of the body illustrating directional terms
Source: Pearson Education

4. **deep** a term meaning further below from the surface

5. **dist/o** + **-al**

   a. pertaining to farthest (away from beginning of structure) _____/_____

6. **dors/o** + **-al**

> **TERMINOLOGY TIDBIT**
> The combining form *dors/o* comes from the Latin word *dorsum* meaning "the back."

   a. pertaining to back (side of the body) _____/_____

7. **infer/o** + **-ior**

   a. pertaining to below _____/_____

8. **later/o** + **-al**

   a. pertaining to the side _____/_____

9. **medi/o** + **-al**

   a. pertaining to the middle _____/_____

10. **poster/o** + **-ior**

   a. pertaining to back (side of body) _____/_____

11. **prone** a term meaning to lie face down (see Figure 4.5A)

> **TERMINOLOGY TIDBIT**
> The term *prone* comes from the Latin word *pronus* meaning "leaning forward."

4.5A The prone position
Source: Pearson Education

12. **proxim/o** + **-al**

   a. pertaining to nearest (to beginning of structure) _____/_____

13. **superficial** a term meaning nearer the surface

14. **super/o** + **-ior**

   a. pertaining to above _____/_____

15. **supine** a term meaning to lie face up (see Figure 4.5B)

> **TERMINOLOGY TIDBIT**
> The term *supine* comes from the Latin word *supinus* meaning "bent backwards."

4.5B The supine position
Source: Pearson Education

16. ventr/o + -al

    a. pertaining to belly (side of body)   _____ / _____

Body Surface Terminology

The different regions of the body are named so that referring to them is easy and accurate. Many are named for a body structure underlying the region. For example, the sternal region overlies the sternum and the abdominal region overlies the abdominal cavity (see Figure 4.6).

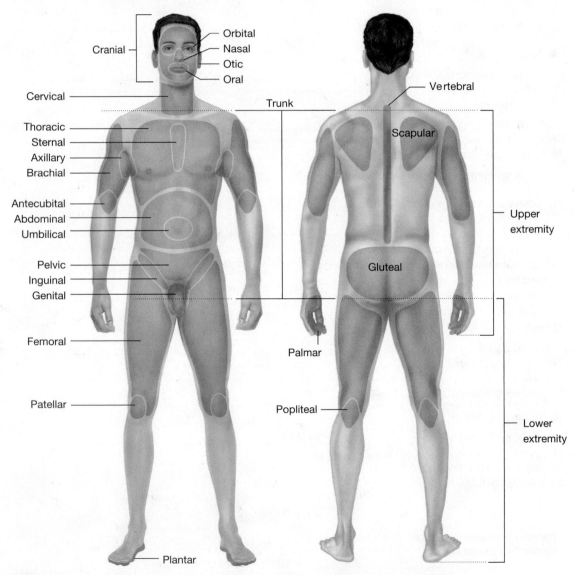

4.6 Anterior and posterior views of the body illustrating the location of various body regions

Building Body Surface Terms

Like directional terms, many body surface terms are Latin-style words consisting of a word root and suffix.

For each of the following combinations of word parts, build the corresponding term for that body surface region. Terms not built from word parts are simply defined. One cautionary note: Some of the following terms may appear to be built from word parts but are not.

1. **abdomin/o + -al**

> **TERMINOLOGY TIDBIT**
> Now that you are learning medical terminology, it is important to use these terms instead of common phrases and terms. Many people commonly say *stomach* (an organ) when they actually mean *abdomen* (a body region).

    a. pertaining to the abdomen   _____ / _____

2. **ante- + cubit/o + -al**

    a. pertaining to in front of the elbow   _____ / _____ / _____

3. **axillary** a term meaning underarm area

4. **brachi/o + -al**

    a. pertaining to the arm   _____ / _____

5. **cervic/o + -al**

    a. pertaining to the neck   _____ / _____

6. **crani/o + -al**

    a. pertaining to the skull   _____ / _____

7. **femor/o + -al**

    a. pertaining to the femur/thigh   _____ / _____

8. **genit/o + -al**

    a. pertaining to the genitals   _____ / _____

9. **glute/o + -al**

    a. pertaining to the buttocks   _____ / _____

10. **inguin/o + -al**

    a. pertaining to the groin   _____ / _____

11. **lower extremity** a phrase used to refer to the entire leg

12. **nas/o + -al**

    a. pertaining to the nose   _____ / _____

13. **orbit/o + -al**

    a. pertaining to the eye socket   _____ / _____

14. **or/o** + **-al**

    a. pertaining to the mouth   /

15. **ot/o** + **-ic**

    a. pertaining to the ear   /

16. **palmar** a term meaning the palm of the hand

17. **patell/o** + **-ar**

    a. pertaining to the kneecap   /

18. **pelv/o** + **-ic**

    a. pertaining to the pelvis   /

19. **plantar** a term meaning the sole of the foot

20. **popliteal** a term meaning the creased area behind the knee

21. **scapul/o** + **-ar**

    a. pertaining to the shoulder blade   /

22. **stern/o** + **-al**

    a. pertaining to the breast bone   /

23. **thorac/o** + **-ic**

    a. pertaining to the chest   /

24. **trunk** a term meaning the torso, excluding the head and extremities

25. **umbilical** a term meaning the region around the navel

26. **upper extremity** a phrase used to refer to the entire arm

27. **vertebr/o** + **-al**

    a. pertaining to the backbone   /

Body Cavities

The majority of the body's internal organs, or **viscera**, are found within one of four body cavities (see Figure 4.7). Two of these cavities, the **cranial cavity** and **spinal cavity**, are on the dorsal side of the body. The other two, the **thoracic cavity** and **abdominopelvic cavity**, are ventral. The organs within the cavities are usually found within protective membrane sacs.

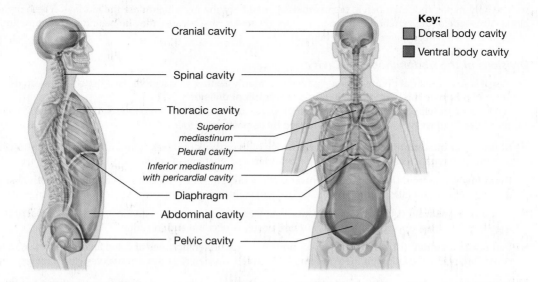

Cranial cavity	Key:
	Dorsal body cavity
Spinal cavity	Ventral body cavity

Thoracic cavity
Superior mediastinum
Pleural cavity
Inferior mediastinum with pericardial cavity
Diaphragm
Abdominal cavity
Pelvic cavity

Lateral view   **Anterior view**

4.7 The dorsal (in red) and ventral (in purple) body cavities

Cavity	Description
Cranial **crani/o** = skull **-al** = pertaining to	Dorsal cavity; lies inside the skull and contains the brain; the brain is protected by a membrane sac called the **meninges**.
Spinal **spin/o** = spine **-al** = pertaining to	Dorsal cavity; formed by a canal through the vertebrae; contains the spinal cord; the spinal cord is also protected by the meninges.
Thoracic **thorac/o** = chest **-ic** = pertaining to	Superior of two ventral cavities; found enclosed by the ribs and separated from the abdominopelvic cavity by the **diaphragm** muscle; contains organs such as the lungs, heart, esophagus, trachea, aorta, and thymus gland; it can be subdivided into one central and two side regions. • **Mediastinum:** central region; contains the heart, trachea, esophagus, aorta, and thymus gland; heart is encased in the **pericardial sac.** • **Pleural cavities:** side regions; each contains a lung; sac protecting the lungs is called the **pleura**.
Abdominopelvic **abdomin/o** = abdomen **pelv/o** = pelvis **-ic** = pertaining to	Inferior of two ventral cavities; large cavity generally subdivided into abdominal and pelvic cavities; however, no clear structure indicating where one cavity stops and the other begins; organs of abdominopelvic cavity are protected by a membrane covering called the **peritoneum**. • **Abdominal cavity:** houses the stomach, liver, gallbladder, spleen, pancreas, and portions of the colon and intestine. • **Pelvic cavity:** contains the urinary bladder, ureters, urethra, and portions of the colon and intestine in both genders; in females also contains the uterus, ovaries, fallopian tubes, and vagina; in males also contains the prostate gland, seminal vesicles, bulbourethral gland, and a portion of the vas deferens.

The only major abdominopelvic organs that lie outside of the peritoneum are the kidneys. These organs lie along either side of the vertebral column just under the lower ribs. Because they lie behind the peritoneum, their position is called *retroperitoneal* (**retro-** = behind).

Divisions of the Abdominopelvic Cavity

Because it is so large, the abdominopelvic cavity is commonly divided into regions. Health personnel can use either of two methods to do this: **clinical divisions** or **anatomical divisions**.

When using the clinical divisions, the abdominopelvic cavity is divided into four equal quadrants that cross at the navel (see Figure 4.8). Each quadrant is named by its position as follows:

- **Right upper quadrant** (RUQ): contains right lobe of liver (bulk of liver), right kidney, upper portion of right ureter, pancreas (small section), gallbladder, and portions of colon and intestine

- **Right lower quadrant** (RLQ): contains lower portion of right ureter, portions of colon and intestine, appendix, right ovary and fallopian tube (in females), and right vas deferens and seminal vesicle (in males)

- **Left upper quadrant** (LUQ): contains stomach, spleen, left lobe of liver (smaller), pancreas (most of the organ), left kidney, upper portion of left ureter, portions of colon and intestine

- **Left lower quadrant** (LLQ): contains lower portion of left ureter, portions of colon and intestine, sigmoid colon, left ovary and fallopian tube (in females), and left vas deferens and seminal vesicle (in males)

The urinary bladder, rectum, uterus (in females), and prostate gland (in males) are midline structures and therefore do not actually fall into any one quadrant.

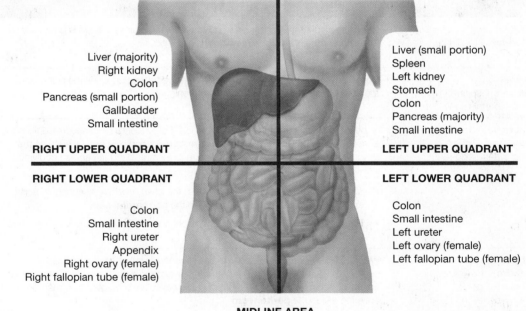

Liver (majority)
Right kidney
Colon
Pancreas (small portion)
Gallbladder
Small intestine

RIGHT UPPER QUADRANT

Liver (small portion)
Spleen
Left kidney
Stomach
Colon
Pancreas (majority)
Small intestine

LEFT UPPER QUADRANT

RIGHT LOWER QUADRANT

Colon
Small intestine
Right ureter
Appendix
Right ovary (female)
Right fallopian tube (female)

LEFT LOWER QUADRANT

Colon
Small intestine
Left ureter
Left ovary (female)
Left fallopian tube (female)

MIDLINE AREA

Rectum - Bladder - Uterus (female) - Prostate (male)

4.8 The clinical divisions of the abdomen; the abdominopelvic cavity is divided into four quadrants

Anatomical divisions are smaller. This system divides the abdominopelvic cavity into nine sections like a tic-tac-toe board (see Figure 4.9). The nine regions are as follows:

- **Right hypochondriac** (**hypo-** = below; **chondr/o** = cartilage; **-iac** = pertaining to): right lateral side of upper row under lower ribs that are connected to the sternum by cartilage

- **Epigastric** (**epi-** = above; **gastr/o** = stomach; **-ic** = pertaining to): middle area of upper row overlying stomach

- **Left hypochondriac:** left lateral side of upper row

- **Right lumbar** (**lumb/o** = low back; **-ar** = pertaining to): right lateral side of middle row near waist

- **Umbilical:** middle area of middle row containing navel (also called *umbilicus*)

- **Left lumbar:** left lateral side of middle row

- **Right iliac** (**ili/o** = ilium; **-ac** = pertaining to): right lateral side of lower row near groin; also called **right inguinal** (**inguin/o** = groin; **-al** = pertaining to)

- **Hypogastric** (**hypo-** = below; **gastr/o** = stomach; **-ic** = pertaining to): middle area of lower row

- **Left iliac:** (**ili/o** = ilium; **-ac** = pertaining to): left lateral side of lower row near groin; also called **left inguinal** (**inguin/o** = groin; **-al** = pertaining to)

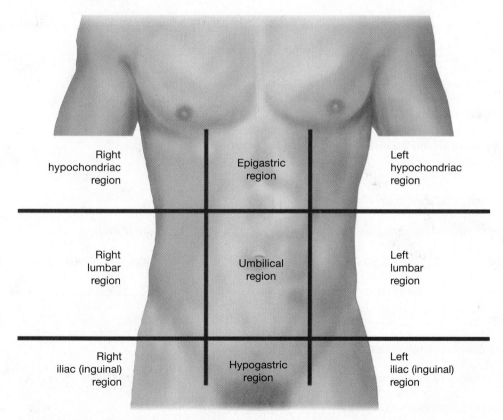

Right
hypochondriac
region

Epigastric
region

Left
hypochondriac
region

Right
lumbar
region

Umbilical
region

Left
lumbar
region

Right
iliac (inguinal)
region

Hypogastric
region

Left
iliac (inguinal)
region

4.9 The anatomical divisions of the abdomen; the abdominopelvic cavity is divided into nine regions

Directional Terms

For each of the following directional terms, write a directional term that could be used to indicate the opposite direction.

1. anterior _____

2. caudal _____

3. cephalic _____

4. deep _____

5. distal _____

6. dorsal _____

7. inferior _____

8. lateral _____

9. medial _____

10. posterior _____

11. proximal _____

12. superficial _____

13. superior _____

14. ventral _____

15. supine _____

Fill in the Blank

Fill in the blank to complete each of the following sentences.

1. The _____ cavity contains the spinal cord.

2. The sac protecting the lungs is called the _____.

3. The cranial and spinal cavities are found on the _____ side of the body.

4. The _____ is the only major abdominopelvic internal organ found outside the peritoneum.

5. The heart, lungs, esophagus, aorta, and thymus gland are found in the _____ cavity.

6. The _____ protects the organs of the abdominopelvic cavity.

7. The cranial cavity contains the _____.

8. The pericardial sac covers the _____.

9. The urinary bladder is found in the _____ cavity.

10. The brain and spinal cord are protected by a sac called the _____.

11. The liver is found in the _____ cavity.

12. The central region of the thoracic cavity is called the _____.

Labeling Exercise—External Surface Anatomy

Write the name of each area on the numbered line.

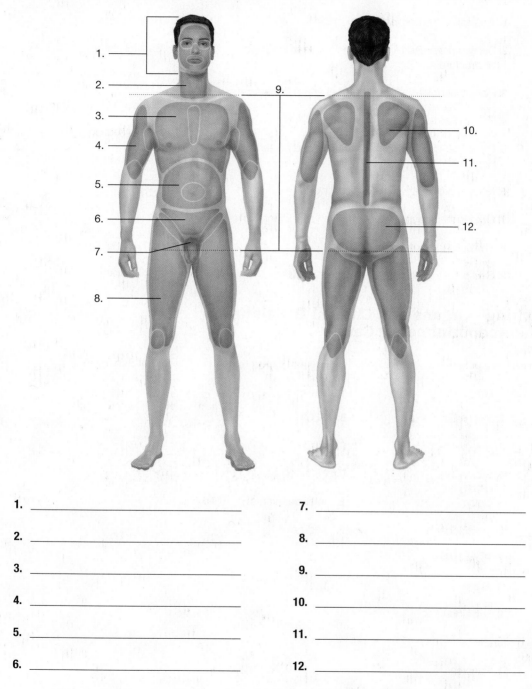

1. _____

2. _____

3. _____

4. _____

5. _____

6. _____

7. _____

8. _____

9. _____

10. _____

11. _____

12. _____

Matching—Planes and Sections

Match each body plane and section to its definition. Answers may be used more than once.

_____ **1.** Also called the *coronal plane*

_____ **2.** Section produced by cut at right angle to long axis of structure

_____ **3.** Plane that divides the body into left and right portions

_____ **4.** The two vertical planes

_____ **5.** Plane that divides body into anterior and posterior portions

_____ **6.** Section produced by the coronal plane

_____ **7.** Divides the body into upper and lower portions

_____ **8.** The only horizontal plane

_____ **9.** Section cut along long axis of the structure

A. Frontal plane

B. Sagittal plane

C. Transverse plane

D. Longitudinal section

E. Frontal section

F. Cross-section

Matching—Organs and Clinical Divisions of the Abdominopelvic Cavity

Match each organ to the quadrant in which you would expect to find the majority of that organ.

_____ **1.** Liver

_____ **2.** Left ureter

_____ **3.** Spleen

_____ **4.** Stomach

_____ **5.** Colon

_____ **6.** Gallbladder

_____ **7.** Right ovary

_____ **8.** Sigmoid colon

_____ **9.** Left kidney

_____ **10.** Uterus

_____ **11.** Pancreas

_____ **12.** Small intestine

_____ **13.** Appendix

A. RUQ

B. RLQ

C. LUQ

D. LLQ

E. In all quadrants

F. Midline

Labeling Exercise—Anatomical Divisions of the Abdominopelvic Cavity

Write the name for each anatomical division of the abdominopelvic cavity on the line provided.

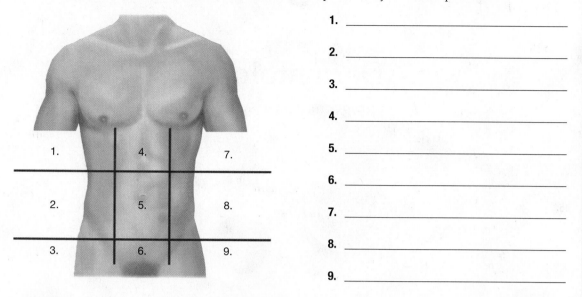

1. _____

2. _____

3. _____

4. _____

5. _____

6. _____

7. _____

8. _____

9. _____

MyMedicalTerminologyLab™

MyMedicalTerminologyLab is a premium online homework management system that includes a host of features to help you study. Registered users will find:

- A multitude of activities and assignments built within the MyLab platform
- Powerful tools that track and analyze your results—allowing you to create a personalized learning experience
- Videos and audio pronunciations to help enrich your progress
- Streaming lesson presentations and self-paced learning modules
- A space where you and your instructors can view and manage your assignments

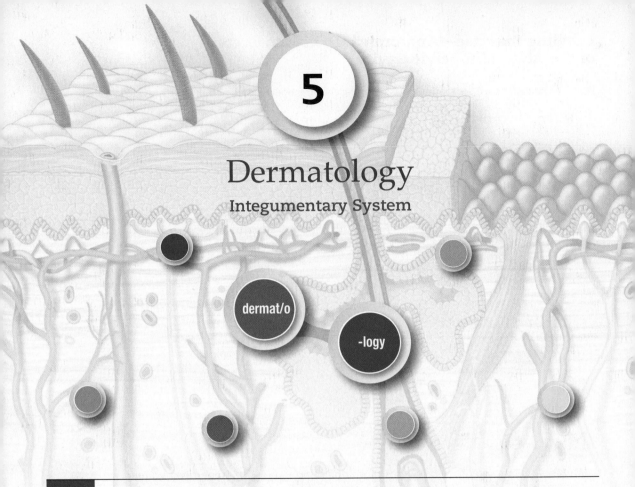

5

Dermatology
Integumentary System

dermat/o

-logy

∨ Learning Objectives

Upon completion of this chapter, you will be able to:

5-1 Describe the medical specialty of dermatology.

5-2 Understand the functions of the skin.

5-3 Define dermatology-related combining forms, prefixes, and suffixes.

5-4 Identify the organs treated in dermatology.

5-5 Build dermatology medical terms from word parts.

5-6 Explain dermatology medical terms.

5-7 Use dermatology abbreviations.

A Brief Introduction to Dermatology

Dermatology is the branch of medicine concerned with the diagnosis and treatment of conditions involving the skin and its accessory structures, **hair** and **nails**. A **dermatologist** specializes in treating skin tumors, damaged skin from trauma and burns, skin infections, inflammatory skin conditions, and cosmetic disorders including hair loss, scars, and skin changes associated with aging.

Plastic surgery is another branch of medicine that treats conditions involving the integumentary system as well as conditions of the musculoskeletal system, head and face, hands, breasts, and external genitalia. **Plastic surgeons** repair, reconstruct, or improve damaged or missing body structures.

The **skin,** or **integument,** is the largest organ in the body, weighing an average of 20 pounds. It serves several important functions.

- **Protection** – Skin is a continuous two-way barrier that prevents pathogens such as bacteria from invading the body and vital substances such as water from leaking out of the body.

- **Temperature regulation** – If the body is too hot, evaporation of sweat from sweat glands and dilation of blood vessels in the skin helps to cool the body; if it needs to conserve heat, blood vessels constrict; additionally, the fatty subcutaneous layer serves as insulation.

- **Sensation** – Skin contains many different sensory receptors that send information to the brain regarding the senses of touch, pressure, temperature, and pain.

- **Waste disposal** – A small amount of waste products, such as excess salt, is excreted from the body in the form of sweat.

Dermatology Combining Forms

The following list presents combining forms closely associated with the skin and used for building and defining dermatology terms.

aden/o	gland		**lip/o**	fat
adip/o	fat		**melan/o**	melanin, black
cutane/o	skin		**onych/o**	nail
cyan/o	blue		**py/o**	pus
derm/o	skin		**seb/o**	sebum, oil
dermat/o	skin		**trich/o**	hair
hidr/o	sweat		**ungu/o**	nail
kerat/o	keratin, hard, hornlike			

The following list presents combining forms that are not specific to the skin but are used for building and defining dermatology terms.

bi/o	life		**myc/o**	fungus
carcin/o	cancer		**necr/o**	death
chem/o	chemical		**scler/o**	hardening
cry/o	cold		**vesic/o**	bladder, sac
erythr/o	red		**xanth/o**	yellow
ichthy/o	scaly		**xer/o**	dry
leuk/o	white			

Suffix Review

These suffixes introduced in Chapter 2 are being reviewed in this chapter because they are especially important for building dermatology terms.

-al	pertaining to	-oid	resembling
-cle	small	-oma	tumor, mass
-cyte	cell	-opsy	view of
-derma	skin condition	-ose	pertaining to
-ectomy	surgical removal	-osis	abnormal condition
-genic	producing	-ous	pertaining to
-ia	state, condition	-pathy	disease
-ic	pertaining to	-phagia	eating, swallowing
-itis	inflammation	-plasty	surgical repair
-logist	one who studies	-rrhea	flow, discharge
-logy	study of	-sclerosis	hardening
-malacia	abnormal softening	-tic	pertaining to
-megaly	enlarged	-tome	instrument used to cut

Prefix Review

These prefixes introduced in Chapter 3 are being reviewed in this chapter because they are especially important for building dermatology terms.

an-	without	pachy-	thick
epi-	above	per-	through
hyper-	excessive	sub-	beneath, under
hypo-	below, insufficient	trans-	across
intra-	within		

Organs Commonly Treated in Dermatology

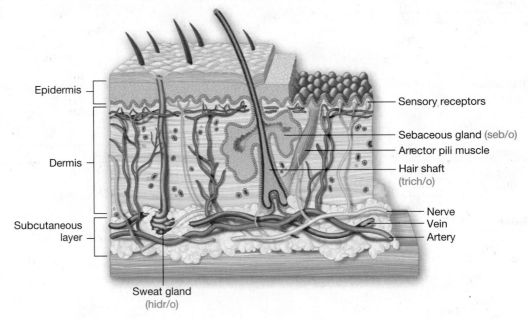

5.1 Structures of the skin

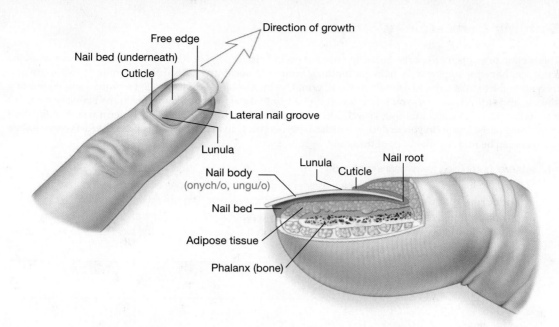

Direction of growth

Free edge

Nail bed (underneath)

Cuticle

Lateral nail groove

Lunula

Lunula

Cuticle

Nail root

Nail body
(onych/o, ungu/o)

Nail bed

Adipose tissue

Phalanx (bone)

5.2 Nail structure

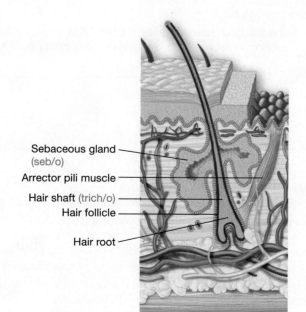

Sebaceous gland
(seb/o)

Arrector pili muscle

Hair shaft (trich/o)

Hair follicle

Hair root

5.3 Hair structure

Building Dermatology Terms

This section presents word parts most often used to build dermatology terms. Following the explanation of the term, you have the opportunity to begin building your own vocabulary. Read the meaning of each term and then fill in the blanks to build a single medical term. Use the slashes to divide prefixes, word roots, combining vowels, and suffixes. To help you out you will find a key to the word parts underneath the blanks: **r** for word root, **p** for prefix, **cv** for combining vowel, and **s** for suffix. Remember that not every term will contain all of these word parts; it is up to you to decide which to use. As you gain experience, this process will become easier. Answers can be found at the back of the book.

1. **aden/o**–combining form meaning **gland**

   A gland is an organ that secretes a substance; the two general types of glands in the body are **endocrine glands** and **exocrine glands**; endocrine glands, like the thyroid gland and pituitary gland, secrete directly into the bloodstream, they are not part of the skin; exocrine glands, like **sweat glands** and **sebaceous glands**, located in the dermis layer of the skin, secrete into a duct

   a. surgical removal of a gland _____/_____
                                                                  _r_   _s_

   b. inflammation of a gland _____/_____
                               _r_   _s_

   c. tumor in a gland _____/_____
                      _r_   _s_

   d. disease of a gland _____/_____/_____
                      _r_   _cv_   _s_

   e. enlarged gland _____/_____/_____
                      _r_   _cv_   _s_

2. **adip/o**–combining form meaning **fat**

   Fat tissue makes up the subcutaneous layer; forms continuous layer over the body underlying the dermis; serves as insulation, energy storage, and protective padding layer (see again Figure 5.1)

   a. pertaining to fat _____/_____
                      _r_   _s_

   b. fat cell _____/_____/_____
                      _r_   _cv_   _s_

   c. tumor made of fat _____/_____
                      _r_   _s_

3. **cutane/o**–combining form meaning **skin**

   Skin is also called the **integument**; protective outer layer of the body; composed of two layers:

   - **Epidermis:** outer layer; composed primarily of overlapping layers of flat, dead keratinized cells that form protective barrier to keep out bacteria and other pathogens; deepest layer of epidermis is **basal layer** composed of living cells that grow and divide to replace dead cells sloughed off from skin surface; lacks a blood supply, depends on dermis for nourishment; location of **melanocytes**
   - **Dermis:** inner layer; strong, flexible connective tissue for strength; houses hair follicles, sweat glands, sebaceous glands, sensory receptors, and blood vessels

   The **subcutaneous layer** is a layer of tissue underlying the dermis; not truly a layer of the skin, but closely associated with and assists in the functions of the skin; primarily composed of fat; insulates the body, provides protective padding, and stores energy (see again Figure 5.1)

a. pertaining to the skin _____/_____
r   s

b. pertaining to beneath the skin _____/_____/_____
p   r   s

c. pertaining to through the skin _____/_____/_____
p   r   s

---

4. cyan/o–combining form meaning **blue**

Skin appears to be a blue color when its blood supply becomes deoxygenated; deoxygenated blood is a very dark red color that makes the skin appear blue when viewed through the layers of the skin

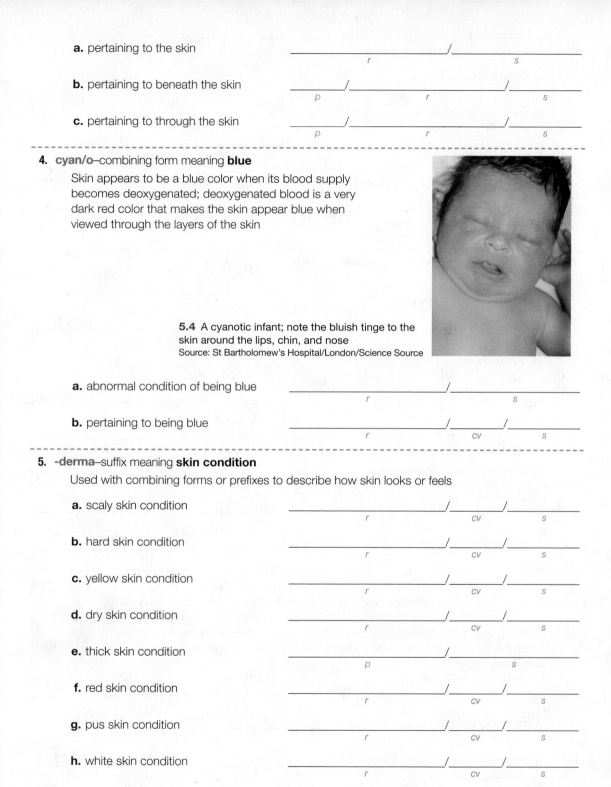

5.4 A cyanotic infant; note the bluish tinge to the skin around the lips, chin, and nose
Source: St Bartholomew's Hospital/London/Science Source

a. abnormal condition of being blue _____/_____
r   s

b. pertaining to being blue _____/_____/_____
r   cv   s

---

5. -derma–suffix meaning **skin condition**

Used with combining forms or prefixes to describe how skin looks or feels

a. scaly skin condition _____/_____/_____
r   cv   s

b. hard skin condition _____/_____/_____
r   cv   s

c. yellow skin condition _____/_____/_____
r   cv   s

d. dry skin condition _____/_____/_____
r   cv   s

e. thick skin condition _____/_____
p   s

f. red skin condition _____/_____/_____
r   cv   s

g. pus skin condition _____/_____/_____
r   cv   s

h. white skin condition _____/_____/_____
r   cv   s

6. derm/o–combining form meaning **skin**

a. pertaining to the skin
_____/_____
r   s

b. pertaining to above the skin
_____/_____/_____
p   r   s

c. pertaining to within the skin
_____/_____/_____
p   r   s

d. pertaining to below the skin
_____/_____/_____
p   r   s

e. pertaining to across the skin
_____/_____/_____
p   r   s

7. dermat/o–combining form meaning **skin**

a. skin inflammation
_____/_____
r   s

b. study of the skin
_____/_____/_____
r   cv   s

c. one who studies the skin
_____/_____/_____
r   cv   s

d. abnormal condition of the skin
_____/_____
r   s

e. surgical repair of the skin
_____/_____/_____
r   cv   s

f. abnormal skin fungus condition
_____/_____/_____/_____
r   cv   r   s

g. disease of the skin
_____/_____/_____
r   cv   s

h. hardened skin condition
_____/_____/_____
r   cv   s

8. hidr/o–combining form meaning **sweat**

Sweat is secreted by sweat glands; primary function is to cool the skin by evaporation; also contains a small amount of waste products such as sodium chloride, urea, and ammonia; sweat glands are tightly coiled structures located in the dermis; sweat is carried to the skin surface by a sweat duct (see again Figure 5.1)

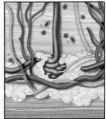

5.5 Sweat gland

a. abnormal condition of sweating
_____/_____
r   s

b. abnormal condition with lack of sweating
_____/_____/_____
p   r   s

c. sweat gland inflammation
_____/_____/_____
r   r   s

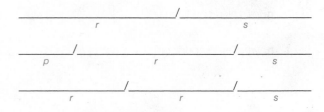

d. abnormal condition of excessive sweating

_____ / _____ / _____
     p   *r*   *s*

---

9. **kerat/o**–combining form meaning **keratin, hard, hornlike**

This hard protein is found in **hair**, **nails**, and the outermost layer of cells in the epidermis; may become overgrown resulting in thick, hornlike layer of skin

    a. hornlike skin condition

_____ / _____ / _____
                       r   *cv*   *s*

    b. hornlike abnormal condition

_____ / _____
                       r   *s*

    c. producing keratin

_____ / _____ / _____
                       r   *cv*   *s*

---

10. **lip/o**–combining form meaning **fat**

    a. surgical removal of fat

_____ / _____
                       r   *s*

    b. resembling fat

_____ / _____
                       r   *s*

    c. fat tumor

_____ / _____
                       r   *s*

    d. fat cell

_____ / _____ / _____
                       r   *cv*   *s*

---

11. **melan/o**–combining form meaning **melanin, black**

Melanin is the black pigment found in melanocytes that gives skin and hair its color; the more melanin present, the darker the hair or skin; provides protection against damage from ultraviolet (UV) ray exposure

    a. black tumor

_____ / _____
                       r   *s*

    b. black cell

_____ / _____ / _____
                       r   *cv*   *s*

    c. pertaining to being black

_____ / _____ / _____
                       r   *cv*   *s*

---

12. **onych/o**–combining form meaning **nail**

Nails are flat plates of keratin, called the **nail body**, that cover ends of fingers and toes; connected to tissue underneath by the **nail bed**; grows longer from the **nail root** located at the base of the nail and covered by the **cuticle**; light-colored half-moon area at the base of the nail is the **lunula**; exposed edge that is trimmed to shorten the nail is the **free edge** (see again Figure 5.2)

5.6 Nail

    a. surgical removal of a nail

_____ / _____
                       r   *s*

    b. inflammation of a nail

_____ / _____
                       r   *s*

c. abnormal softening of a nail

_____/_____/_____
r   cv   s

d. abnormal nail fungus condition

_____/_____/_____/_____
r   cv   r   s

e. nail eating (biting)

_____/_____/_____
r   cv   s

f. state of excessive nail (growth)

_____/_____/_____
p   r   s

---

13. **py/o**–combining form meaning **pus**

   Pus is a semisolid fluid associated with certain bacterial infections; consists of tissue fluid, dead bacteria, debris from damaged cells, and dead white blood cells

   a. producing pus

   _____/_____/_____
   r   cv   s

   b. discharge of pus

   _____/_____/_____
   r   cv   s

---

14. **seb/o**–combining form meaning **oil, sebum**

   Sebum is the oily secretion of sebaceous glands; released directly into a hair follicle and serves to lubricate the skin to keep it soft and prevent it from cracking (see again Figure 5.3)

   a. flow of oil

   _____/_____/_____
   r   cv   s

---

15. **trich/o**–combining form meaning **hair**

   A hair is a shaft of keratinized cells growing up through the layers of the skin; **hair shaft** grows longer from the **hair root** and extends toward the skin surface within a **hair follicle**; sebaceous glands secrete sebum directly into hair follicle; a slender slip of smooth muscle, the **arrector pili**, attaches to the hair follicle and causes the hair shaft to stand up when it contracts (goose bumps) (see again Figure 5.3)

   5.7 Hair

   a. abnormal hair fungus condition

   _____/_____/_____/_____
   r   cv   r   s

   b. hair eating (chewing/biting)

   _____/_____/_____
   r   cv   s

---

16. **ungu/o**–combining form meaning **nail**

   a. pertaining to a nail

   _____/_____
   r   s

   b. pertaining to under a nail

   _____/_____/_____
   p   r   s

Dermatology Vocabulary

The dermatology terms presented in this section include eponyms, modern English words, and those that contain Latin or Greek word parts but are not constructed solely from these word parts. When you recognize word parts within a term, they will give you a hint about the word's meaning. In these instances, look for the word parts to follow the term.

Term	Explanation
abrasion	Skin injury that scrapes away surface of the skin
abscess	A collection of pus in the skin
alopecia	Absence or loss of hair, especially of head
basal cell carcinoma (BCC) **carcin/o** = cancer **-oma** = tumor	Skin cancer in basal cell layer of epidermis; very common cancer caused by sun exposure but rarely metastasizes or spreads
biopsy (BX, bx) **bi/o** = life **-opsy** = view of	Surgical procedure to remove a piece of tissue by needle, knife, punch, or brush to examine under a microscope in order to make a diagnosis
boil	Bacterial infection of a hair follicle; also called a *furuncle*
burn, first-degree (1st degree)	Mild burn that damages epidermis only; results in erythema but no blisters; generally, there is no scarring
burn, second-degree (2nd degree)	Burn damage that extends through the epidermis and into the dermis, causing blisters to form; scarring may occur
burn, third-degree (3rd degree)	Burn damage to the full thickness of skin and into underlying tissues; infection and fluid loss are major concerns; usually requires skin grafts to cover burned areas; scarring will occur
cauterization	Intentional destruction of tissue by a caustic chemical, electric current, laser, or freezing

TERMINOLOGY TIDBIT
The term *alopecia* comes from the Greek word *alopekia* meaning "fox mange," a condition that causes hair to fall out.

5.8 Basal cell carcinoma
Source: Centers for Disease Control and Prevention

First-degree burn
Second-degree burn
Third-degree burn

Epidermis
Dermis
Subcutaneous layer

5.9 Illustration comparing the depth of the three types of burns

Term	Explanation
cellulitis	Inflammation of connective tissue cells of skin
chemabrasion chem/o = chemical	Removal of superficial layers of skin using chemicals; also called a *chemical peel*
contusion	Blunt trauma to skin that results in bruising but no break in the skin **TERMINOLOGY TIDBIT** The term *contusion* comes from the Latin word *contusion* meaning "to bruise or crush."
cryosurgery cry/o = cold	Using extreme cold to freeze and destroy tissue
culture and sensitivity (C&S)	Laboratory test that grows a colony of bacteria removed from infected area in order to identify the specific type of bacteria and then determine its sensitivity to a variety of antibiotics
cyst	Fluid-filled sac under the skin
debridement	Removal of foreign material and dead or damaged tissue from a wound
decubitus ulcer (decub)	Open sore caused by pressure over bony prominences obstructing blood flow; can appear in bedridden patients who lie in one position too long and can be difficult to heal; commonly called a *bedsore* or a *pressure sore* **TERMINOLOGY TIDBIT** The term *decubitus* comes from the Latin word *decumbo*, meaning "lying down," which leads to the use of the term for a bedsore or pressure sore.
dermabrasion derm/o = skin	Scraping skin with rotating wire brushes or sandpaper; used to remove acne scars

dermatome
  derm/o = skin
  -tome = instrument to cut
	Instrument that cuts out a small section of skin or a thin slice of skin to be used for a graft

ecchymosis	"Black-and-blue" skin bruise caused by blood collecting under skin after trauma **5.10** Man lying supine on the ground with a large ecchymosis on his left lateral rib cage Source: Pearson Education
erythema erythr/o = red	Redness of skin
fissure	Cracklike break in skin
gangrene	Tissue necrosis caused by loss of blood supply **TERMINOLOGY TIDBIT** The term *gangrene* comes from the Greek word *gangraina* meaning "an eating sore," which describes how this condition progresses by growing deeper and wider.

Term	Explanation
herpes simplex	Infection by herpes simplex virus (HSV) causing painful blisters around lips and nose; commonly called *fever blisters* **5.11** Herpes simplex infection, commonly called *fever blisters* Source: Sokolenok/Shutterstock
herpes zoster	Viral infection of a nerve root that causes the appearance of very painful blisters along the path of a nerve; commonly called *shingles* **5.12** Herpes zoster Source: Phadungsak photo/Shutterstock
impetigo	Inflammatory skin disease with pustules that rupture and become crusted
laceration	Jagged-edged skin wound caused by tearing of the skin; does not mean a skin cut
laser surgery	Removal of skin lesions and birthmarks using laser beam
lesion	General term that indicates the presence of some type of tissue abnormality, wound, or injury
macule	Flat, discolored spot on the skin surface; example is a freckle or birthmark
malignant melanoma (MM) **melan/o** = black **-oma** = tumor	Aggressive form of skin cancer that originates in a melanocyte; prone to metastasize or spread **5.13** Malignant melanoma Source: National Cancer Institute
necrosis **necr/o** = death **-osis** = abnormal condition	Area of tissue death **5.14** Necrosis Source: Myibean/Shutterstock
nevus	Pigmented skin blemish, birthmark, or mole
nodule	Solid, raised clump of skin cells
onychia **onych/o** = nail	Inflamed nail bed

> **TERMINOLOGY TIDBIT**
> The term *lesion* comes from the Latin word *laedere* meaning "to injure."

Term	Explanation
papule	Small, solid, raised lesion on surface of the skin
petechiae	Flat, pinpoint, purplish spots from bleeding under the skin
pruritus	Severe itching
psoriasis	Chronic inflammatory condition consisting of crusty papules forming patches with circular borders **5.15** Psoriasis Source: Hriana/Shutterstock
purpura	Purplish-red bruises usually occurring in people with thin, easily damaged skin **5.16** Purpura Source: Scimat/Science Source
pustule	Raised spot on the skin containing pus
skin graft (SG)	Transfer of the skin from a normal area to cover another site; used to treat burn victims and after some surgical procedures
squamous cell carcinoma (SCC) **carcin/o** = cancer **-oma** = tumor	Skin cancer that begins in the epidermis but may grow into deeper tissue; does not generally metastasize to other areas of the body **5.17** Squamous cell carcinoma Source: National Cancer Institute
tinea	Fungal skin disease resulting in itching, scaling lesions **5.18** Illustration of fungal infection on a foot (athlete's foot). Source: Justyle/Shutterstock
ulcer	Open sore or lesion in the skin or mucous membrane
urticaria	Skin eruption of pale reddish wheals with severe itching; usually associated with food allergy, stress, or drug reactions; also called *hives*

TERMINOLOGY TIDBIT
The term *urticaria* comes from the Latin word *urtica* meaning "nettle."

Term	Explanation
varicella	Highly contagious viral infection with skin rash; commonly called *chickenpox* 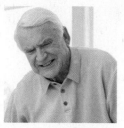 **5.19** Characteristic blistered rash of varicella (chickenpox) Source: Centers for Disease Control and Prevention
vesicle vesic/o = bladder, sac -cle = small	Small, fluid-filled raised spot on the skin
wheal	Small, round, raised area on the skin that may be accompanied by itching; usually seen in allergic reactions

Dermatology Abbreviations

The following list presents common dermatology abbreviations.

BCC	basal cell carcinoma	**ID**	intradermal
BX, bx	biopsy	**MM**	malignant melanoma
C&S	culture and sensitivity	**SCC**	squamous cell carcinoma
decub	decubitus ulcer	**SG**	skin graft
Derm, derm	dermatology	**STSG**	split-thickness skin graft
HSV	herpes simplex virus	**Subc, Subq**	subcutaneous
I&D	incision and drainage	**ung**	ointment

CASE STUDY

History of Present Illness

A 71-year-old male was referred to a dermatologist for evaluation of right foot ulcers that had not healed for three years. The ulcers first began as a tender, reddened pustule on the lateral aspect of the right foot. The first ulcer appeared three months later and was quickly followed by the development of two additional ulcers. The lesions have not improved with treatment with oral antibiotics, topical anti-inflammatory cream, or whirlpool regimen.

Past Medical History

Source: Monkey Business Images/Shutterstock

Patient was diagnosed with thromboangiitis obliterans eight years ago. He had a vascular bypass for the right lower leg five years ago and for the left lower leg two years ago. He tests negative for diabetes mellitus.

Family and Social History

Patient is a retired night watchman. He is active and engages in extensive landscaping of his yard for a hobby. He smoked two packs of cigarettes per week beginning in his teenage years but stopped smoking at the time thromboangiitis obliterans was diagnosed. He denies alcohol or illicit drug use. He has been married for 49 years and has three married children. His mother died at age 75 following complications of type II diabetes mellitus necessitating bilateral below-the-knee amputations. His father is still alive at age 93 and in reasonable health for his age. He has no siblings.

Physical Examination

There are three ulcers on the lateral aspect of the right foot and ankle. Each measures approximately 3 × 4 cm. The ulcers are covered by necrotic tissue, and there are copious amounts of pus drainage from each. Erythema is noted in the skin around the edge of each ulcer.

Diagnostic Tests

C&S of drainage from each ulcer revealed staphylococcus bacterial infections that were found to be resistant to penicillin and sensitive to vancomycin, which is available only in IV form. Fungal scrapings were negative.

Diagnosis

Gangrene ulcers right lower leg.

Plan of Treatment

1. Admit to hospital for IV antibiotic therapy, whirlpool, and surgical debridement of ulcers
2. Schedule patient for skin graft in the future when infection has cleared up and if lower leg circulation is sufficient to support healing of grafts

Critical Thinking Questions

Answer the following questions regarding this case study. Do not just copy words out of the case study but translate all medical terms. In order to answer some of these questions, you may need to look up information in another chapter of this text, in a medical dictionary, or online. Answers can be found at the back of the book.

1. Describe how the ulcers first appeared before they were actual ulcers.

   _____

   _____

2. Describe the treatments that have not healed the ulcers.

   _____

   _____

3. What medical condition does this patient not have that his mother did have?

   _____

   _____

4. Which of the following regarding the ulcers is NOT true?

   a. edges of ulcers are blue in color

   b. no fungi are present

   c. ulcers are covered by dead tissue

   d. a lot of pus is present

5. Explain what a C&S is. What does it mean that the bacteria are resistant to penicillin and sensitive to vancomycin?

   _____

   _____

6. The ulcers are infected by staphylococcus bacteria. Go to www.mayoclinic.com; type "staph infections" in the search box; and write a brief description about where this bacterium is found and how it causes serious infections.

   _____

   _____

7. This patient has ulcers that are caused by gangrene. What is the root cause of gangrene?

_____

_____

8. Explain each of the treatments planned when this patient is admitted to the hospital.

_____

_____

PRACTICE

Sound It Out

The following are some of the key terms from this chapter written as their phonetic spelling. Sound out each term and write it in the blank. Pronunciations for all terms are included in the audio glossary at www.mymedicalterminologylab.com.

1. ah-BRAY-zhun _____
2. add-eh-POH-ma _____
3. SIST _____
4. an-hi-DROH-sis _____
5. BYE-op-see _____
6. sell-you-LYE-tis _____
7. ULL-ser _____
8. AB-sess _____
9. DER-mah-tohm _____
10. FISH-er _____
11. sigh-ah-NO-sis _____
12. GANG-green _____
13. high-poh-DER-mik _____

14. VESS-ikl _____
15. lip-OH-mah _____
16. NOD-yool _____
17. MACK-yool _____
18. neh-KROH-sis _____
19. PAP-yool _____
20. soh-RYE-ah-sis _____
21. der-mah-TALL-oh-jee _____
22. seb-or-EE-ah _____
23. sub-kyoo-TAY-nee-us _____
24. TIN-ee-ah _____
25. UNG-gwal _____

Transcription Practice

Each of the following sentences is written in common English. Underline any words or phrases that can be replaced by a medical term. Then rewrite the entire sentence using medical terms. Answers can be found at the back of the book.

1. The specialist in treating skin conditions removed a sample of skin with a knife and examined it under a microscope to determine if the patient has a pigmented congenital skin blemish rather than aggressive skin cancer beginning in a melanocyte.

   _____

   _____

2. A laboratory test that grows a colony of bacteria to identify the type was performed to determine how best to treat the infected open sore.

   _____

   _____

3. The patient had a very large hair follicle with a bacterial infection surrounded by a large area of inflamed connective tissue skin cells around it.

   _____

   _____

4. Ms. Marks was lucky; when she tripped off the curb, she received only skin trauma that scraped away a layer of skin and blunt trauma to the skin resulting in bruises.

   _____

   _____

5. Mr. Brown's chronic exposure to toxins at work had left him with dry skin, scaly skin, and thick skin.

   _____

   _____

6. After years of nail biting, the patient developed a soft nail condition and an abnormal fungus nail condition that required surgical removal of the nail.

   _____

   _____

7. To repair the areas of full-thickness burns, a transfer of skin from a normal area to cover another site was necessary.

   _____

   _____

8. Mr. Strong was concerned that the lump he could feel under his skin was a gland tumor, but it turned out to be only a fat tumor and was removed with a surgical removal of the fat.

   _____

   _____

9. The surgeon who uses surgery to improve the appearance of damaged skin helped Mr. Marsh decide whether to have abrasion using chemicals or abrasion using a rotating wire brush for his face-lift.

   _____

   _____

10. New medical students often have difficulty telling the difference between a flat discolored spot, a raised solid lesion, and a fluid-filled sac under the skin.

_____

_____

Labeling Exercise

Write the name of each structure on the numbered line. Also use this space to write the combining form where appropriate.

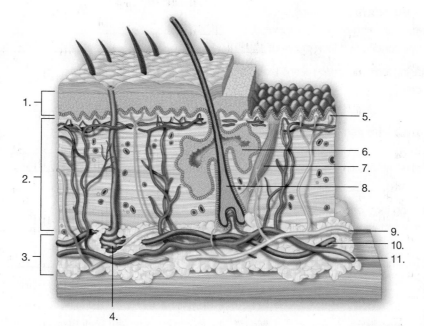

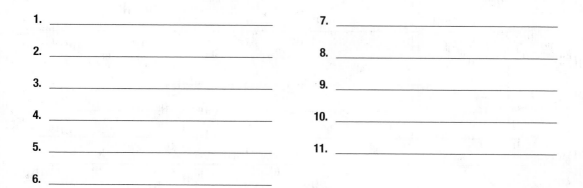

1. _____

2. _____

3. _____

4. _____

5. _____

6. _____

7. _____

8. _____

9. _____

10. _____

11. _____

Build Medical Terms

Use each of the following word parts to build the indicated medical terms.

1. The suffix –*derma* means skin condition.
   a. dry skin condition _____
   b. red skin condition _____
   c. pus skin condition _____
   d. hard skin condition _____
   e. thick skin condition _____

2. The combining form *hidr/o* means sweat.
   a. abnormal condition of excessive sweat _____
   b. abnormal condition of lack of sweat _____

3. The combining form *melan/o* means black.
   a. black cell _____
   b. black tumor _____

4. The combining form *dermat/o* means skin.
   a. skin disease _____
   b. surgical repair of skin _____
   c. study of skin _____

5. The combining form *onych/o* means nail.
   a. abnormal softening of nail _____
   b. abnormal condition of nail fungus _____
   c. surgical removal of nail _____

Spelling

Some of the following terms are misspelled. Identify the incorrect terms and spell them correctly in the blank provided.

1. empetigo _____
2. urticaria _____
3. wheel _____
4. psoriasis _____
5. fissure _____
6. tenia _____
7. peteckiae _____
8. gangreen _____
9. cauterization _____
10. necrowsis _____

Fill in the Blank

Fill in the blank to complete each of the following sentences.

1. A(n) _____ is a cracklike break in the skin while a(n) _____ is a jagged-edged skin wound.

2. Infection by the _____ virus causes painful blisters around the lips.

3. Ms. Branch had her acne scars removed with _____.

4. A diagnosis of _____ burn was made when the physician noted that the full thickness of skin was burned away.

5. A freckle is an example of a(n) _____.

6. The severe area of necrosis required _____ to remove the dead and damaged tissue.

7. A(n) _____ is a typical black-and-blue bruise from trauma.

8. The physician performed a(n) _____ to obtain a sample of the infected tissue to examine under a microscope.

9. A raised skin lesion that is solid is a(n) _____, but if it contains pus, it is a(n) _____.

10. Unfortunately, the bedridden patient developed a(n) _____ from being in one position too long.

Abbreviation Matching

Match each abbreviation with its definition.

_____ **1.** bx	**A.**	skin graft
_____ **2.** MM	**B.**	basal cell carcinoma
_____ **3.** Subq	**C.**	intradermal
_____ **4.** SCC	**D.**	split-thickness skin graft
_____ **5.** C&S	**E.**	biopsy
_____ **6.** BCC	**F.**	ointment
_____ **7.** SG	**G.**	squamous cell carcinoma
_____ **8.** STSG	**H.**	subcutaneous
_____ **9.** ung	**I.**	malignant melanoma
_____ **10.** ID	**J.**	culture and sensitivity

Medical Term Analysis

Examine each of the following terms. Begin by dividing each into its word parts and writing them in the indicated blanks (*P = prefix*; *WR = word root*; *CF = combining form*; *S = suffix*). Follow with the definition of each word part and then finally the meaning of the full term.

1. **adenomegaly**

   CF _____

   means _____

   S _____

   means _____

   Term meaning: _____

   _____

2. **adipocyte**

   CF _____

   means _____

   S _____

   means _____

   Term meaning: _____

   _____

3. **cyanosis**

   WR _____

   means _____

   S _____

   means _____

   Term meaning: _____

   _____

4. **hypodermic**

   P _____

   means _____

   WR _____

   means _____

   S _____

   means _____

   Term meaning: _____

   _____

5. **keratogenic**

   CF _____

   means _____

   S _____

   means _____

   Term meaning: _____

   _____

6. **lipectomy**

   WR _____

   means _____

   S _____

   means _____

   Term meaning: _____

   _____

7. **pyorrhea**

   CF _____

   means _____

   S _____

   means _____

   Term meaning: _____

   _____

8. **erythroderma**

   CF _____

   means _____

   S _____

   means _____

   Term meaning: _____

   _____

9. **trichomycosis**

   CF _____

   means _____

   WR _____

   means _____

   S _____

   means _____

   Term meaning: _____

   _____

10. **subcutaneous**

    P _____

    means _____

    WR _____

    means _____

    S _____

    means _____

    Term meaning: _____

    _____

MyMedicalTerminologyLab™

MyMedicalTerminologyLab is a premium online homework management system that includes a host of features to help you study. Registered users will find:

- A multitude of activities and assignments built within the MyLab platform
- Powerful tools that track and analyze your results—allowing you to create a personalized learning experience
- Videos and audio pronunciations to help enrich your progress
- Streaming lesson presentations and self-paced learning modules
- A space where you and your instructors can view and manage your assignments

Photomatch Challenge

Match each skin lesion with its picture.

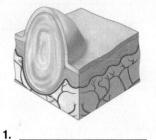

1. _____

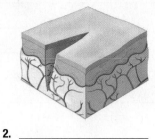

2. _____

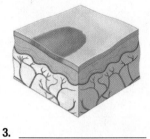

3. _____

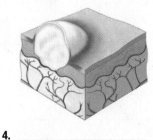

4. _____

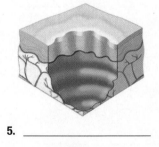

5. _____

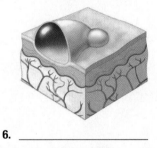

6. _____

Word Bank:

ulcer	macule	pustule
fissure	cyst	vesicle

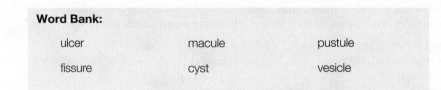

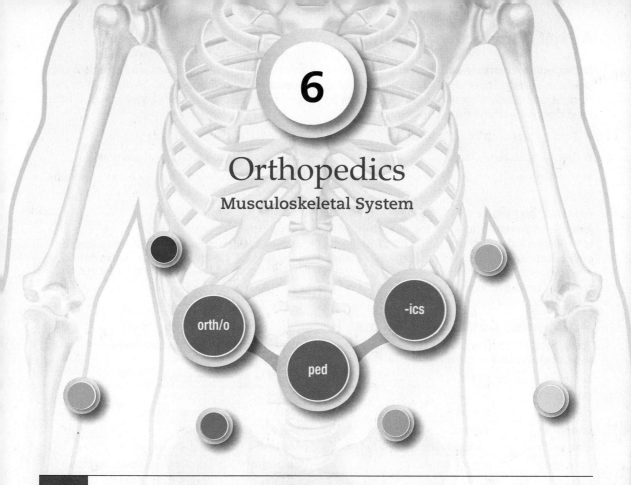

6

Orthopedics

Musculoskeletal System

∨ Learning Objectives

Upon completion of this chapter, you will be able to:

6-1 Describe the medical specialty of orthopedics.

6-2 Understand the function of the musculoskeletal system.

6-3 Define orthopedic-related combining forms, prefixes, and suffixes.

6-4 Identify the organs treated in orthopedics.

6-5 Build orthopedic medical terms from word parts.

6-6 Explain orthopedic medical terms.

6-7 Use orthopedic abbreviations.

A Brief Introduction to Orthopedics

Orthopedics, or **orthopedic surgery**, is the medical specialty that treats disorders involving the musculoskeletal system. Physicians in this specialty, called **orthopedists** or **orthopedic surgeons**, use medical, surgical, and physical means to correct defects and improve the function of bones, joints, and muscles. Examples of conditions treated by orthopedists are:

- Birth defects such as spina bifida
- Trauma such as fractures
- Infections such as osteomyelitis
- Tumors such as osteogenic sarcoma
- Inflammatory conditions such as arthritis
- Muscular problems such as muscular dystrophy

The musculoskeletal system consists of the **bones**, **muscles**, and **joints** of the body. The bones are joined by **ligaments** to form the **skeleton**, which is the framework of the body. The place where two bones meet is called a joint and provides flexibility for movement. Muscles, attached to the skeleton by **tendons**, cross over joints. These muscles contract to move the bones at each joint.

> **TERMINOLOGY TIDBIT**
> The term *skeleton* comes from the Greek word *skeltos* meaning "dried up." It was originally used to refer to a dried-up mummified body, but over time came to be used for bones.

Orthopedic Combining Forms

The following list presents combining forms closely associated with the musculoskeletal system and used for building and defining orthopedic terms.

arthr/o	joint		**muscul/o**	muscle
burs/o	bursa		**my/o**	muscle
carp/o	carpus (wrist)		**myel/o**	bone marrow
chondr/o	cartilage		**oste/o**	bone
clavicul/o	clavicle (collar bone)		**patell/o**	patella (kneecap)
coccyg/o	coccyx (tailbone)		**phalang/o**	phalanges (fingers and toes)
cost/o	rib		**pub/o**	pubis (part of pelvis)
crani/o	skull		**radi/o**	radius (part of forearm)
femor/o	femur (thigh bone)		**sacr/o**	sacrum
fibul/o	fibula (thinner lower leg bone)		**scapul/o**	scapula (shoulder blade)
humer/o	humerus (upper arm bone)		**scoli/o**	crooked, bent
ili/o	ilium (part of pelvis)		**spondyl/o**	vertebra
ischi/o	ischium (part of pelvis)		**stern/o**	sternum (breast bone)
kyph/o	hump		**tars/o**	tarsus (ankle)
lord/o	bent backward		**ten/o**	tendon
mandibul/o	mandible (lower jaw)		**tendin/o**	tendon
maxill/o	maxilla (upper jaw)		**tibi/o**	tibia (shin, larger lower leg bone)
metacarp/o	metacarpus (hand bones)		**uln/o**	ulna (part of forearm)
metatars/o	metatarsus (foot bones)		**vertebr/o**	vertebra (backbone)

The following list presents combining forms that are not specific to orthopedics but are also used for building and defining orthopedic terms.

cutane/o	skin		**orth/o**	straight
electr/o	electricity		**path/o**	disease
fibr/o	fibrous			

Suffix Review

These suffixes introduced in Chapter 2 are being reviewed in this chapter because they are especially important for building orthopedic terms.

-ac	pertaining to		-itis	inflammation
-al	pertaining to		-kinesia	movement
-algia	pain		-malacia	abnormal softening
-ar	pertaining to		-metry	process of measuring
-ary	pertaining to		-oma	tumor
-asthenia	weakness		-osis	abnormal condition
-centesis	puncture to withdraw fluid		-otomy	cutting into
-clasia	surgical breaking		-ous	pertaining to
-cyte	cell		-pathy	disease
-desis	surgical fusion		-plasty	surgical repair
-dynia	pain		-porosis	porous
-eal	pertaining to		-rrhaphy	suture
-ectomy	surgical removal		-rrhexis	rupture
-genic	producing		-scope	instrument for viewing
-gram	record		-scopy	process of visually examining
-graphy	process of recording		-tome	instrument to cut
-ic	pertaining to		-trophy	development

Prefix Review

These prefixes introduced in Chapter 3 are being reviewed here because they are especially important for building orthopedic terms.

a-	without		intra-	within
brady-	slow		per-	through
dys-	painful, difficult, abnormal		sub-	under
hyper-	excessive		supra-	above
inter-	between			

Organs Commonly Treated in Orthopedics

Skull　　　　　　**Pelvis**　　　　　　**Hand**

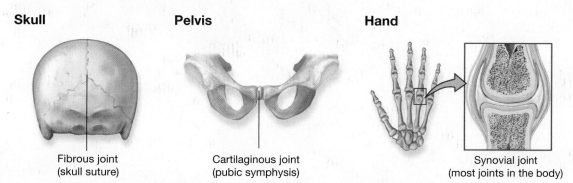

Fibrous joint
(skull suture)

Cartilaginous joint
(pubic symphysis)

Synovial joint
(most joints in the body)

6.1 Examples of three types of joints found in the body

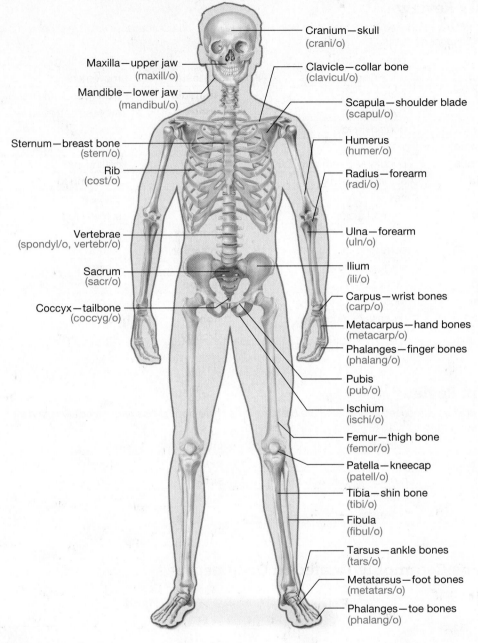

Cranium—skull
(crani/o)

Maxilla—upper jaw
(maxill/o)

Mandible—lower jaw
(mandibul/o)

Clavicle—collar bone
(clavicul/o)

Scapula—shoulder blade
(scapul/o)

Sternum—breast bone
(stern/o)

Humerus
(humer/o)

Rib
(cost/o)

Radius—forearm
(radi/o)

Vertebrae
(spondyl/o, vertebr/o)

Ulna—forearm
(uln/o)

Sacrum
(sacr/o)

Ilium
(ili/o)

Coccyx—tailbone
(coccyg/o)

Carpus—wrist bones
(carp/o)

Metacarpus—hand bones
(metacarp/o)

Phalanges—finger bones
(phalang/o)

Pubis
(pub/o)

Ischium
(ischi/o)

Femur—thigh bone
(femor/o)

Patella—kneecap
(patell/o)

Tibia—shin bone
(tibi/o)

Fibula
(fibul/o)

Tarsus—ankle bones
(tars/o)

Metatarsus—foot bones
(metatars/o)

Phalanges—toe bones
(phalang/o)

6.2 The skeleton

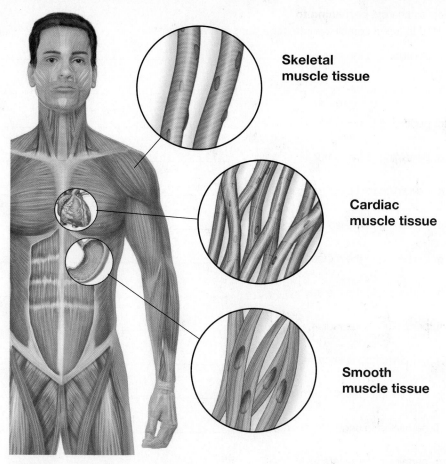

Skeletal muscle tissue

Cardiac muscle tissue

Smooth muscle tissue

6.3 Types of muscle tissue in the body

Building Orthopedic Terms

This section presents word parts most often used to build orthopedic terms. Following the explanation of the term, you have the opportunity to begin building your own vocabulary. Read the meaning for each term and then fill in the blanks to build a single medical term. Use the slashes to divide prefixes, word roots, combining vowels, and suffixes. To help you out you will find a key to the word parts underneath the blanks: **r** for word roots, **p** for prefix, **cv** for combining vowel, and **s** for suffix. Remember that not every term will contain all these word parts; it's up to you to decide which to use. As you gain experience, this process becomes easier. Answers can be found at the back of the book.

1. **-ac**–suffix meaning **pertaining to**
   Used to turn a combining form for a bone into an adjective

   a. pertaining to the ilium

   _____/_____
                  r   *s*

   b. pertaining to under the ilium

   _____/_____/_____
        p   *r*   *s*

2. **-al**–suffix meaning **pertaining to**
    Used to turn a combining form for a bone into an adjective

    a. pertaining to the carpus   _____/_____
                                                                                       r   s

    b. pertaining to the rib   _____/_____
                                                                                       r   s

    c. pertaining to between the ribs   _____/_____/_____
                             p   r   s

    d. pertaining to the femur   _____/_____
                                                                               r   s

    e. pertaining to the humerus   _____/_____
                                              r   s

    f. pertaining to the ischium   _____/_____
                                              r   s

    g. pertaining to the metacarpus   _____/_____
                                              r   s

    h. pertaining to the metatarsus   _____/_____
                                              r   s

    i. pertaining to the radius   _____/_____
                                              r   s

    j. pertaining to the sacrum   _____/_____
                                              r   s

    k. pertaining to the sternum   _____/_____
                                              r   s

    l. pertaining to under the sternum   _____/_____/_____
                             p   r   s

    m. pertaining to the tarsus   _____/_____
                                              r   s

    n. pertaining to the tibia   _____/_____
                                              r   s

    o. pertaining to the vertebrae   _____/_____
                                              r   s

    p. pertaining to between the vertebrae   _____/_____/_____
                             p   r   s

- -

3. **-ar**–suffix meaning **pertaining to**
    Used to turn a combining form for a bone into an adjective

    a. pertaining to the clavicle   _____/_____
                                              r   s

    b. pertaining to the fibula   _____/_____
                                              r   s

    c. pertaining to the mandible   _____/_____
                                              r   s

    d. pertaining to under the mandible   _____/_____/_____
                             p   r   s

e. pertaining to the patella

_____ /_____
                r   s

f. pertaining to the scapula

_____ /_____
                r   s

g. pertaining to under the scapula

_____ /_____ /_____
       p   r   s

h. pertaining to the ulna

_____ /_____
                r   s

---

4. **arthr/o**–combining form meaning **joint**

A joint is formed where two or more bones meet; also called an **articulation**; there are three types of joints in the body based on the amount of movement between the bones: (see again Figure 6.1)

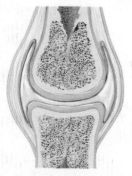

- **fibrous joints** - bones are united by fibrous tissue that allows essentially no movement between the bones; examples are the sutures between the skull bones
- **cartilaginous joints** - bones are connected by cartilage that allows a small amount of shifting; example is the pubic symphysis
- **synovial joints** - bones are encased in an elastic joint capsule that allows the greatest range of motion; most common joint type in the body; examples are the shoulder and knee

6.4 Typical synovial joint

a. puncture to withdraw fluid from a joint

_____ /_____ /_____
                r   cv   s

b. surgically break a joint

_____ /_____ /_____
                r   cv   s

c. surgical fusion of a joint

_____ /_____ /_____
                r   cv   s

d. process of recording a joint

_____ /_____ /_____
                r   cv   s

e. record of a joint

_____ /_____ /_____
                r   cv   s

f. joint inflammation

_____ /_____
                r   s

g. process of visually examining a joint

_____ /_____ /_____
                r   cv   s

h. instrument for viewing a joint

_____ /_____ /_____
                r   cv   s

i. surgical repair of a joint

_____ /_____ /_____
                r   cv   s

j. joint pain

_____ /_____
                r   s

---

5. **-ary**–suffix meaning **pertaining to**
   Used to turn a combining form for a bone into an adjective

   a. pertaining to the maxilla   _____/_____
                                              r   s

   b. pertaining to above the maxilla   _____/_____/_____
                                               p   r   s

---

6. **burs/o**–combining form meaning **bursa**
   A bursa is a fluid-filled sac typically found between tendon and bone to reduce friction

   a. pertaining to a bursa   _____/_____
                                         r   s

   b. bursa inflammation   _____/_____
                                      r   s

   c. surgical removal of a bursa   _____/_____
                                               r   s

---

7. **chondr/o**–combining form meaning **cartilage**
   Cartilage is tough, flexible connective tissue that covers ends of bones in joint; serves as shock absorber

   a. pertaining to cartilage   _____/_____
                                           r   s

   b. cartilage inflammation   _____/_____
                                          r   s

   c. surgical removal of cartilage   _____/_____
                                                 r   s

   d. abnormal cartilage softening   _____/_____/_____
                                                r   cv   s

   e. cartilage tumor   _____/_____
                                   r   s

   f. surgical repair of cartilage   _____/_____/_____
                                                r   cv   s

---

8. **crani/o**–combining form meaning **skull**
   Skull consists of frontal, parietal, temporal, ethmoid, sphenoid, occipital, mandible, maxilla, zygomatic, vomer, palatine, nasal, and lacrimal bones; protects the brain, eyes, and ears; provides attachment sites for muscles for chewing, facial expression, and moving the head

   6.5 Skull

   a. pertaining to the skull   _____/_____
                                           r   s

   b. pertaining to within the skull   _____/_____/_____
                                              p   r   s

c. cutting into the skull

_____/_____
                    r   s

d. surgical repair of the skull

_____/_____/_____
        r   cv   s

---

9. -eal–suffix meaning **pertaining to**
  Used to turn a combining form for a bone
  into an adjective

  a. pertaining to the coccyx

_____/_____
                    r   s

  b. pertaining to the phalanges

_____/_____
                    r   s

---

10. -ic–suffix meaning **pertaining to**
  Used to turn a combining form for a bone into an adjective

  a. pertaining to the pubis

_____/_____
                    r   s

  b. pertaining to above the pubis

_____/_____/_____
     p   r   s

---

11. -kinesia–suffix meaning **movement**

  a. slow movement

_____/_____
                    p   s

  b. difficult movement

_____/_____
                    p   s

  c. excessive movement

_____/_____
                    p   s

---

12. muscul/o–combining form meaning **muscle**
  Contraction of muscle tissue produces movement in the body; three types of
  muscles: (see again Figure 6.3)

  • **skeletal muscle**: attached to bone; contracts to move skeleton; voluntary
    muscle
  • **smooth muscle**: located in internal organs (such as urinary bladder and
    stomach); contracts to produce movement of the organ; involuntary muscle
  • **cardiac muscle**: found only in the heart; contracts to push blood through the
    heart chambers; involuntary muscle

6.6 Muscles

  a. pertaining to muscle

_____/_____
                    r   s

  b. pertaining to within muscle

_____/_____/_____
     p   r   s

---

13. myel/o–combining form meaning **bone marrow**

There are two types of bone marrow inside bones:
- **red bone marrow**: located in the small spaces of spongy bone; produces all blood cells
- **yellow bone marrow**: located within the hollow shaft of bones; composed of adipose tissue

a. bone marrow tumor

_____ / _____
r   s

b. producing bone marrow

_____ / _____ / _____
r   cv   s

c. disease of bone marrow

_____ / _____ / _____
r   cv   s

- -

14. my/o–combining form meaning **muscle**

a. muscle pain

_____ / _____
r   s

b. muscle weakness

_____ / _____
r   s

c. record of muscle's electricity

_____ / _____ / _____ / _____ / _____
r   cv   r   cv   s

d. process of recording muscle's electricity

_____ / _____ / _____ / _____ / _____
r   cv   r   cv   s

e. muscle disease

_____ / _____ / _____
r   cv   s

f. suture a muscle

_____ / _____ / _____
r   cv   s

g. ruptured muscle

_____ / _____ / _____
r   cv   s

- -

15. oste/o–combining form meaning **bone**

Bone is a hard, calcified connective tissue; functions include supporting and moving the body; providing vital protection to underlying organs such as heart, lungs, liver, and bladder; housing bone marrow; and serving as storehouse for important minerals such as calcium

Two types of bone tissue:
- **compact bone**: dense, hard exterior surface of bones; also called *cortical* bone
- **spongy bone**: found inside bones; has numerous, small spaces within that house red bone marrow; also called *cancellous* bone

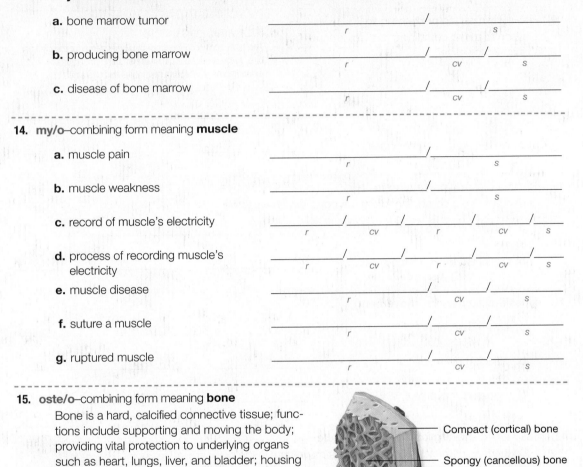

Compact (cortical) bone

Spongy (cancellous) bone

6.7 Bone.

a. bone pain

_____ / _____
r   s

b. bone cell

_____ / _____ / _____
r   cv   s

c. producing bone

_____ / _____ / _____
r   cv   s

d. bone and joint inflammation

_____ / _____ / _____ / _____
      r   *cv*   *r*   *s*

e. bone and cartilage inflammation

_____ / _____ / _____ / _____
      r   *cv*   *r*   *s*

f. bone and cartilage tumor

_____ / _____ / _____ / _____
      r   *cv*   *r*   *s*

g. surgical breaking of a bone

_____ / _____ / _____
      r   *cv*   *s*

h. bone and bone marrow inflammation

_____ / _____ / _____ / _____
      r   *cv*   *r*   *s*

i. bone disease

_____ / _____ / _____
      r   *cv*   *s*

j. instrument to cut bone

_____ / _____ / _____
      r   *cv*   *s*

k. abnormal softening of bone

_____ / _____ / _____
      r   *cv*   *s*

l. porous bone

_____ / _____ / _____
      r   *cv*   *s*

---

16. spondyl/o–combining form meaning **vertebra**

    a. abnormal condition of a vertebra

_____ / _____
      r   *s*

    b. vertebra inflammation

_____ / _____
      r   *s*

---

17. ten/o–combining form meaning **tendon**

A tendon is a strong band of connective tissue that anchors muscle to bone

    a. tendon pain

_____ / _____
      r   *s*

    b. tendon pain

_____ / _____ / _____
      r   *cv*   *s*

    c. surgical fusion of a tendon

_____ / _____ / _____
      r   *cv*   *s*

    d. suture of a tendon

_____ / _____ / _____
      r   *cv*   *s*

---

18. tendin/o–combining form meaning **tendon**

    a. pertaining to a tendon

_____ / _____
      r   *s*

    b. tendon inflammation

_____ / _____
      r   *s*

    c. surgical repair of a tendon

_____ / _____ / _____
      r   *cv*   *s*

    d. abnormal condition of a tendon

_____ / _____
      r   *s*

Orthopedic Vocabulary

The orthopedic terms presented in this section include eponyms, modern English words, and those that contain Latin or Greek word parts but are not constructed solely from these word parts. When you recognize word parts within a term, they will give you a hint about the word's meaning. In these instances, look for the word parts to follow the term.

Term	Explanation
bone graft	Surgical procedure that uses a piece of bone to replace lost bone or to fuse two bones together
bone scan	Nuclear medicine scan using radioactive dye to visualize bones; especially useful for finding stress fractures and bone cancer
carpal tunnel syndrome (CTS) **carp/o** = wrist **-al** = pertaining to	Repetitive motion disorder caused by pressure on tendons and nerves as they pass through carpal tunnel of wrist **6.8** Nerves and blood vessels enclosed by carpal tunnel formed by wrist bones and tendons
closed fracture	Broken bone with no open skin wound; also called *simple fracture*

6.8 Nerves and blood vessels enclosed by carpal tunnel formed by wrist bones and tendons

Inflamed median nerve

Tendons crossing the wrist

Carpal tunnel

Carpal bones

Blood vessel

6.9 (A) Closed (or simple) fracture and (B) open (or compound) fracture

A

B

Term	Explanation
comminuted fracture	Bone break where bone shatters into many small fragments

TERMINOLOGY TIDBIT
The term *comminuted* comes from the Latin word *comminuere* meaning "to break into pieces." |
compound fracture	Broken bone with open skin wound; also called *open fracture* (see Figure 6.9)
compression fracture	Bone break causing loss of height of vertebral body; may result from trauma, but in older persons, especially women, may occur in a bone weakened by osteoporosis
contracture	Abnormal shortening of muscle fibers, tendons, or connective tissue making it difficult to stretch muscle
creatine kinase (CK)	Muscle enzyme found in skeletal and cardiac muscle; elevated blood levels associated with heart attack, muscular dystrophy, and other skeletal muscle pathologies
deep tendon reflex (DTR)	Involuntary muscle contraction in response to striking muscle tendon with reflex hammer; test used to determine whether muscles respond properly

6.10 Testing patellar reflex with a reflex hammer
Source: Image Point Fr/Shutterstock |
| **dislocation** | Occurs when bones in joint are displaced from normal alignment and ends of bones are no longer in contact with each other

6.11 The large bump on the top of the shoulder is caused by the upward dislocation of the humerus
Source: Pearson Education |
| **dual-energy absorptiometry** (DXA)
-metry = process of measuring | Test using low-dose X-ray beams to measure bone density; used to diagnose osteoporosis |
| **fibromyalgia**
fibr/o = fibrous
my/o = muscle
-algia = pain | Chronic condition with widespread aching and pain in the muscles and fibrous soft tissue |

Term	Explanation
fixation	Procedure to stabilize fractured bone while it heals; *external fixation* includes casts, splints, and pins inserted through skin; *internal fixation* includes pins, plates, rods, screws, and wires that are put into place during a surgical procedure called *open reduction*
fracture (FX, Fx)	Broken bone
greenstick fracture	Fracture with incomplete break; one side of the bone breaks and other side only bends; commonly seen in children because their bones are still pliable

TERMINOLOGY TIDBIT

The term *fracture* comes from the Latin word *fractura* meaning "to break."

Term	Explanation
herniated nucleus pulposus (HNP)	Protrusion of intervertebral disk between two vertebrae, which puts pressure on spinal nerves; also called *herniated disk* or *ruptured disk;* may require surgery

Cross–section showing compression of nerve root

Intervertebral disk

Spinal nerve

Spinal cord

6.12 Protruding intervertebral disk putting pressure on a spinal nerve

Term	Explanation
impacted fracture	Fracture in which one bone fragment is pushed into another
kyphosis **kyph/o** = hump **-osis** = abnormal condition	Abnormal increase in normal outward curvature of thoracic spine; also called *hunchback* or *humpback*

Kyphosis
(excessive posterior thoracic curvature—hunchback)

Lordosis
(excessive anterior lumbar curvature—swayback)

Scoliosis
(lateral curvature)

6.13 Abnormal spinal curvatures: kyphosis, lordosis, and scoliosis

Term	Explanation
lordosis **lord/o** = bent backward **-osis** = abnormal condition	Abnormal increase in normal forward curvature of lumbar spine; also called *swayback* (see Figure 6.13)
magnetic resonance imaging (MRI)	Diagnostic imaging technique that uses electromagnetic energy to produce an image; especially useful for viewing soft tissues, such as spinal cord and intervertebral disks **6.14** MRI showing a sagittal view of the vertebral column and intervertebral disks Source: Deymos. Hr/Shutterstock
muscle atrophy **a-** = without **-trophy** = development	Loss of muscle bulk due to muscle disease, nervous system disease, or lack of use; commonly called *muscle wasting*
muscular dystrophy (MD) **muscul/o** = muscle **-ar** = pertaining to **dys-** = abnormal **-trophy** = development	One of a group of inherited diseases involving progressive muscle degeneration, weakness, and atrophy
nonsteroidal anti-inflammatory drugs (NSAIDs)	Large group of drugs that provide mild pain relief and anti-inflammatory benefits for conditions such as arthritis
oblique fracture	Bone break in which fracture line runs along an angle to shaft of the bone
orthosis **orth/o** = straight	Externally applied brace or splint used to prevent or correct deformities; *orthotist* is person skilled in making and adjusting orthoses **6.15** A stroke patient with an orthotic brace on her right arm Source: Michal Heron/Pearson Education

Term	Explanation
osteoarthritis (OA) **oste/o** = bone **arthr/o** = joint **-itis** = inflammation	Arthritis caused by loss of cartilage cushion covering bones in joint; most common in weight-bearing joints; results in bone rubbing against bone
osteoporosis **oste/o** = bone **-porosis** = porous	Condition that develops due to a decrease in bone mass; results in a thinning and weakening of the bone; may lead to pathologic fractures; most commonly seen in older women
osteogenic sarcoma **oste/o** = bone **-genic** = producing **-oma** = tumor	Most common type of bone cancer; usually begins in osteocytes found at ends of bones; most frequently occurs in persons 10–25 years old
pathologic fracture **path/o** = disease	Broken bone caused by diseased or weakened bone, not trauma
percutaneous diskectomy **per-** = through **cutane/o** = skin **-ous** = pertaining to **-ectomy** = surgical removal	Thin catheter tube is inserted into intervertebral disk through skin to suck out pieces of herniated or ruptured disk; or laser is used to vaporize disk
prosthesis	Any artificial device used as substitute for body part that is either missing from birth or lost as the result of an accident or disease; example: artificial leg; *prosthetist* is person trained in making prostheses

> **TERMINOLOGY TIDBIT**
> The term *prosthesis* comes from the Greek word *prostithenai* meaning "an addition."

Term	Explanation
radiography **-graphy** = process of recording	Diagnostic imaging procedure using X-rays to see internal structure of body; especially useful for visualizing bones and joints

6.16 X-ray of lower leg showing fractures in the tibia and fibula
Source: Itsmejust/Shutterstock

Term	Explanation
reduction	Correcting fracture or dislocation by realigning bone; *closed reduction* moves bones externally; *open reduction* manipulates bones through a surgical incision; open reduction usually performed before *internal fixation* of bone fragments

> **TERMINOLOGY TIDBIT**
> The term *reduction* comes from the Latin word *reductio* meaning "to lead back."

Term	Explanation
repetitive motion disorder	Group of chronic disorders with tendon, muscle, joint, and nerve damage caused by prolonged periods of pressure, vibration, or repetitive movements
rheumatoid arthritis (RA) **arthr/o** = joint **-itis** = inflammation	Arthritis with swelling, stiffness, pain, and degeneration of cartilage in joints caused by chronic soft tissue inflammation; may result in crippling deformities; an autoimmune disease **6.17** Typical hand and wrist deformities of rheumatoid arthritis Source: Michal Heron/Pearson Education
scoliosis **scoli/o** = crooked **-osis** = abnormal condition	Abnormal lateral curvature of spine (see Figure 6.13)
spasm	Sudden, involuntary, strong muscle contraction
spina bifida	Birth defect that occurs when vertebra fails to fully form around spinal cord; ranges from mild to severe; if spinal cord is damaged, some degree of paralysis results
spiral fracture	Bone break in which fracture line spirals around shaft of the bone; caused by twisting injury; often slower to heal than other types of fractures
sprain	Ligament injury from overstretching, but without joint dislocation or bone fracture
strain	Damage to the muscle or tendons from overuse or overstretching
stress fracture	A slight bone break caused by repetitive low-impact forces, such as running, rather than single forceful impact
total hip arthroplasty (THA) **arthr/o** = joint **-plasty** = surgical repair	Surgical reconstruction of hip with artificial hip joint; also called *total hip replacement (THR)* **6.18** (A) A fractured femur, (B) repaired with a total hip arthroplasty **A** **B**
total knee arthroplasty (TKA) **arthr/o** = joint **-plasty** = surgical repair	Surgical reconstruction of knee joint with artificial knee joint; also called *total knee replacement (TKR)*
transverse fracture	Bone break with fracture line straight across shaft of bone

Orthopedic Abbreviations

The following list presents common orthopedic abbreviations.

AE	above elbow	LE	lower extremity
AK	above knee	LLE	left lower extremity
BDT	bone density testing	LUE	left upper extremity
BE	below elbow	MD	muscular dystrophy
BK	below knee	MRI	magnetic resonance imaging
BMD	bone mineral density	NSAID	nonsteroidal anti-inflammatory drug
C1, C2, etc.	first cervical vertebra, second cervical vertebra, etc.	OA	osteoarthritis
		ORIF	open reduction–internal fixation
Ca	calcium		
CK	creatine kinase	Orth, ortho	orthopedics
CTS	carpal tunnel syndrome	RA	rheumatoid arthritis
DJD	degenerative joint disease	RLE	right lower extremity
DTR	deep tendon reflex	RUE	right upper extremity
DXA	dual-energy absorptiometry	T1, T2, etc.	first thoracic vertebra, second thoracic vertebra, etc.
EMG	electromyogram		
FX, Fx	fracture	THA	total hip arthroplasty
HNP	herniated nucleus pulposus	THR	total hip replacement
IM	intramuscular	TKA	total knee arthroplasty
JRA	juvenile rheumatoid arthritis	TKR	total knee replacement
L1, L2, etc.	first lumbar vertebra, second lumbar vertebra, etc.	UE	upper extremity

CASE STUDY

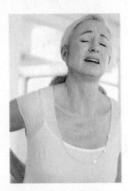

Source: Monkey Business Images/Shutterstock

History of Present Illness

A 68-year-old female presents at the orthopedic clinic for an initial evaluation of severe low back pain that radiates into the posterior RLE and into her foot. Patient has experienced intermittent mild symptoms for the past six months. She states these symptoms typically last only one day and are gone when she wakes up the next morning. Current episode of severe pain began two days ago. She reports that there was no lifting or injury immediately preceding the pain but notes that both her husband and youngest son require physical assistance due to their medical conditions. She struggles to provide this assistance due to her history of carpal tunnel syndrome and compression fracture.

Past Medical History

Osteoporosis and compression Fx of T10 four years ago, treated with an orthotic to support thoracic spine. She continues to take NSAIDs if experiences any thoracic back pain. Breast cancer, mastectomy, and chemotherapy with no reoccurrence in 12 years. Carpal tunnel syndrome requiring carpal tunnel release surgery when she was 52.

Family and Social History

Patient is married. Her husband, 85, has moderate Alzheimer's disease but is still able to remain at home. She was a line worker at a battery factory where she was required to lift 5-pound boxes of batteries at a rate of 60 per hour. She retired on disability following carpal tunnel release. Patient smoked cigarettes for 45 years, but quit 14 years ago. Father died at age 72 from myocardial infarction; mother died at 84 from renal failure; one sister is alive and well; three living children, no miscarriages, two children, oldest son and daughter are healthy, youngest son, 40, has spina bifida. He is confined to a wheelchair and lives at home with parents.

Physical Examination

Well-nourished, well-developed cooperative Caucasian female in obvious pain sitting on examination table. She has tenderness over lower spinal muscles on both sides of lumbar spine with right more tender than left. LE muscle strength is normal and there is no apparent muscle atrophy. DTRs are normal on left and reduced on right.

Diagnostic Tests

Lumbar X-ray revealed mild spondylosis at L4-5 but no appreciable spinal arthritis. MRI confirms HNP at L4-5 level.

Diagnosis

L4-5 HNP

Plan of Treatment

1. Conservative treatment with physical therapy for pain relief, traction, and back-strengthening exercises
2. Consider percutaneous diskectomy if conservative treatment fails to improve symptoms
3. Meet with patient and family to plan alternative strategies so that she may avoid having to lift other family members

Critical Thinking Questions

Answer the following questions regarding this case study. Do not just copy words out of the case study but translate all medical terms. To answer some of these questions, you may need to look up information from another chapter of this text, in a medical dictionary, or online. Answers are found at the back of the book.

1. Use a medical reference source to give more information on osteoporosis. Why do you think that osteoporosis commonly leads to compression fractures?

   _____

   _____

2. Go to www.drugs.com and click on "Drugs by Condition." Then search for drugs that treat osteoporosis. Describe two different drugs that treat this condition.

   _____

   _____

3. List all abbreviations used and what each stands for.

   _____

   _____

4. Which of the following is NOT part of this patient's previous medical diagnoses?
   a. collapse of 10th thoracic vertebra
   b. radiation treatment for cancer
   c. a repetitive motion disorder
   d. wearing a brace

5. Define the medical conditions of her parents, husband, and son. Use the index of your text to find these conditions.

   _____

   _____

6. List and describe the two diagnostic imaging procedures this patient underwent. What were their results?

_____

_____

7. What are the PT plans for this patient?

_____

_____

8. Describe the planned surgical treatment if the conservative treatment does not improve her symptoms.

_____

_____

PRACTICE

Sound It Out

The following are some of the key terms from this chapter written as their phonetic spelling. Sound out each term and write it in the blank. Pronunciations for all terms are included in the audio glossary at www.mymedicalterminologylab.com

1. figh-broh-my-AL-jee-ah _____

2. KON-droh-plas-tee _____

3. ee-lek-troh-MY-oh-gram _____

4. FEM-or-all _____

5. ar-thro-PLAS-tee _____

6. ILL-ee-ack _____

7. in-ter-VER-teh-bral _____

8. in-tra-MUSS-kew-lar _____

9. lor-DOH-sis _____

10. man-DIB-yoo-lar _____

11. ber-SIGH-tis _____

12. met-ah-CAR-pal _____

13. FIB-yoo-lar _____

14. my-ah-LOH-mah _____

15. ar-thro-sen-TEE-sis _____

16. skoh-lee-OH-sis _____

17. pa-TELL-ar _____

18. pross-THEE-sis _____

19. PYOO-bik _____

20. ray-dee-OG-rah-fee _____

21. kon-DROH-mah _____

22. oss-tee-oh-por-ROH-sis _____

23. ten-oh-DIN-ee-ah _____

24. kon-TRACK-chur _____

25. TIB-ee-all _____

Transcription Practice

Each of the following sentences is written in common English. Underline any words or phrases that can be replaced by a medical term. Then rewrite the entire sentence using medical terms. Answers can be found at the back of the book.

1. The shattered bone break required manipulation through a surgical incision and a surgical procedure to stabilize.

   _____

   _____

2. Diagnostic imaging procedure to visualize bones revealed a pertaining to the femur bone and cartilage tumor.

   _____

   _____

3. The patient's chronically inflamed bursa eventually required surgical removal of the bursa.

   _____

   _____

4. Mary's hand deformities from an autoimmune type of arthritis were improved by wearing an external brace or splint.

   _____

   _____

5. When Otto's loss of cartilage cushion arthritis in his knee prevented him from walking, he had a surgical reconstruction with an artificial knee.

   _____

   _____

6. What first appeared to be a fracture with an angled fracture line turned out to be a fracture that spirals down the bone shaft.

   _____

   _____

7. A nuclear medicine scan of the bone was necessary to identify the slight fracture caused by repetitive low-impact forces.

   _____

   _____

8. Jean's pertaining to the vertebrae porous bones was diagnosed by low-dose X-ray beams that measure bone density.

   _____

   _____

9. The child's abnormal movements caused the physician to suspect an inherited disease with progressive muscle degeneration and weakness.

   _____

   _____

10. The ankle damage to the tendons from overstretching was severe enough to require surgical fusion of the tendon.

    _____

    _____

Labeling Exercise

Write the name of each bone on the numbered line. Also use this space to write the common name and combining form where appropriate.

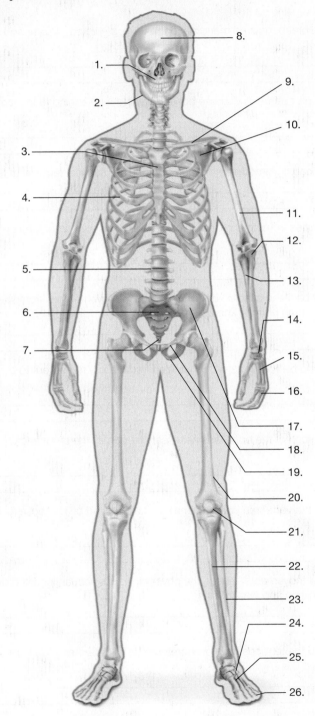

1. _____

2. _____

3. _____

4. _____

5. _____

6. _____

7. _____

8. _____

9. _____

10. _____

11. _____

12. _____

13. _____

14. _____

15. _____

16. _____

17. _____

18. _____

19. _____

20. _____

21. _____

22. _____

23. _____

24. _____

25. _____

26. _____

1. _____

2. _____

3. _____

4. _____

5. _____

6. _____

7. _____

8. _____

9. _____

10. _____

11. _____

12. _____

13. _____

14. _____

15. _____

16. _____

17. _____

18. _____

19. _____

20. _____

21. _____

22. _____

23. _____

24. _____

25. _____

26. _____

Build Medical Terms

Use each of the following word parts to build the indicated medical terms.

The combining form *arthr/o* means joint.

1. puncture to withdraw fluid from joint _____

2. joint inflammation _____

3. instrument for viewing joint _____

4. surgical repair of joint _____

5. process of recording joint _____

The combining form *my/o* means muscle.

6. muscle weakness _____

7. muscle suture _____

The suffix *-kinesia* means movement.

8. excessive movement _____

9. slow movement _____

The combining form *oste/o* means bone.

10. instrument to cut bone _____

11. porous bone _____

12. bone producing _____

The combining form *chondr/o* means cartilage.

13. abnormal softening of cartilage _____

14. cartilage tumor _____

15. surgical repair of cartilage _____

Fill in the Blank

Fill in the blank to complete each of the following sentences.

1. In a _____ fracture there is no open skin wound.

2. DXA is a diagnostic test for _____.

3. The common name for _____ is hunchback.

4. Braces and splints are examples of a(n) _____.

5. _____ is an example of a repetitive motion disorder affecting the wrist.

6. A(n) _____ is any medical device used to substitute for a body part.

7. _____ fractures are most commonly seen in children.

8. Bones are held together by _____, while _____ anchor muscles to bones.

9. Pins, plates, and rods are examples of _____.

10. A(n) _____ is a sudden, strong, involuntary muscle contraction.

Abbreviation Matching

Match each abbreviation with its definition.

_____ **1.** LLE   **A.** rheumatoid arthritis

_____ **2.** OA   **B.** fracture

_____ **3.** MD   **C.** second lumbar vertebra

_____ **4.** CTS   **D.** left lower leg

_____ **5.** RA   **E.** total hip arthroplasty

_____ **6.** L2   **F.** muscular dystrophy

_____ **7.** ORIF   **G.** osteoarthritis

_____ **8.** Fx   **H.** intramuscular

_____ **9.** IM   **I.** open reduction, internal fixation

_____ **10.** THA   **J.** carpal tunnel syndrome

MyMedicalTerminologyLab™

MyMedicalTerminologyLab is a premium online homework management system that includes a host of features to help you study. Registered users will find:

- A multitude of activities and assignments built within the MyLab platform
- Powerful tools that track and analyze your results—allowing you to create a personalized learning experience
- Videos and audio pronunciations to help enrich your progress
- Streaming lesson presentations and self-paced learning modules
- A space where you and your instructors can view and manage your assignments

Medical Term Analysis

Examine each of the following terms. Begin by dividing it into its word parts and writing them in the indicated blanks (*P = prefix*; *WR = word root*; *CF = combining form*; *S = suffix*). Follow with the definition of each word part and finally the meaning of the full term.

1. **arthrodesis**

   CF _____

   means _____

   S _____

   means _____

   Term meaning: _____

   _____

2. **bursectomy**

   WR _____

   means _____

   S _____

   means _____

   Term meaning: _____

   _____

3. **electromyogram**

   CF _____

   means _____

   CF _____

   means _____

   S _____

   means _____

   Term meaning: _____

   _____

4. **intracranial**

   P _____

   means _____

   WR _____

   means _____

   S _____

   means _____

   Term meaning: _____

   _____

5. **osteomyelitis**

   CF _____

   means _____

   WR _____

   means _____

   S _____

   means _____

   Term meaning: _____

   _____

6. **tenalgia**

   WR _____

   means _____

   S _____

   means _____

   Term meaning: _____

   _____

7. spondylosis

WR _____

means _____

S _____

means _____

Term meaning: _____

_____

8. substernal

P _____

means _____

WR _____

means _____

S _____

means _____

Term meaning: _____

_____

9. intervertebral

P _____

means _____

WR _____

means _____

S _____

means _____

Term meaning: _____

_____

10. supramaxillary

P _____

means _____

WR _____

means _____

S _____

means _____

Term meaning: _____

_____

Spelling

Some of the following terms are misspelled. Identify the incorrect terms and spell them correctly in the blank provided.

1. contracture _____

2. bursektomy _____

3. lordosis _____

4. nonsteroidal _____

5. orthosis _____

6. arthrocentesis _____

7. chondroectomy _____

8. coxygeal _____

9. diskinesia _____

10. spondilosis _____

Photomatch Challenge

Match each fracture with its name in the Word Bank.

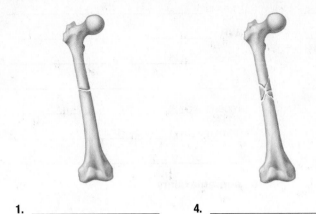

1. _____

4. _____

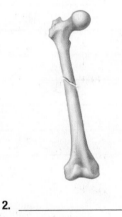

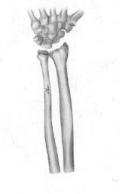

Word Bank:

Comminuted fracture

Compression fracture

Greenstick fracture

Oblique fracture

Spiral fracture

Transverse fracture

2. _____

5. _____

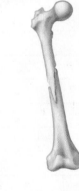

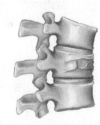

3. _____

6. _____

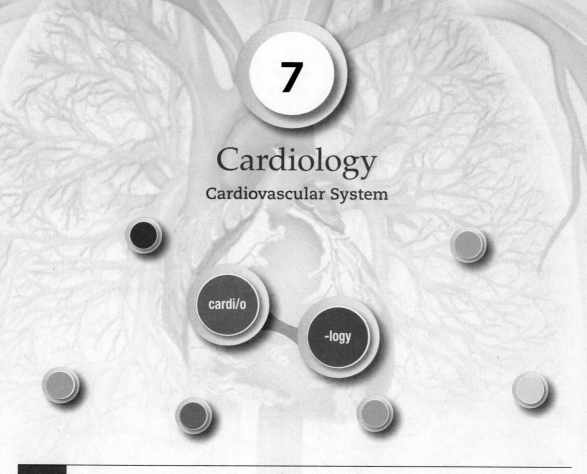

7

Cardiology

Cardiovascular System

cardi/o   -logy

Learning Objectives

Upon completion of this chapter, you will be able to:

7-1   Describe the medical specialty of cardiology.

7-2   Understand the functions of the cardiovascular system.

7-3   Define cardiology-related combining forms, prefixes, and suffixes.

7-4   Identify the organs treated in cardiology.

7-5   Build cardiology medical terms from word parts.

7-6   Explain cardiology medical terms.

7-7   Use cardiology abbreviations.

A Brief Introduction to Cardiology

Cardiology is the diagnosis and treatment of diseases and conditions affecting the cardiovascular system. **Cardiologists** are responsible for treating conditions such as coronary artery disease, cardiac arrhythmias, hypertension, heart valve disease, congenital heart defects, cardiomyopathy, congestive heart failure, myocardial infarction, heart transplants, and peripheral vascular diseases.

   Cardiovascular technologists are allied health professionals who work alongside the cardiologist. These technologists perform or assist in a variety of diagnostic and therapeutic procedures including electrocardiography, echocardiography, exercise stress testing, and cardiac catheterization.

   The cardiovascular system consists of the **heart** and **blood vessels**. The heart, composed of cardiac muscle tissue, contracts to push blood through the blood vessels to transport substances such as oxygen, nutrients, and waste products to all areas of the body. The three types of blood vessels are the **arteries**, **veins**, and **capillaries**. Blood is carried away from the heart by arteries, which deliver it to capillary beds. Capillaries are the narrowest blood vessels and the point at which oxygen and nutrients are delivered to and wastes are picked up from the local tissues. After exiting capillary beds, blood travels back to the heart through veins.

Cardiology Combining Forms

The following list presents combining forms closely associated with the cardiovascular system and used for building and defining cardiology terms.

angi/o	vessel		sphygm/o	pulse
aort/o	aorta		steth/o	chest
arteri/o	artery		thromb/o	clot
arteriol/o	arteriole		valv/o	valve
ather/o	fatty substance, plaque		valvul/o	valve
atri/o	atrium		varic/o	dilated vein
cardi/o	heart		vas/o	blood vessel
coron/o	heart		vascul/o	blood vessel
embol/o	plug		ven/o	vein
isch/o	to hold back		ventricul/o	ventricle
phleb/o	vein		venul/o	venule

The following list presents combining forms that are not specific to the cardiovascular system but are also used for building and defining cardiology terms.

cutane/o	skin		my/o	muscle
electr/o	electricity		pulmon/o	lung
esophag/o	esophagus		son/o	sound

Suffix Review

These suffixes introduced in Chapter 2 are being reviewed in this chapter because they are especially important for building cardiology terms.

-ac	pertaining to		-emia	blood condition
-al	pertaining to		-genic	producing
-ar	pertaining to		-gram	record
-ary	pertaining to		-graphy	process of recording
-dynia	pain		-ia	condition
-eal	pertaining to		-ic	pertaining to
-ectomy	surgical removal		-ism	state of

-itis	inflammation	-otomy	cutting into
-logist	one who studies	-ous	pertaining to
-logy	study of	-pathy	disease
-lysis	to destroy	-plasty	surgical repair
-lytic	destruction	-rrhaphy	suture
-manometer	instrument to measure pressure	-rrhexis	rupture
-megaly	enlarged	-sclerosis	hardening
-ole	small	-scope	instrument for viewing
-oma	tumor, mass	-spasm	involuntary muscle contraction
-ose	pertaining to	-stenosis	narrowing
-osis	abnormal condition	-tic	pertaining to
		-ule	small

Prefix Review

These prefixes introduced in Chapter 3 are being reviewed in this chapter because they are especially important for building cardiology terms.

a-	without	per-	through
brady-	slow	peri-	around
endo-	within, inner	poly-	many
hyper-	excessive	tachy-	fast
hypo-	below, insufficient	trans-	across
inter-	between	ultra-	excess
intra-	within		

Organs Commonly Treated in Cardiology

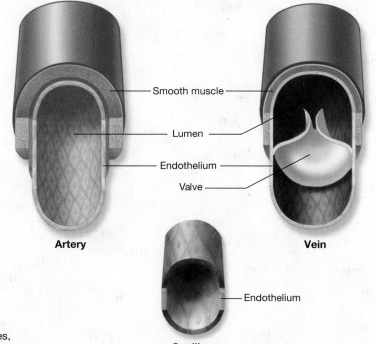

Artery   Smooth muscle   Lumen   Endothelium   Valve   **Vein**

Capillary   Endothelium

7.1 Comparative structure of arteries, capillaries, and veins

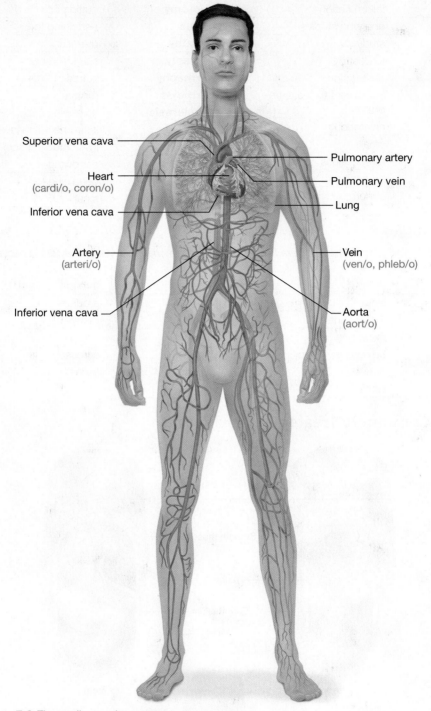

Superior vena cava

Heart
(cardi/o, coron/o)

Inferior vena cava

Artery
(arteri/o)

Inferior vena cava

Pulmonary artery

Pulmonary vein

Lung

Vein
(ven/o, phleb/o)

Aorta
(aort/o)

7.2 The cardiovascular system

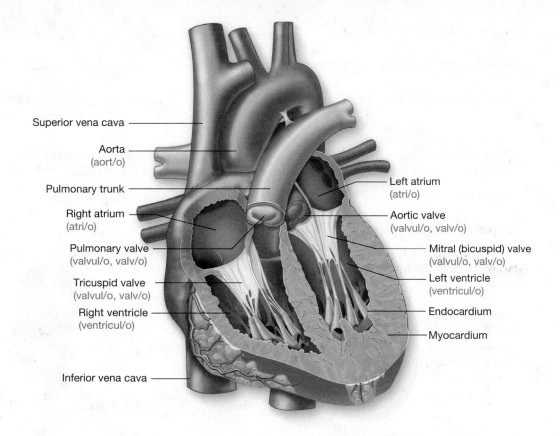

Superior vena cava

Aorta
(aort/o)

Pulmonary trunk

Right atrium
(atri/o)

Pulmonary valve
(valvul/o, valv/o)

Tricuspid valve
(valvul/o, valv/o)

Right ventricle
(ventricul/o)

Inferior vena cava

Left atrium
(atri/o)

Aortic valve
(valvul/o, valv/o)

Mitral (bicuspid) valve
(valvul/o, valv/o)

Left ventricle
(ventricul/o)

Endocardium

Myocardium

7.3 Structures of the heart

Building Cardiology Terms

This section presents word parts most often used to build cardiology terms. Following the explanation of the term, you have the opportunity to begin building your own vocabulary. Read the meaning for each term and then fill in the blanks to build a single medical term. Use the slashes to divide prefixes, word roots, combining vowels, and suffixes. To help you out you will find a key to the word parts underneath the blanks: **r** for word roots, **p** for prefix, **cv** for combining vowel, and **s** for suffix. Remember that not every term will contain all these word parts; it's up to you to decide which to use. As you gain experience, this process becomes easier. Answers can be found at the back of the book.

1. **angi/o**–combining form meaning **vessel**

    May be used to refer to either blood vessels or lymph vessels; it does not indicate a specific type of blood vessel, such as artery, vein, or capillary

    a. record of a vessel

    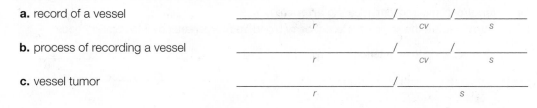
    _____/_____/_____
    r   cv   s

    b. process of recording a vessel

    _____/_____/_____
    r   cv   s

    c. vessel tumor

    _____/_____
    r   s

d. surgical repair of a vessel   _____ / _____ / _____
                                                    r   cv   s

e. involuntary muscle spasm in a vessel _____ / _____ / _____
                                                    r   cv   s

f. inflammation of many vessels   _____ / _____ / _____
                                          p   r   s

- -

2. **aort/o**–combining form meaning **aorta**

   The aorta is the largest artery in the body; receives oxygenated blood from left ventricle and delivers it to all other arteries for distribution to the entire body (see again Figures 7.2 and 7.3)

   a. pertaining to the aorta   _____ / _____
                                                    r   s

   b. surgical repair of the aorta   _____ / _____ / _____
                                                    r   cv   s

- -

3. **arteri/o**–combining form meaning **artery**

   Arteries are blood vessels that carry blood away from the heart and toward a capillary bed; the arterial wall contains a thick layer of **smooth muscle** that contracts or relaxes to change size of **lumen**, the channel through which blood flows; smooth inner lining is **endothelium**; arteries to the lungs carry deoxygenated blood and arteries to the body carry oxygenated blood (see again Figure 7.1)

   7.4 Artery

   a. pertaining to an artery   _____ / _____
                                                    r   s

   b. record of an artery   _____ / _____ / _____
                                          r   cv   s

   c. process of recording an artery   _____ / _____ / _____
                                                    r   cv   s

   d. suture of an artery   _____ / _____ / _____
                                          r   cv   s

   e. ruptured artery   _____ / _____ / _____
                                    r   cv   s

   f. narrowing of an artery   _____ / _____ / _____
                                            r   cv   s

   g. small artery   _____ / _____
                                  r   s

- -

4. **arteriol/o**–combining form meaning **arteriole**

   Arterioles are the smallest arteries; carry blood from larger arteries into capillary beds

   a. pertaining to an arteriole   _____ / _____
                                                     r   s

- -

5. **ather/o**–combining form meaning **fatty substance, plaque**

Refers to soft, yellow, fatty deposits that build up along inner wall of blood vessels; these deposits, referred to as *plaques*, narrow blood vessel lumen and reduce amount of blood vessel can deliver

   a. hardening of plaque

   _____ / _____ / _____
                        r   *cv*   *s*

   b. surgical removal of plaque

   _____ / _____
                      r   *s*

---

6. **atri/o**–combining form meaning **atrium**

Atria are upper chambers of the heart; receive blood returning to the heart; left atrium receives oxygenated blood from lungs via **pulmonary veins** and right atrium receives deoxygenated blood from body via **superior vena cava** and **inferior vena cava**; **interatrial septum** separates left and right atria (see again Figures 7.2 and 7.3)

   a. pertaining to the atrium

   _____ / _____
                    r   *s*

   b. pertaining to between the atria

   _____ / _____ / _____
        p   *r*   *s*

   c. pertaining to the atrium and ventricle

   _____ / _____ / _____ / _____
          r   *cv*   *r*   *s*

---

7. **cardi/o**–combining form meaning **heart**

The heart is composed of cardiac muscle tissue called **myocardium** that contracts to develop pressure needed to push blood through blood vessels; divided into left and right halves by **septum**; right side of heart pumps blood to lungs for oxygenation; left side of heart pumps oxygenated blood to the body; upper chambers are **atria** that receive blood returning to heart; lower chambers are **ventricles** that contract to force blood out of heart and into arteries; inner lining is **endocardium**, a thin, smooth layer of tissue to reduce friction as blood passes through heart chambers; four heart **valves** open and close to ensure that blood flows only in forward direction (see again Figure 7.3)

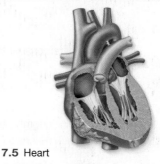

7.5 Heart

   a. pertaining to the heart

   _____ / _____
                r   *s*

   b. heart pain

   _____ / _____ / _____
          r   *cv*   *s*

   c. record of heart's electrical (activity)

   _____ / _____ / _____ / _____ / ____
       r   *cv*   *r*   *cv*   *s*

   d. process of recording heart's electrical (activity)

   _____ / _____ / _____ / _____ / ____
       r   *cv*   *r*   *cv*   *s*

   e. one who studies the heart

   _____ / _____ / _____
          r   *cv*   *s*

   f. study of the heart

   _____ / _____ / _____
          r   *cv*   *s*

   g. enlarged heart

   _____ / _____ / _____
          r   *cv*   *s*

h. disease of the heart muscle

_____/_____/_____/_____/_____/_____
r   cv   r   cv   s

i. ruptured heart

_____/_____/_____
r   cv   s

j. pertaining to around the heart

_____/_____/_____
p   r   s

k. pertaining to inner (lining) of the heart

_____/_____/_____
p   r   s

l. pertaining to heart muscle

_____/_____/_____/_____
r   cv   r   s

---

8. coron/o–combining form meaning **heart**

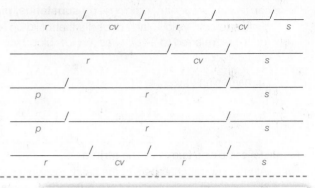

a. pertaining to the heart

_____/_____
r   s

---

9. embol/o–combining form meaning **plug, embolus**

An embolus is a piece broken off from a clot or a mass of fat or bacteria that floats through blood vessels until it plugs up a small blood vessel, blocking blood flow; if this occurs in a coronary artery supplying heart muscle, a heart attack may result

a. surgical removal of an embolus

_____/_____
r   s

b. condition of having an embolus

_____/_____
r   s

---

10. isch/o–combining form meaning **to hold back**

To hold back means to stop, as in blood flow

a. condition of blood being held back

_____/_____
r   s

---

11. phleb/o–combining form meaning **vein**

Veins are blood vessels that carry blood back to the heart from capillary beds; venous wall has only a thin layer of smooth muscle; veins contain **valves** that ensure blood moves only toward the heart and does not flow backward and pool; veins from body carry deoxygenated blood and veins from lungs carry oxygenated blood; largest veins are **superior vena cava** returning blood from upper body to heart, and **inferior vena cava** returning blood from lower body to heart (see again Figures 7.1 and 7.2)

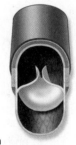

7.6 Vein

a. vein inflammation

_____/_____
r   s

b. cutting into a vein

_____/_____/_____
r   cv   s

c. record of a vein
_____/_____/_____
　　　　　　　　　　　　_r_　　　　　_cv_　　　　　_s_

d. process of recording a vein
_____/_____/_____
　　　　　　　　　　　　_r_　　　　　_cv_　　　　　_s_

- -

12. -sclerosis–suffix meaning **hardening**
　　Used in the cardiovascular system to describe a blood vessel becoming hard and inflexible due to buildup of cholesterol plaques along vessel wall

a. hardening of an artery
_____/_____/_____
　　　　　　　　　　　　_r_　　　　　_cv_　　　　　_s_

- -

13. steth/o–combining form meaning **chest**

> **TERMINOLOGY TIDBIT**
> As you have learned, _-scope_ means instrument for viewing. In this case, it is a misnomer since this is an instrument for _listening_.

a. instrument for viewing the chest
_____/_____/_____
　　　　　　　　　　　　_r_　　　　　_cv_　　　　　_s_

- -

14. thromb/o–combining form meaning **blood clot**, **thrombus**
　　Refers to a blood clot forming in blood vessel; if large enough, it will partially or completely block blood flow through blood vessel

a. pertaining to a clot
_____/_____/_____
　　　　　　　　　　　　_r_　　　　　_cv_　　　　　_s_

b. abnormal condition of (having) clots
_____/_____
　　　　　　　　　　　　_r_　　　　　　　　_s_

c. vessel inflammation with clots
_____/_____/_____/_____
　　　_r_　　　　_cv_　　　　_r_　　　　　_s_

d. inflammation of vein with clots
_____/_____/_____/_____
　　　_r_　　　　_cv_　　　　_r_　　　　　_s_

e. producing a clot
_____/_____/_____
　　　　　　　　　　　　_r_　　　　　_cv_　　　　　_s_

f. to destroy a clot
_____/_____/_____
　　　　　　　　　　　　_r_　　　　　_cv_　　　　　_s_

- -

15. valv/o–combining form meaning **valve**
　　Valves are flaplike structures that close tightly to prevent backflow of blood; ensures that blood always flows in forward direction; there are four valves in heart (**tricuspid**, **mitral**, **pulmonary**, and **aortic**) and many valves in veins (see again Figure 7.3)

a. surgical repair of a valve
_____/_____/_____
　　　　　　　　　　　　_r_　　　　　_cv_　　　　　_s_

b. cutting into a valve
_____/_____/_____
　　　　　　　　　　　　_r_　　　　　_cv_　　　　　_s_

c. small valve
_____/_____
　　　　　　　　　　　　_r_　　　　　　　　_s_

- -

16. valvul/o–combining form meaning **valve**

    a. pertaining to a valve   _____ / _____
                                                                   r   *s*

    b. inflammation of a valve   _____ / _____
                                                                     r   *s*

---

17. varic/o–combining form meaning **dilated vein, varicosity**

Condition in which a vein becomes dilated and tortuous; most common in superficial leg veins; caused by any circumstance that leads to blood pooling, such as ineffective valves, pregnancy, or an occupation requiring long periods of standing; blood flow through varicosity becomes very slow and sluggish

    a. abnormal condition of   _____ / _____
       (having a) varicosity   *r*   *s*

    b. pertaining to a varicosity   _____ / _____
                                                        r   *s*

---

18. vas/o–combining form meaning **blood vessel**

    a. involuntary muscle contraction   _____ / _____ / _____
       of a blood vessel   *r*   *cv*   *s*

---

19. vascul/o–combining form meaning **blood vessel**

    a. pertaining to a blood vessel   _____ / _____
                                                 r   *s*

    b. pertaining to the heart and blood   _____ / _____ / _____ / _____
       vessels   *r*   *cv*   *r*   *s*

---

20. ven/o–combining form meaning **vein**

    a. pertaining to a vein   _____ / _____
                                                r   *s*

    b. record of a vein   _____ / _____ / _____
                                         r   *cv*   *s*

    c. process of recording a vein   _____ / _____ / _____
                                         r   *cv*   *s*

    d. pertaining to within a vein   _____ / _____ / _____
                                      p   *r*   *s*

    e. small vein   _____ / _____
                                              r   *s*

---

21. ventricul/o–combining form meaning **ventricle**

The ventricles are large, very muscular pumping chambers of the heart; left ventricle pumps oxygenated blood into the **aorta** for body and right ventricle pumps deoxygenated blood into **pulmonary trunk** and **pulmonary arteries** toward lungs; **interventricular septum** separates left and right ventricles (see again Figures 7.2 and 7.3)

> **TERMINOLOGY TIDBIT**
>
> The term *ventricle* comes from the Latin term *venter,* meaning "little belly." Although it originally referred to the abdomen and then the stomach, it came to stand for any hollow region inside an organ.

a. pertaining to a ventricle

_____/_____
                 r   s

b. pertaining to between the ventricles

_____/_____/_____
   p   r   s

----

22. venul/o–combining form meaning **venule**

Venules are the smallest veins; receive blood from capillaries and carry it to larger veins

a. pertaining to a venule

_____/_____
                 r   s

Cardiology Vocabulary

The cardiology terms presented in this section include eponyms, modern English words, and those that contain Latin or Greek word parts but are not constructed solely from these word parts. When you recognize word parts within a term, they will give you a hint about the word's meaning. In these instances, look for the word parts to follow the term.

Term	Explanation
aneurysm	Localized widening of artery due to weakness in arterial wall; may develop in any artery, but common sites are abdominal aorta and cerebral arteries **7.7** Illustration of a large aneurysm in the abdominal aorta that has ruptured
angina pectoris	Severe chest pain caused by myocardial ischemia **TERMINOLOGY TIDBIT** The term _angina_ comes from the Latin word _angere_ meaning "to strangle, cause pain, press tight." This describes the sensation that occurs during angina pectoris.
arrhythmia a- = without	Irregular heartbeat
auscultation	Listening to sounds within body, such as heart or lungs, by using _stethoscope_ **TERMINOLOGY TIDBIT** The term _auscultation_ comes from the Latin word _auscultare_ meaning "to listen to."

Term	Explanation
bacterial endocarditis endo- = inner cardi/o = heart -itis = inflammation	Inflammation of inner lining of heart (the endocardium) caused by bacteria; may result in visible accumulation of bacteria called *vegetation*
blood pressure (BP)	Measurement of pressure exerted by blood against walls of blood vessel
bradycardia brady- = slow cardi/o = heart -ia = condition	Abnormally slow heart rate below 60 beats per minute (bpm)
cardiac arrest cardi/o = heart -ac = pertaining to	Complete stoppage of all heart activity, both electrical signals and muscle contractions
cardiac catheterization (CC) cardi/o = heart -ac = pertaining to	Passage of thin tube (catheter) through veins or arteries leading into heart; used to detect heart abnormalities, to collect cardiac blood samples, and to determine pressure within heart
cardiac enzymes cardi/o = heart -ac = pertaining to	Complex proteins released by heart muscle when it is damaged; taken by blood sample to determine amount of heart disease or damage; most common cardiac enzymes are creatine kinase (CK), glutamic oxaloacetic transaminase (GOT), and lactate dehydrogenase (LDH)
cardiopulmonary resuscitation (CPR) cardi/o = heart pulmon/o = lungs -ary = pertaining to	Combination of external compressions to sternum and rescue breathing to maintain blood flow and air movement in and out of lungs during cardiac and respiratory arrest
congenital septal defect (CSD)	Birth defect in wall separating two chambers of heart allowing blood to pass between two chambers; there can be atrial septal defect (ASD) or ventricular septal defect (VSD)
congestive heart failure (CHF)	Condition that develops when heart muscle is not able to pump blood forcefully enough, reducing blood flow to body; results in weakness, dyspnea, and edema

> **TERMINOLOGY TIDBIT**
> The term *congenital* comes from the Latin word *congenitus* meaning "born with."

Term	Explanation
coronary artery bypass graft (CABG) **coron/o** = heart **-ary** = pertaining to	Open-heart surgery in which blood vessel, often leg vein, is grafted to route blood around occluded coronary artery

7.8 Illustration of a triple coronary artery bypass graft; one end of the vein grafts is connected to the aorta, and the other end is grafted into coronary arteries after the location of the blocked area

Term	Explanation
coronary artery disease (CAD) **coron/o** = heart **-ary** = pertaining to	Chronic heart disease caused by arteriosclerosis or atherosclerosis of coronary arteries; also called *arteriosclerotic heart disease* (ASHD)

7.9 Formation of an atherosclerotic plaque within a coronary artery that may lead to coronary artery disease, angina pectoris, and myocardial infarction

Term	Explanation
deep vein thrombosis (DVT) **thromb/o** = clot **-osis** = abnormal condition	Formation of blood clots in deep veins; usually occurs in legs; pieces of clot may break away forming *emboli*

Term	Explanation
defibrillation	Using instrument called *defibrillator* to give electrical shock to heart for purpose of converting arrhythmia back to normal heartbeat; also called *cardioversion* **7.10** An emergency medical technician positions defibrillator paddles on the chest of a supine male patient Source: Floyd Jackson/Pearson Education
Doppler ultrasonography **ultra-** = excess **son/o** = sound **-graphy** = process of recording	Imaging technique using ultrasound to create moving image; utilized to evaluate blood flow through blood vessels, movement of heart valves, and movement of heart muscle during contraction
electrocardiography **electr/o** = electricity **cardi/o** = heart **-graphy** = process of recording	Diagnostic procedure that records electrical activity of heart; used to diagnose damage to heart tissue from coronary heart disease or myocardial infarction
endarterectomy **endo-** = inner **arteri/o** = artery **-ectomy** = surgical removal	Surgical removal of inner lining of artery in order to remove plaques
fibrillation	Abnormal quivering or contractions of heart fibers; occurrence within fibers of ventricle of heart may result in cardiac arrest and death; emergency equipment to defibrillate, or convert heart to normal beat, is necessary
heart murmur	Abnormal heart sound such as soft blowing sound or harsh click; may be soft and heard only with stethoscope or so loud it can be heard several feet away
heart transplantation	Replacement of diseased or malfunctioning heart with donor's heart
heart valve prolapse	Cusps or flaps of heart valve are too loose and fail to shut tightly, allowing blood to flow backward (regurgitation) through valve when heart chamber contracts; most commonly occurs in mitral valve, but may affect any heart valve
heart valve stenosis **-stenosis** = narrowing	Cusps or flaps of heart valve are too stiff and unable to open fully, making it difficult for blood to flow through; condition may affect any of heart valves but most often affects mitral valve

Term	Explanation
Holter monitor	Portable ECG monitor worn by patient for period of few hours to few days to assess heart and pulse activity as person goes through activities of daily living; used to assess patient who experiences chest pain and unusual heart activity during exercise and normal activities **7.11** Patient being set up with Holter monitor; electrodes placed on chest are connected to small monitor that he will wear Source: Craig X. Sotres/Pearson Education
hypertension (HTN) **hyper-** = excessive	Blood pressure above normal range; usually systolic pressure above 140 mmHg or diastolic pressure above 90 mmHg
hypotension **hypo-** = insufficient	Decrease in blood pressure; can occur in shock, infection, cancer, anemia, or as death approaches
implantable cardioverter defibrillator (ICD) **cardi/o** = heart	Electrical device implanted in chest cavity with electrodes to heart; applies shock to heart to stop potentially life-threatening arrhythmias such as fibrillation
infarct	Area of tissue necrosis (death) that develops from ischemia
intravascular thrombolytic therapy **intra-** = within **vascul/o** = blood vessel **-ar** = pertaining to **thromb/o** = clot **-lytic** = destruction	Treatment for clots occluding blood vessel; drugs, such as streptokinase (SK) or tissue plasminogen activator (tPA), are injected into blood vessels to chemically dissolve clots; commonly referred to as *clot-busters*

Term	Explanation

myocardial infarction (MI)
  my/o = muscle
  cardi/o = heart
  -al = pertaining to

Infarct of heart muscle caused by occlusion of one or more of coronary arteries; symptoms include angina pectoris and shortness of breath; also referred to as *heart attack*

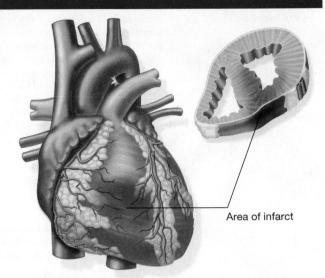

Area of infarct

7.12 External and cross-sectional view of an infarct caused by a myocardial infarction

myocardial ischemia
  my/o = muscle
  cardi/o = heart
  -al = pertaining to
  isch/o = hold back
  -emia = blood condition

Loss of blood supply to heart muscle tissue of myocardium due to occlusion of coronary artery; may cause angina pectoris or myocardial infarction

occlusion

Blockage of blood vessel or other hollow structure; may be caused by thrombus, plaque, or embolus

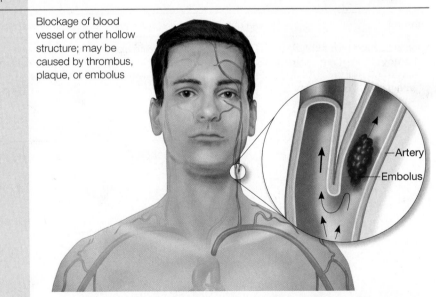

Artery

Embolus

7.13 Illustration of an embolus floating in an artery; the embolus will eventually lodge in an artery that is smaller than it is, resulting in occlusion of that artery

Term	Explanation
pacemaker	Electrical device that artificially stimulates contraction of heart muscle; treatment for bradycardia Pacemaker **7.14** Placement of a pacemaker under the skin between the heart and shoulder; electrode wires then run to the heart muscle
percutaneous transluminal coronary angioplasty (PTCA) **per-** = through **cutane/o** = skin **-ous** = pertaining to **trans-** = across **coron/o** = heart **-ary** = pertaining to **angi/o** = vessel **-plasty** = surgical repair	Method for treating coronary artery narrowing; balloon catheter is inserted into coronary artery and inflated to dilate narrow blood vessel
peripheral vascular disease (PVD) **vascul/o** = blood vessel **-ar** = pertaining to	Disease of blood vessels away from central region of body, most typically in legs; symptoms include pain, numbness, and impaired circulation
sphygmomanometer **sphygm/o** = pulse **-manometer** = instrument to measure pressure	Instrument for measuring blood pressure; also referred to as *blood pressure cuff* **7.15** Using a sphygmomanometer to measure blood pressure Source: Michal Heron/Pearson Education

Term	Explanation
stent	Stainless steel tube placed within blood vessel or duct to widen lumen; may be placed in coronary artery to treat myocardial ischemia due to atherosclerosis **7.16** The process of placing a stent in a blood vessel: (A) catheter is used to place a collapsed stent next to an atherosclerotic plaque; (B) stent is expanded; (C) catheter is removed, leaving the expanded stent behind
stress test	Method for evaluating cardiovascular fitness; patient is placed on treadmill or bicycle and then subjected to steadily increasing levels of work; EKG and oxygen levels are taken while patient exercises; test is stopped if abnormalities occur on EKG
tachycardia **tachy-** = fast **cardi/o** = heart **-ia** = condition	Abnormally fast heart rate greater than 100 beats per minute (bpm)
transesophageal echocardiography (TEE) **trans-** = across **esophag/o** = esophagus **-eal** = pertaining to **cardi/o** = heart **-graphy** = process of recording	Specialized echocardiography procedure in which patient swallows ultrasound head in order to better visualize internal cardiac structures, especially cardiac valves
varicose veins **varic/o** = dilated vein	Swollen and distended veins, most commonly in legs **TERMINOLOGY TIDBIT** The term *varicose* comes from the Latin word *varix* meaning "dilated vein." **7.17** Varicose veins develop when their valves fail to control blood flow, which allows more than the normal amount of blood to collect in superficial leg veins

Term	Explanation
venipuncture **ven/o** = vein	Puncture into vein to withdraw blood or inject medication or fluids

Cardiology Abbreviations

The following list presents common cardiology abbreviations.

ACG	angiocardiography	**HTN**	hypertension
AF	atrial fibrillation	**ICD**	implantable
AS	arteriosclerosis		cardioverter defibrillator
ASCVD	arteriosclerotic cardiovascular	**ICU**	intensive care unit
	disease	**IV**	intravenous
ASD	atrial septal defect	**LDH**	lactate dehydrogenase
ASHD	arteriosclerotic heart disease	**LVH**	left ventricular hypertrophy
AV, A-V	atrioventricular	**MI**	myocardial infarction
BP	blood pressure	**mmHg**	millimeters of mercury
bpm	beats per minute	**MS**	mitral stenosis
CABG	coronary artery bypass graft	**MVP**	mitral valve prolapse
CAD	coronary artery disease	**NSR**	normal sinus rhythm
cath	catheterization	**P**	pulse
CC	cardiac catheterization	**PTCA**	percutaneous transluminal
CCU	coronary care unit		coronary angioplasty
CHD	congestive heart disease	**PVC**	premature ventricular contraction
CHF	congestive heart failure	**PVD**	peripheral vascular disease
CK	creatine kinase	**SA, S-A**	sinoatrial
CP	chest pain	**SGOT**	serum glutamic oxaloacetic
CPR	cardiopulmonary resuscitation		transaminase
CSD	congenital septal defect	**SK**	streptokinase
CV	cardiovascular	**SOB**	shortness of breath
DVT	deep vein thrombosis	**TEE**	transesophageal echocardiogram
ECG	electrocardiogram	**tPA**	tissue plasminogen activator
ECHO	echocardiogram	**V Fib**	ventricular fibrillation
EKG	electrocardiogram	**VSD**	ventricular septal defect
GOT	glutamic oxaloacetic transaminase	**VT, V-tach**	ventricular tachycardia
HR	heart rate		

CASE STUDY

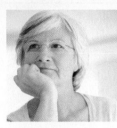

Source: Shutterstock

History of Present Illness

Patient is a 56-year-old female, referred to the cardiology clinic by her family physician for increasingly severe SOB. She denies angina pectoris. Symptoms first appeared five years ago following an acute episode of viral bronchitis. At that time, the SOB was attributed to the lung infection. However, symptoms continued to gradually worsen rather than improve. Adult-onset asthma and emphysema have been ruled out by a pulmonologist. At this time, the patient is experiencing severe SOB with mild activity. She has recently noticed swelling in her feet, and her family physician has now diagnosed CHF, prescribed digoxin, and referred her for further diagnosis and treatment.

Past Medical History

Appendectomy at age eight. Rheumatic fever at age 16. Three pregnancies, all children delivered vaginally and are healthy. Left breast lumpectomy at age 45 with no reoccurrence of malignancy.

Family and Social History

Patient drinks one or two alcoholic beverages weekly. She has not ever smoked, but husband smokes one pack/day. She is a school teacher. No exposure to environmental toxins. Family history is negative for heart disease. Mother died at age 26 from complications of childbirth. Father died at age 60 from lung cancer. She has one sister, age 60, who is healthy except for rheumatoid arthritis.

Physical Examination

Pt is mildly SOB sitting in exam room. HR is 153 bpm, rhythm is normal. BP is 180/90 in left arm while sitting. No cyanosis is noted. Weight is within normal range, but she does have noticeable edema in bilateral feet but not in her hands or face. Abdomen is mildly distended with fluid, but no organomegaly is palpated. Chest auscultation reveals a clearly audible heart murmur during ventricular contraction.

Diagnostic Tests

EKG: tachycardia at rate of 153 bpm but normal rhythm and no evidence of an MI. Transesophageal echocardiography is consistent with mitral prolapse with regurgitation of blood into left atrium from left ventricle.

Diagnosis

Mitral valve prolapse and CHF secondary to rheumatic heart disease.

Plan of Treatment

1. Schedule patient for mitral valvoplasty with prosthetic valve

Critical Thinking Questions

Answer the following questions regarding this case study. Do not just copy words out of the case study but translate all medical terms. To answer some of these questions, you may need to look up information from another chapter of this text, in a medical dictionary, or online. Answers are found at the back of the book.

1. Name and define the symptom that brought this patient to the cardiologist. Name and define the symptoms that the patient denies having.

   _____

   _____

2. Name and describe the family physician's diagnosis. What new symptom led this physician to make this diagnosis?

   _____

   _____

3. This patient takes digoxin. Look this up, and describe why it is prescribed.

_____

_____

4. Explain the results of the EKG.

_____

_____

5. What is edema? Where does this patient have and not have edema?

_____

_____

6. *Cyanosis* means:
   a. an abnormal breath sound
   b. blue color to the skin
   c. dizziness
   d. yellow color to the whites of the eyes

7. Explain the final diagnosis. What diagnostic test best supported this diagnosis? Justify your conclusion.

_____

_____

_____

8. Explain the treatment planned for this patient.

_____

_____

PRACTICE

Sound It Out

The following are some of the key terms from this chapter written as their phonetic spelling. Sound out each term and write it in the blank. Pronunciations for all terms are included in the audio glossary at www.mymedicalterminologylab.com.

1. VAY-zoh-spazm _____

2. AN-jee-oh-plas-tee _____

3. in-trah-VEE-nus _____

4. car-dee-oh-my-OP-ah-thee _____

5. ath-er-oh-skleh-ROH-sis _____

6. brad-ee-CAR-dee-ah _____

7. CAR-dee-oh-VAS-kyoo-lar _____

8. dee-fib-rih-LAY-shun _____

9. ee-lek-troh-car-dee-OG-rah-fee _____

10. em-boh-LIZ-em _____

11. end-ar-teh-REK-toh-mee _____

12. fih-brill-AY-shun _____

13. high-per-TEN-shun _____

14. IN-farkt _____

15. my-oh-CAR-dee-all _____

16. fleh-BYE-tis _____

17. en-doh-car-DYE-tis _____

18. sfig-moh-mah-NOM-eh-ter _____

19. tak-ee-CAR-dee-ah _____

20. throm-boh-LYE-sis _____

21. AN-yoo-rizm _____

22. car-dee-oh-MEG-ah-lee _____

23. pol-ee-an-jee-EYE-tis _____

24. throm-BOH-sis _____

25. STETH-oh-scope _____

Transcription Practice

Each of the following sentences is written in common English. Underline any words or phrases that can be replaced by a medical term. Then rewrite the entire sentence using medical terms. Answers can be found at the back of the book.

1. Dr. Jones suspected his patient had had a heart attack, so he ordered a record of the heart's electrical (activity) and a blood test to look for proteins released into the blood by damaged heart muscle.

   _____

   _____

2. The paramedics applied an electrical shock to the patient's heart because abnormal quivering was detected.

   _____

   _____

3. The patient developed an abnormally slow heartbeat and required surgery to implant an electrical device to artificially stimulate the heart to beat.

   _____

   _____

4. Susan wore a portable ECG monitor for 24 hours to further evaluate her severe chest pain caused by myocardial ischemia.

   _____

   _____

5. The patient had an ultrasound imaging technique to create a moving image of her heart valves to assess whether she had heart valves that were too loose and failed to shut tightly or heart valves that were too stiff and unable to open fully.

   _____

   _____

   _____

6. While listening to the sounds within the body, the nurse detected an abnormal heart sound caused by mitral valve flaps that are too loose.

   _____

   _____

7. The patient suffered tissue necrosis because of an area losing its blood supply when a floating clot broke off a soft, yellow, fatty deposit.

_____

_____

8. A procedure to pass a thin tube through veins leading into the heart was ordered to determine whether the patient requires a balloon procedure to widen a narrow coronary artery.

_____

_____

9. The patient experiences severe chest pain due to severe hardening of the coronary arteries.

_____

_____

10. This patient's high blood pressure eventually caused him to develop a condition in which the heart muscle is not able to pump forcefully enough.

_____

_____

Spelling

Some of the following terms are misspelled. Identify the incorrect terms and spell them correctly in the blank provided.

1. tackycardia _____

2. arrhythmia _____

3. phlebotomy _____

4. awscultation _____

5. atheriosclerosis _____

6. defibrillation _____

7. thrombophlebitis _____

8. anurysm _____

9. angiohma _____

10. occlusion _____

Labeling Exercise

Write the name of each structure on the numbered line. Also use this space to write the combining form where appropriate.

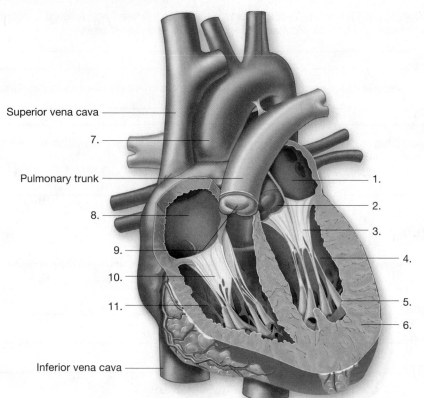

Superior vena cava

7.

Pulmonary trunk

8.

9.

10.

11.

Inferior vena cava

1.

2.

3.

4.

5.

6.

1. _____   7. _____

2. _____   8. _____

3. _____   9. _____

4. _____   10. _____

5. _____   11. _____

6. _____

Build Medical Terms

Use each of the following word parts to build the indicated medical terms.

The combining form *cardi/o* means heart.

1. study of heart _____

2. enlarged heart _____

3. heart rupture _____

4. heart record _____

The combining form *valv/o* means valve.

5. surgical repair of valve _____

6. cutting into valve _____

The suffix *-sclerosis* means hardening.

7. artery hardening _____

8. plaque hardening _____

The combining form *angi/o* means blood vessel.

9. blood vessel tumor _____

10. involuntary muscle spasm in a blood vessel _____

The combining form *arteri/o* means artery.

11. suture of an artery _____

12. pertaining to an artery _____

13. process of recording an artery _____

The combining form *thromb/o* means clot.

14. clot vein inflammation _____

15. to destroy a clot _____

Fill in the Blank

Fill in the blank to complete each of the following sentences.

1. A(n) _____ is a localized wide spot in an artery.

2. Complete stoppage of all heart activity is called _____.

3. Auscultation uses an instrument called a(n) _____.

4. A(n) _____ is a portable EKG monitor worn by a person for several hours to a few days.

5. A baby born with a(n) _____ has a birth defect in the wall separating two chambers of the heart.

6. A(n) _____ is performed to withdraw blood or inject medication into a vein.

7. Endocarditis may result in the visible growth of bacteria called _____.

8. Drugs such as streptokinase are commonly called _____.

9. A(n) _____ is an abnormal heart sound such as soft blowing or harsh clicking.

10. The paramedics performed _____ by compressing the sternum to maintain blood flow.

Abbreviation Matching

Match each abbreviation with its definition.

_____ **1.** ASHD	**A.** coronary artery disease
_____ **2.** ACG	**B.** electrocardiogram
_____ **3.** HTN	**C.** myocardial infarction
_____ **4.** EKG	**D.** arteriosclerotic heart disease
_____ **5.** VSD	**E.** chest pain
_____ **6.** CHF	**F.** hypertension
_____ **7.** CAD	**G.** ventricular septal defect
_____ **8.** PVC	**H.** angiocardiography
_____ **9.** CP	**I.** congestive heart failure
_____ **10.** MI	**J.** premature ventricular contraction

Medical Term Analysis

Examine each of the following terms. Begin by dividing it into its word parts and writing them in the indicated blanks (*P = prefix*; *WR = word root*; *CF = combining form*; *S = suffix*). Follow with the definition of each word part and then finally the meaning of the full term.

1. **aortoplasty**

   CF _____

   means _____

   S _____

   means _____

   Term meaning: _____

   _____

2. **embolectomy**

   WR _____

   means _____

   S _____

   means _____

   Term meaning: _____

   _____

3. **cardiomyopathy**

   CF _____

   means _____

   CF _____

   means _____

   S _____

   means _____

   Term meaning: _____

   _____

4. **endocardial**

   P _____

   means _____

   WR _____

   means _____

   S _____

   means _____

   Term meaning: _____

   _____

5. **thromboangiitis**

   CF _____

   means _____

   WR _____

   means _____

   S _____

   means _____

   Term meaning: _____

   _____

6. **atherosclerosis**

   CF _____

   means _____

   S _____

   means _____

   Term meaning: _____

   _____

7. **valvulotomy**

    WR _____

    means _____

    S _____

    means _____

    Term meaning: _____

    _____

8. **interventricular**

    P _____

    means _____

    WR _____

    means _____

    S _____

    means _____

    Term meaning: _____

    _____

9. **cardiovascular**

    CF _____

    means _____

    WR _____

    means _____

    S _____

    means _____

    Term meaning: _____

    _____

10. **stethoscope**

    CF _____

    means _____

    S _____

    means _____

    Term meaning: _____

    _____

MyMedicalTerminologyLab™

MyMedicalTerminologyLab is a premium online homework management system that includes a host of features to help you study. Registered users will find:

- A multitude of activities and assignments built within the MyLab platform
- Powerful tools that track and analyze your results—allowing you to create a personalized learning experience
- Videos and audio pronunciations to help enrich your progress
- Streaming lesson presentations and self-paced learning modules
- A space where you and your instructors can view and manage your assignments

Photomatch Challenge

Match each procedure illustrated below with its name in the Word Bank.

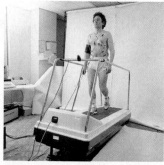

Source: Susanna Price © Dorling Kindersley

1. _____

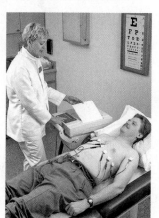

Source: Craig X. Sotres/Pearson Education

3. _____

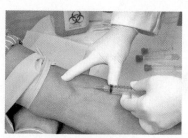

Source: Michal Heron/Pearson Education

2. _____

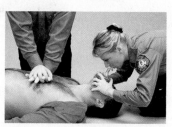

Source: Michal Heron/Pearson Education

4. _____

Word Bank:

Cardiopulmonary resuscitation

Venipuncture

Stress test

Electrocardiography

Prefixes can help you tell apart these two EKG strips.

One is bradycardia and the other is tachycardia.

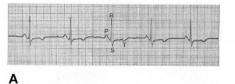

A

Source: Pearson Education

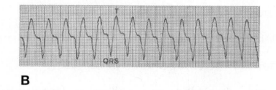

B

5. What does the prefix **brady-** mean, and which strip is bradycardia?

_____

6. What does the prefix **tachy-** mean, and which strip is tachycardia?

_____

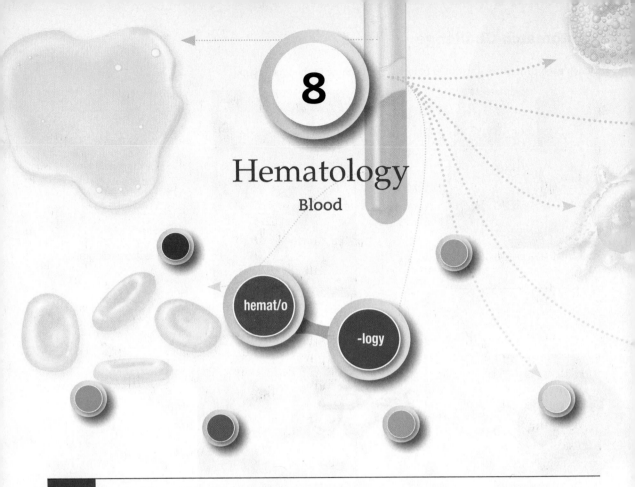

8

Hematology

Blood

hemat/o — -logy

⌄ Learning Objectives

Upon completion of this chapter, you will be able to:

8-1 Describe the medical specialty of hematology.

8-2 Understand the functions of blood.

8-3 Define hematology-related combining forms, prefixes, and suffixes.

8-4 Identify the components of blood.

8-5 Build hematology medical terms from word parts.

8-6 Explain hematology medical terms.

8-7 Use hematology abbreviations.

A Brief Introduction to Hematology

Hematology is the diagnosis and treatment of disorders of the blood and blood-forming tissues. A **hematologist** specializes in the treatment of bleeding disorders, cancers of the blood-forming tissues, and anemia as well as in interpreting blood tests and the science of blood transfusions.

Blood is the fluid found inside of blood vessels. Approximately 55% of blood is a watery fluid called **plasma**. Many important substances such as **glucose**, **amino acids**, **hormones**, and **electrolytes** are transported in the plasma. The remaining 45% of blood consists of the **formed elements**, which are cells (or cell fragments) floating in the plasma. The formed elements include **erythrocytes** (red blood cells), **leukocytes** (white blood cells), and **platelets** (formerly called *thrombocytes*). Erythrocytes contain **hemoglobin** (protein that transports oxygen); leukocytes provide protection against pathogens (there are five specialized types: **neutrophils**, **basophils**, **eosinophils**, **monocytes**, **lymphocytes**); platelets are small platelike fragments of a larger cell and initiate **hemostasis** (blood-clotting process). All of the formed elements are produced in red bone marrow by a process called **hematopoiesis**.

Hematology Combining Forms

The following list presents combining forms closely associated with blood and used for building and defining hematology terms.

bas/o	base		**hemat/o**	blood
coagul/o	clotting		**leuk/o**	white
eosin/o	rosy red		**lymph/o**	lymph
erythr/o	red		**neutr/o**	neutral
hem/o	blood		**thromb/o**	clot

The following list presents combining forms that are not specific to hematology but are also used for building and defining hematology terms.

cyt/o	cell		**path/o**	disease
embol/o	plug		**phleb/o**	vein
glyc/o	sugar		**septic/o**	infection
lip/o	fat			

Suffix Review

These suffixes introduced in Chapter 2 are being reviewed in this chapter because they are especially important for building hematology terms.

-cyte	cell		**-meter**	instrument for measuring
-cytosis	abnormal cell condition (too many)		**-metry**	process of measuring
			-oma	mass, tumor
-ectomy	surgical removal		**-osis**	abnormal condition
-emia	blood condition		**-otomy**	cutting into
-globin	protein		**-penia**	too few
-ia	condition		**-phil**	attracted to
-ic	pertaining to		**-plasm**	formation
-logist	one who studies		**-poiesis**	formation
-logy	study of		**-rrhage**	excessive, abnormal flow
-lysis	to destroy		**-stasis**	stopping
-lytic	destruction		**-tic**	pertaining to

Prefix Review

These prefixes introduced in Chapter 3 are being reviewed in this chapter because they are especially important for building hematology terms.

a-	without	hypo-	below, insufficient
an-	without	mono-	one
anti-	against	pan-	all
auto-	self	poly-	many
hyper-	excessive		

Components of Blood

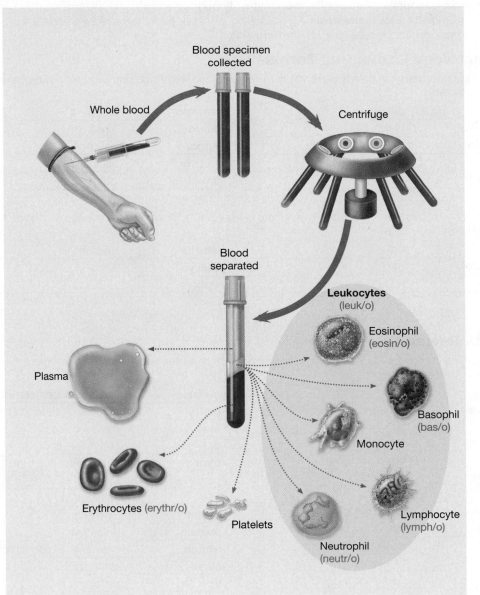

Blood specimen collected

Whole blood

Centrifuge

Blood separated

Leukocytes (leuk/o)

Eosinophil (eosin/o)

Plasma

Basophil (bas/o)

Monocyte

Erythrocytes (erythr/o)

Platelets

Lymphocyte (lymph/o)

Neutrophil (neutr/o)

8.1 Components of whole blood

Building Hematology Terms

This section presents word parts most often used to build hematology terms. Following the explanation of the term, you have the opportunity to begin building your own vocabulary. Read the meaning for each term and then fill in the blanks to build a single medical term. Use the slashes to divide prefixes, word roots, combining vowels, and suffixes. To help you out you will find a key to the word parts underneath the blanks: **r** for word roots, **p** for prefix, **cv** for combining vowel, and **s** for suffix. Remember that not every term will contain all these word parts; it's up to you to decide which to use. As you gain experience, this process becomes easier. Answers can be found at the back of the book.

1. **-cyte**–suffix meaning **cell**
   Refers to formed elements

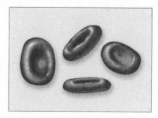

8.2 Erythrocytes

   a. red cell

                                   _____ / _____ / _____
                                           r   cv   s

   b. white cell

      _____ / _____ / _____
                            r   cv   s

   c. clotting cell

      _____ / _____ / _____
                            r   cv   s

   d. one cell

      _____ / _____
                            p   s

   e. lymph cell

      _____ / _____ / _____
                            r   cv   s

2. **-cytosis**–suffix meaning **abnormal cell condition**
   Typically used to indicate an abnormal increase in cell numbers

   a. abnormal condition in red cells

      _____ / _____ / _____
                            r   cv   s

   b. abnormal condition in white cells

      _____ / _____ / _____
                            r   cv   s

   c. abnormal condition in clotting cells

      _____ / _____ / _____
                            r   cv   s

3. **-emia**–suffix meaning **blood condition**

   a. condition of being without blood

      _____ / _____
                            p   s

   b. blood condition with excessive sugar

      _____ / _____ / _____
                p   r   s

   c. blood condition with insufficient sugar

      _____ / _____ / _____
                p   r   s

   d. blood condition with excessive fat

      _____ / _____ / _____
                p   r   s

4. hem/o–combining form meaning **blood**

a. blood cell

_____/_____/_____
r   CV   s

b. blood protein

_____/_____/_____
r   CV   s

c. stopping of blood

_____/_____/_____
r   CV   s

d. excessive, abnormal flow of blood

_____/_____/_____
r   CV   s

e. to destroy blood

_____/_____/_____
r   CV   s

f. to destroy blood cells

_____/_____/_____/_____/_____
r   CV   r   CV   s

g. blood cell mass

_____/_____/_____/_____
r   CV   r   s

h. instrument for measuring blood cells

_____/_____/_____/_____/_____
r   CV   r   CV   s

i. process of measuring blood cells

_____/_____/_____/_____/_____
r   CV   r   CV   s

- -

5. hemat/o–combining form meaning **blood**

a. study of blood

_____/_____/_____
r   CV   s

b. one who studies blood

_____/_____/_____
r   CV   s

c. pertaining to blood

_____/_____
r   s

d. blood mass

_____/_____
r   s

e. study of blood diseases

_____/_____/_____/_____/_____
r   CV   r   CV   s

f. too few blood cells

_____/_____/_____/_____/_____
r   CV   r   CV   s

g. blood formation

_____/_____/_____
r   CV   s

- -

6. -penia–suffix meaning **too few**

Typically used to indicate that there are too few cells

a. too few red (cells)

_____/_____/_____
r   CV   s

b. too few white (cells)

_____/_____/_____
r   CV   s

c. too few clotting cells

_____/_____/_____/_____/_____
r   CV   r   CV   s

d. too few of all cells

_____/_____/_____/_____
p   r   cv   s

e. too few rosy red (cells)

_____/_____/_____.
r   cv   s

f. too few neutral (cells)

_____/_____/_____
r   cv   s

---

7. -phil–suffix meaning **attracted to**

Used to name three types of white blood cells based on type of stain they attract (chemically bind with)

8.3 Eosinophil

a. attracted to rosy red (stain)

_____/_____/_____
r   cv   s

b. attracted to basic (stain)

_____/_____/_____
r   cv   s

c. attracted to neutral (stain)

_____/_____/_____
r   cv   s

---

8. -poiesis–suffix meaning **formation**

Used to indicate process that produces new blood cells

a. formation of red (cells)

_____/_____/_____
r   cv   s

b. formation of white (cells)

_____/_____/_____
r   cv   s

c. formation of clotting (cells)

_____/_____/_____
r   cv   s

---

9. thromb/o–combining form meaning **clot**

A clot is a hard collection of fibrin, blood cells, and tissue debris that is the end result of hemostasis or blood-clotting process

a. to destroy a clot

_____/_____/_____
r   cv   s

b. surgical removal of a clot

_____/_____
r   s

c. abnormal condition of clots

_____/_____
r   s

Hematology Vocabulary

The hematology terms presented in this section include eponyms, modern English words, and those that contain Latin or Greek word parts but are not constructed solely from these word parts. When you recognize word parts within a term, they will give you a hint about the word's meaning. In these instances, look for the word parts to follow the term.

Term	Explanation
anemia an- = without -emia = blood condition	Group of blood disorders involving either a reduction in number of circulating erythrocytes or amount of hemoglobin in red blood cells; results in decreased oxygen delivery to tissues **TERMINOLOGY TIDBIT** The term *anemia* is built by combining the Greek prefix *an-* meaning "without" and *haima* meaning "blood." The *h* has been lost over time.
anticoagulant anti- = against coagul/o = clotting	Any substance that prevents clot formation
aplastic anemia a- = without -plasm = formation -tic = pertaining to an- = without -emia = blood condition	Severe form of anemia caused by loss of functioning red bone marrow; results in decrease in number of all blood cells; may require bone marrow transplant
autotransfusion auto- = self	Collecting and storing one's own blood to use to replace blood lost during surgery
blood culture and sensitivity (C&S)	Blood specimen incubated to check for bacterial growth; if bacteria are present, they are identified and best antibiotic treatment is determined **TERMINOLOGY TIDBIT** The term *culture* comes from the Latin word *cultura* meaning "to grow or cultivate." This part of a lab test involves growing bacteria from an infection.
blood transfusion	Transfer of blood from one person to another

8.4 A blood bag prepared for a transfusion; bag is clearly labeled with blood type and identification number
Source: Michal Heron/Pearson Education

Term	Explanation
bone marrow aspiration	Removal of small sample of bone marrow by needle and examined for diseases such as leukemia or aplastic anemia **8.5** Bone marrow is being aspirated from leg of an infant to test for leukemia Source: Nathan Eldridge/Pearson Education
bone marrow transplant (BMT)	Patient receives red bone marrow donation after own bone marrow is destroyed by radiation or chemotherapy
coagulate coagul/o = clotting	Formation of blood clot **TERMINOLOGY TIDBIT** The term *coagulate* comes from the Latin word *coagulare* meaning "to curdle."
complete blood count (CBC)	Comprehensive blood test that includes red blood cell count (RBC), white blood cell count (WBC), hemoglobin (Hgb), hematocrit (Hct), white blood cell differential, and platelet count
embolus embol/o = plug	Commonly called *floating clot;* usually piece of thrombus breaks away and floats through bloodstream until it lodges in a smaller blood vessel and blocks blood flow
erythrocyte sedimentation rate (ESR, SR, sed rate) erythr/o = red -cyte = cell	Blood test that measures rate at which red blood cells settle out of blood to form sediment in bottom of test tube; indicates presence of inflammatory disease
hematocrit (HCT, Hct, crit) hemat/o = blood	Blood test that measures volume of red blood cells within total volume of blood
hematoma hemat/o = blood -oma = mass, tumor	Collection of blood under skin as a result of blood escaping into tissue from damaged blood vessel; commonly called *bruise* **TERMINOLOGY TIDBIT** The term *hematoma* can be confusing. Its simple translation is "blood tumor"; however, it is used to refer to blood that has leaked out of a blood vessel and pooled in the tissues. For example, a bruise is a type of hematoma. **8.6** A large hematoma on the forehead of a young man
hemoglobin (Hgb, Hb, HGB) hem/o = blood -globin = protein	Blood test that measures amount of hemoglobin present in given volume of blood
hemophilia hem/o = blood -phil = attracted to	Inherited lack of a vital clotting factor; results in almost complete inability to stop bleeding

Term	Explanation

iron-deficiency anemia
  an- = without
  -emia = blood condition
	Anemia resulting when there is not enough iron to build hemoglobin for red blood cells

leukemia
  leuk/o = white
  -emia = blood condition
	Cancer of leukocyte-forming red bone marrow; patient has large number of abnormal and immature leukocytes circulating in blood

pernicious anemia (PA)
  an- = without
  -emia = blood condition
	Anemia resulting when digestive system absorbs insufficient amount of vitamin B_{12}; vitamin B_{12} is necessary for erythrocyte production
	
	TERMINOLOGY TIDBIT
	The term *pernicious* comes from the Latin word *perniciosus* meaning "destructive."

phlebotomy
  phleb/o = vein
  -otomy = cutting into
	Removal of blood specimen from vein for laboratory tests; also called *venipuncture*

platelet count	Blood test that determines number of platelets in given volume of blood

polycythemia vera
  poly- = many
  cyt/o = cell
  hem/o = blood
  -ia = condition
	Condition characterized by too many erythrocytes; blood becomes too thick to flow easily through blood vessels

prothrombin time (pro-time, PT)	Blood test that measures how long it takes for clot to form after prothrombin, a blood-clotting protein, is activated
red blood cell count (RBC)	Blood test that determines number of erythrocytes in volume of blood; decrease may indicate anemia; increase may indicate polycythemia vera

septicemia
  septic/o = infection
  -emia = blood condition
	Presence of bacteria or their toxins in bloodstream; commonly called *blood poisoning*

sequential multiple analyzer computer (SMAC)	Machine that performs multiple blood chemistry tests automatically
serum	Blood that has had formed elements and clotting factors removed

sickle cell anemia
  an- = without
  -emia = blood condition
	Inherited blood cell disorder in which erythrocytes take on an abnormal curved or "sickle" shape; cells are fragile and easily damaged resulting in anemia; occurs almost exclusively in persons of African descent

Normal red blood cells   **Sickled cells**

8.7 Comparison of normal-shaped and abnormal sickle-shaped red blood cells

Term	Explanation
thalassemia **-emia** = blood condition	Inherited blood disorder in which body is unable to correctly make hemoglobin, resulting in anemia
thrombolytic therapy **thromb/o** = clot **-lytic** = destruction	Administering medication to dissolve blood clot and restore normal circulation
white blood cell count (WBC)	Blood test that determines number of leukocytes in volume of blood; increase may indicate infection or leukemia; decrease may be caused by some diseases, radiation therapy, or chemotherapy
white blood cell differential (diff)	Blood test determines number of each type of leukocyte

TERMINOLOGY TIDBIT

The term *thalassemia* comes from the Greek word *thalassa* meaning "sea." This name came about because this condition was first known around the Mediterranean Sea.

Hematology Abbreviations

The following list presents common hematology abbreviations.

basos	basophils
BMT	bone marrow transplant
CBC	complete blood count
C&S	blood culture and sensitivity
diff	differential
eosins, eos	eosinophils
ESR, SR, sed rate	erythrocyte sedimentation rate
HCT, Hct, crit	hematocrit
Hgb, Hb, HGB	hemoglobin
lymphs	lymphocytes
monos	monocytes
PA	pernicious anemia
PMN, polys	polymorphonuclear neutrophil
PT, pro-time	prothrombin time
RBC	red blood cell, red blood cell count
Rh+	Rh-positive
Rh−	Rh-negative
segs	segmented neutrophils
SMAC	sequential multiple analyzer computer
WBC	white blood cell, white blood cell count

CASE STUDY

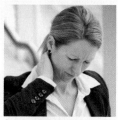

Source: Shutterstock

History of Present Illness

A 42-year-old woman is referred to the hematology clinic by her family physician. She reports experiencing increasing fatigue and dyspnea. It was initially associated only with intense physical activity, but now she cannot walk up a flight of stairs without becoming short of breath. She has had three episodes of sinusitis and pharyngitis in the last six months. She has noticed that she bruises more easily than usual and in the last week has had two spontaneous episodes of epistaxis. A CBC performed by her family physician reveals marked pancytopenia prompting the hematology referral.

Past Medical History

Past medical history is unremarkable. She had an appendectomy at age 12 and cholecystectomy at age 35. She has been pregnant three times and has two healthy children and had one miscarriage. She reports normal and regular menstrual periods, no signs of menopause. Patient currently takes no regular medications.

Family and Social History

Patient is married. She works as a chemical researcher for a company producing pesticides. She has no travel outside the country. Parents are alive. Father has hypertension; mother is healthy. Patient is an only child.

Physical Examination

Patient is a thin but well-nourished female who appears older than her stated age. She appears pale and has multiple dime-sized bruises scattered across her arms and lower legs. Respiratory rate is 22 breaths/minute, heart rate is 102 bpm, and blood pressure is 140/78.

Laboratory Findings

Due to already established pancytopenia, a bone marrow aspiration was performed for a bone marrow biopsy. Results of biopsy revealed that bone marrow contained fewer of all cell types than normal. The cells that are present are normal, no evidence of cancer.

Diagnosis

Aplastic anemia

Plan of Treatment

1. Blood transfusion to restore normal erythrocyte and platelet counts and relieve current symptoms
2. Long-term antibiotics to prevent recurring infection
3. Bone marrow–stimulating medication
4. If cell counts do not improve following bone marrow–stimulating medication or if cell counts continue to drop, patient will need a bone marrow transplant
5. Patient is advised to avoid strenuous exercise, refrain from contact sports, practice good handwashing, and to avoid sick people

Critical Thinking Questions

Answer the following questions regarding this case study. Do not just copy words out of the case study but translate all medical terms. To answer some of these questions, you may need to look up information from another chapter of this text, in a medical dictionary, or online. Answers are found at the back of the book.

1. Summarize the complaints that brought this patient to her family physician. Look up and define all medical terms used to describe her symptoms.

   _____

   _____

2. What test did the family physician perform? What does this test entail?

   _____

   _____

3. What was the result of the CBC? How does this explain each of the patient's symptoms?

   _____

   _____

4. What is this patient's medical history in nonmedical terms?

   _____

   _____

5. Carefully review the patient's family and social history. Is there some factor that might be the cause of her bone marrow dysfunction?

   _____

   _____

6. What are the patient's respiratory rate and heart rate? Measure your own breathing rate and pulse and compare them with the patient's results. Go to National Institutes of Health Medline Plus Medical Encyclopedia at www.nlm.nih.gov. Click on V, and scroll down the list and click on Vital Signs. Are her values high, low, or normal?

_____

_____

7. What is a biopsy? What tissue was biopsied in this patient? Summarize the results.

_____

_____

8. List the treatments planned for this patient and indicate which treats her current symptoms and which treat the underlying cause of her condition.

_____

_____

PRACTICE

Sound It Out

The following are some of the key terms from this chapter written as their phonetic spelling. Sound out each term and write it in the blank. Pronunciations for all terms are included in the audio glossary at www.mymedicalterminologylab.com.

1. hee-MAT-oh-krit _____

2. loo-koh-poy-EE-sis _____

3. koh-ag-YOO-late _____

4. EM-boh-lus _____

5. an-NEE-mee-ah _____

6. hee-mat-oh-path-ALL-oh-jee _____

7. HEE-moe-sigh-toh-LYE-sis _____

8. throm-boh-LYE-sis _____

9. AW-toh-trans-FYOO-zhun _____

10. hee-MALL-ih-sis _____

11. ee-RITH-row-PEE-nee-ah _____

12. loo-KEE-mee-ah _____

13. ee-RITH-row-sigh-toe-sis _____

14. LOO-koh-sigh-toh-sis _____

15. throm-BOH-sis _____

16. PAN-sigh-toe-PEE-nee-ah _____

17. hee-mah-TOH-mah _____

18. fleh-BOT-oh-mee _____

19. sep-tih-SEE-mee-ah _____

20. thal-ah-SEE-mee-ah _____

21. HIGH-poh-gly-SEE-me-ah _____

22. noo-troh-PEE-nee-ah _____

23. throm-boh-sigh-TOH-sis _____

24. hee-moh-FILL-ee-ah _____

25. LOO-koh-PEE-nee-ah _____

Transcription Practice

Each of the following sentences is written in common English. Underline any words or phrases that can be replaced by a medical term. Then rewrite the entire sentence using medical terms. Answers can be found at the back of the book.

1. The formed elements of blood are red blood cells, white blood cells, and clotting cells.

   _____

   _____

2. The patient had a small sample of bone marrow removed to determine whether she had cancer of the bone marrow that forms white blood cells.

   _____

   _____

3. The blood vessel was blocked by a floating clot.

   _____

   _____

4. Elena received medication to dissolve a blood clot during her heart attack.

   _____

   _____

5. Because he had diabetes, Ted monitored his blood for an excessive sugar blood condition.

   _____

   _____

6. The patient suffered excessive, abnormal flow of blood and a blood mass as a result of an auto accident.

   _____

   _____

7. The blood specialist determined that Genevieve had developed anemia due to vitamin B_{12} deficiency.

   _____

   _____

8. Following heart surgery, Tran received a blood transfusion of his own blood.

   _____

   _____

9. A comprehensive blood test including six different tests revealed that Marco had too few of all cells.

   _____

   _____

10. Because blood poisoning was suspected, a test to check for bacterial growth in the blood was ordered.

    _____

    _____

Abbreviation Matching

Match each abbreviation with its definition.

_____ **1.** ESR

_____ **2.** PT

_____ **3.** CBC

_____ **4.** RBC

_____ **5.** diff

_____ **6.** HCT

_____ **7.** BMT

_____ **8.** Hgb

_____ **9.** SMAC

_____ **10.** PA

A. red blood cell

B. hemoglobin

C. pernicious anemia

D. bone marrow transplant

E. complete blood count

F. sequential multiple analyzer computer

G. erythrocyte sedimentation rate

H. hematocrit

I. differential

J. prothrombin time

Fill in the Blank

Fill in the blank to complete each of the following sentences.

1. _____ anemia is caused by loss of functioning red bone marrow.

2. The medical term for *floating clot* is _____.

3. Receiving medication to dissolve a blood clot is called _____ therapy.

4. Polycythemia vera is a condition marked by _____ erythrocytes.

5. Another term for *phlebotomy* is _____.

6. A blood _____ is a test to check for bacterial growth.

7. A(n) _____ is a test that measures the volume of red blood cells.

8. Cancer of the leukocyte-forming bone marrow is called _____.

9. Pernicious anemia is caused by insufficient _____.

10. Septicemia is commonly called _____.

Labeling Exercise

Write the name of each blood cell on the numbered line. Also use this space to write the combining form where appropriate.

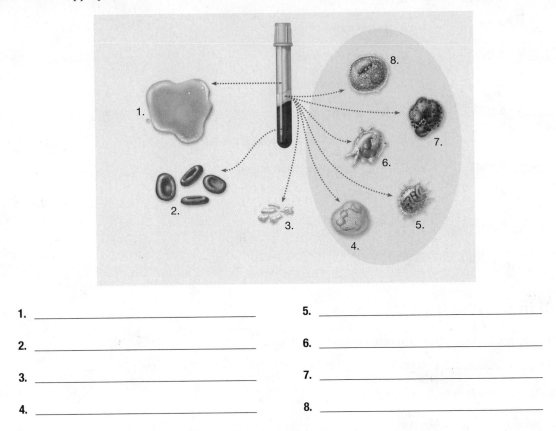

1. _____
2. _____
3. _____
4. _____

5. _____
6. _____
7. _____
8. _____

MyMedicalTerminologyLab™

MyMedicalTerminologyLab is a premium online homework management system that includes a host of features to help you study. Registered users will find:

- A multitude of activities and assignments built within the MyLab platform
- Powerful tools that track and analyze your results—allowing you to create a personalized learning experience
- Videos and audio pronunciations to help enrich your progress
- Streaming lesson presentations and self-paced learning modules
- A space where you and your instructors can view and manage your assignments

Build Medical Terms

Use each of the following word parts to build the indicated medical terms.

The combining form *cyt/o* means cell.

1. red cell _____

2. white cell _____

3. clotting cell _____

The combining form *hemat/o* means blood.

4. study of blood _____

5. blood formation _____

6. pertaining to blood _____

7. blood mass _____

The suffix *-emia* means blood condition.

8. excessive sugar blood condition _____

9. without blood condition _____

The combining form *hem/o* means blood.

10. stopping of blood _____

11. excessive, abnormal flow of blood _____

12. to destroy blood _____

The suffix *-phil* means attracted to.

13. attracted to rosy red _____

14. attracted to basic _____

15. attracted to neutral _____

Medical Term Analysis

Examine each of the following terms. Begin by dividing it into its word parts and writing them in the indicated blanks (*P = prefix*; *WR = word root*; *CF = combining form*; *S = suffix*). Follow with the definition of each word part and then finally the meaning of the full term.

1. **erythrocytosis**

   CF _____

   means _____

   S _____

   means _____

   Term meaning: _____

   _____

2. **hematologist**

   CF _____

   means _____

   S _____

   means _____

   Term meaning: _____

   _____

3. **hematopathology**

   CF _____

   means _____

   CF _____

   means _____

   S _____

   means _____

   Term meaning: _____

   _____

4. **hyperlipemia**

   P _____

   means _____

   WR _____

   means _____

   S _____

   means _____

   Term meaning: _____

   _____

5. **hemocytometer**

   CF _____

   means _____

   CF _____

   means _____

   S _____

   means _____

   Term meaning: _____

   _____

6. **leukopoiesis**

   CF _____

   means _____

   S _____

   means _____

   Term meaning: _____

   _____

7. lymphocyte

CF _____

means _____

S _____

means _____

Term meaning: _____

_____

8. hemoglobin

CF _____

means _____

S _____

means _____

Term meaning: _____

_____

9. pancytopenia

P _____

means _____

CF _____

means _____

S _____

means _____

Term meaning: _____

_____

10. thrombectomy

WR _____

means _____

S _____

means _____

Term meaning: _____

_____

Spelling

Some of the following terms are misspelled. Identify the incorrect terms and spell them correctly in the blank provided.

1. hypoglysemia _____

2. pernicious _____

3. anticoagulant _____

4. septecemia _____

5. thalassemia _____

6. platlet _____

7. polycytemia vera _____

8. phlebotomy _____

9. thrombocytopenia _____

10. eyrthropoiesis _____

Photomatch Challenge

Put the following phlebotomy photos in order by placing the appropriate letter beside the corresponding number in the blanks below.

A

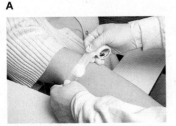

Source: Pearson Education

B

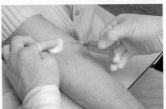

Source: Pearson Education

C

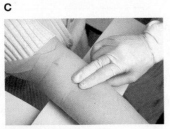

Source: Pearson Education

D

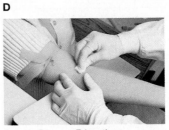

Source: Pearson Education

E

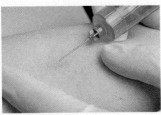

Source: Pearson Education

F

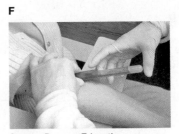

Source: Pearson Education

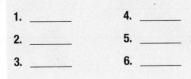

1. _____   4. _____

2. _____   5. _____

3. _____   6. _____

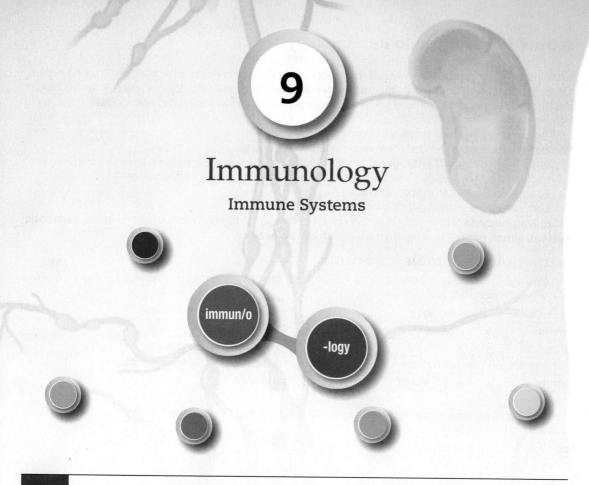

9

Immunology

Immune Systems

immun/o

-logy

Upon completion of this chapter, you will be able to:

9-1 Describe the medical specialty of immunology.

9-2 Understand the function of the immune and lymphatic systems.

9-3 Define immunology-related combining forms, prefixes, and suffixes.

9-4 Identify the organs treated in immunology.

9-5 Build immunology medical terms from word parts.

9-6 Explain immunology medical terms.

9-7 Use immunology abbreviations.

A Brief Introduction to Immunology

Immunology is the branch of medicine that diagnoses and treats conditions involving the immune system. Conditions that **immunologists** often treat include allergies, immunodeficiency disorders, autoimmune diseases, and cancers of the immune system. An **allergist** is an immunologist who has specialized training in treating allergies.

The **immune system** is a network of cells, tissues, and organs throughout the body that work together to protect the body against **pathogens**, anything that can damage the body including viruses, bacteria, toxins, or cancerous cells. Many of the functions of the immune system are carried out by white blood cells called **lymphocytes**. These cells are concentrated throughout the body in the organs of the **lymphatic system**: **lymph nodes**, **tonsils**, **thymus gland**, and **spleen**.

> **TERMINOLOGY TIDBIT**
> The term *immune* is from the Latin word *immunis* meaning "free." It is used to mean freedom from disease.

Immunology Combining Forms

The following list presents combining forms closely associated with the immune system and used for building and defining immunology terms.

adenoid/o	adenoids		**path/o**	disease
immun/o	protection, immunity		**phag/o**	eating
lymph/o	lymph		**splen/o**	spleen
lymphaden/o	lymph node		**thym/o**	thymus gland
lymphangi/o	lymph vessel		**tonsill/o**	tonsils

The following list presents combining forms that are not specific to the immune system but are also used for building and defining immunology terms.

cortic/o	cortex
cyt/o	cell
system/o	system

Suffix Review

These suffixes introduced in Chapter 2 are being reviewed in this chapter because they are especially important for building immunology terms.

-ar	pertaining to		**-logist**	one who studies
-atic	pertaining to		**-logy**	study of
-cyte	cell		**-malacia**	abnormal softening
-ectasis	dilated		**-megaly**	enlarged
-ectomy	surgical removal		**-oid**	resembling
-edema	swelling		**-oma**	tumor, mass
-gen	that which produces		**-osis**	abnormal condition
-genic	producing		**-pathy**	disease
-globulin	protein		**-pexy**	surgical fixation
-gram	record		**-plasty**	surgical repair
-graphy	process of recording		**-rrhaphy**	suture
-iasis	abnormal condition		**-stasis**	stopping
-ic	pertaining to		**-therapy**	treatment
-ist	specialist		**-toxic**	poison
-itis	inflammation			

Prefix Review

These prefixes introduced in Chapter 3 are being reviewed here because they are especially important for building immunology terms.

anti-	against
auto-	self
mono-	one

Organs Commonly Treated in Immunology

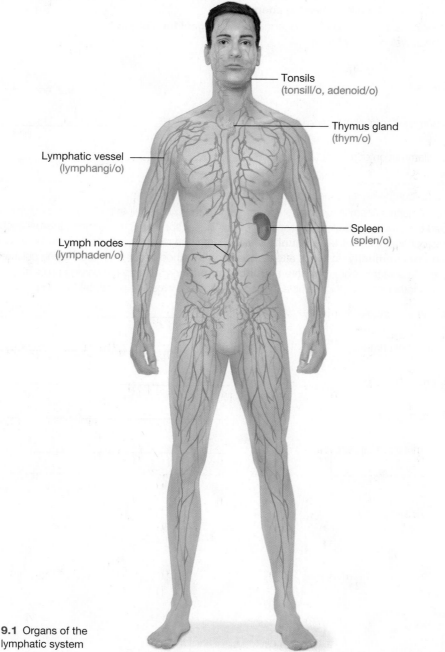

Tonsils
(tonsill/o, adenoid/o)

Thymus gland
(thym/o)

Lymphatic vessel
(lymphangi/o)

Spleen
(splen/o)

Lymph nodes
(lymphaden/o)

9.1 Organs of the lymphatic system

Building Immunology Terms

This section presents word parts most often used to build immunology terms. Following the explanation of the term, you have the opportunity to begin building your own vocabulary. Read the meaning for each term and then fill in the blanks to build a single medical term. Use the slashes to divide prefixes, word roots, combining vowels, and suffixes. To help you out you will find a key to the word parts underneath the blanks: **r** for word roots, **p** for prefix, **cv** for combining vowel, and **s** for suffix. Remember that not every term will contain all these word parts; it's up to you to decide which to use. As you gain experience, this process becomes easier. Answers can be found at the back of the book.

1. **adenoid/o**–combining form meaning **adenoids**

   Adenoids is the commonly used term for **pharyngeal tonsils**, located on back wall of upper throat

   9.2 Adenoid

   a. surgical removal of adenoids _____ / _____
                                                         _r_   _s_

   b. inflammation of adenoids _____ / _____
                                                          _r_   _s_

---

2. **immun/o**–combining form meaning **protection, immunity**

   The immune system is responsible for protecting the body against pathogens and removing damaged cells; **natural immunity** consists of body's nonspecific defense mechanisms (such as macrophages); **acquired immunity** results in immune responses to specific pathogens; **active acquired immunity** develops after exposure to a pathogen (for example, having chickenpox or receiving a vaccination); **passive acquired immunity** results from receiving protective substances from another source (for example, maternal antibodies crossing placenta)

   a. one who studies immunity _____ / _____ / _____
                  _r_   _cv_   _s_

   b. study of immunity _____ / _____ / _____
                  _r_   _cv_   _s_

   c. protection protein _____ / _____ / _____
                  _r_   _cv_   _s_

   d. producing protection _____ / _____ / _____
                  _r_   _cv_   _s_

   e. immunity treatment _____ / _____ / _____
                  _r_   _cv_   _s_

---

3. **lymph/o**–combining form meaning **lymph**

Lymph is the clear fluid collected from body tissues by lymphatic vessels; flows through lymphatic vessels to be returned to venous circulation

> **TERMINOLOGY TIDBIT**
> The term *lymph* comes from the Latin word *lympha*, which means "clear spring water."

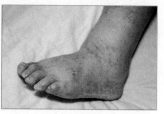

9.3 Lymphedema very commonly occurs in the lower leg
Source: Jan Mika/ Shutterstock

a. pertaining to lymph

_____ / _____
r   s

b. lymph tumor

_____ / _____
r   s

c. lymph swelling

_____ / _____
r   s

d. lymph cell

_____ / _____ / _____
r   cv   s

e. pertaining to a lymph cell

_____ / _____ / _____ / _____
r   cv   r   s

f. lymph cell tumor

_____ / _____ / _____ / _____
r   cv   r   s

g. producing lymph

_____ / _____ / _____
r   cv   s

h. resembling lymph

_____ / _____
r   s

i. stopping lymph

_____ / _____ / _____
r   cv   s

4. **lymphaden/o**–combining form meaning **lymph node**

Simple translation of this word part is "lymph gland," however these organs are not actually glands; lymph nodes are small roundish organs located along the path of lymphatic vessels that house lymphocytes and other white blood cells; as lymph passes through the lymph nodes, these white blood cells remove pathogens and damaged cells (see again Figure 9.1)

9.4 Lymph node

a. surgical removal of a lymph node

_____ / _____
r   s

b. disease of lymph nodes

_____ / _____ / _____
r   cv   s

c. process of recording lymph nodes

_____ / _____ / _____
r   cv   s

d. record of lymph nodes

_____ / _____ / _____
r   cv   s

e. lymph node inflammation

_____ / _____
r   s

f. abnormal condition of the lymph nodes _____ / _____
r   s

5. **lymphangi/o**–combining form meaning **lymph vessel**

A network of vessels that pick up excess fluid from tissues and return it to circulatory system (see again Figure 9.1)

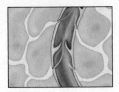

9.5 Lymphatic vessel

a. lymph vessel inflammation _____/_____
r   s

b. disease of lymph vessel _____/_____/_____
r   cv   s

c. lymph vessel tumor _____/_____
r   s

d. process of recording lymph vessels _____/_____/_____
r   cv   s

e. record of a lymph vessel _____/_____/_____
r   cv   s

f. surgical removal of a lymph vessel _____/_____
r   s

g. dilated lymph vessel _____/_____
r   s

h. surgical repair of a lymph vessel _____/_____/_____
r   cv   s

6. **path/o**–combining form meaning **disease**

> **TERMINOLOGY TIDBIT**
> The combining form *path/o* comes from the Greek word *pathos* meaning "suffering."

a. disease producing _____/_____/_____
r   cv   s

b. that which produces disease _____/_____/_____
r   cv   s

c. study of disease _____/_____/_____
r   cv   s

d. one who studies disease _____/_____/_____
r   cv   s

7. **phag/o**–combining form meaning **eating**

Some leukocytes, such as **monocytes**, are important to the immune system because they are able to engulf or "eat" pathogens or damaged cells; monocytes cross blood vessel walls and enter spaces around tissue; at this point, they are called **macrophages** and continue to function by engulfing pathogens

a. eating cell _____/_____/_____
r   cv   s

b. pertaining to an eating cell _____/_____/_____/_____
r   cv   r   s

8. splen/o–combining form meaning **spleen**

The spleen is an organ in the lymphatic system; located on left side of upper abdomen; houses leukocytes responsible for filtering pathogens from blood and destroying worn-out red blood cells (see again Figure 9.1)

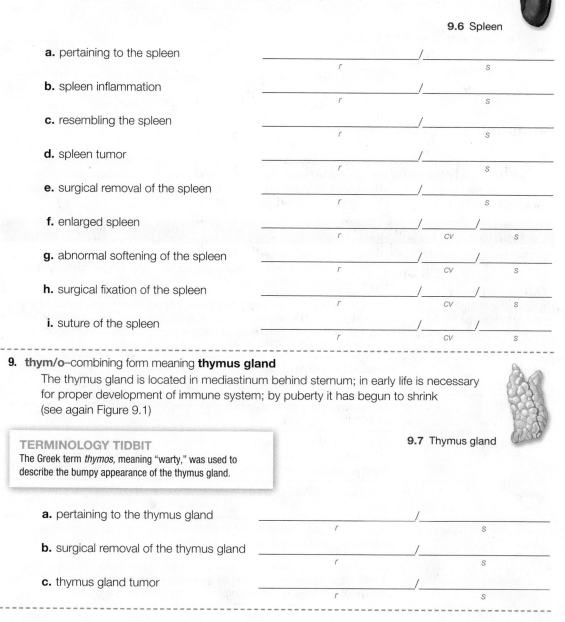

9.6 Spleen

    a. pertaining to the spleen   _____ / _____
                                                r   *s*

    b. spleen inflammation   _____ / _____
                                                r   *s*

    c. resembling the spleen   _____ / _____
                                                r   *s*

    d. spleen tumor   _____ / _____
                                                 r   *s*

    e. surgical removal of the spleen   _____ / _____
                                                r   *s*

    f. enlarged spleen   _____ / _____ / _____
                                          r   *cv*   *s*

    g. abnormal softening of the spleen   _____ / _____ / _____
                                          r   *cv*   *s*

    h. surgical fixation of the spleen   _____ / _____ / _____
                                          r   *cv*   *s*

    i. suture of the spleen   _____ / _____ / _____
                                          r   *cv*   *s*

---

9. thym/o–combining form meaning **thymus gland**

The thymus gland is located in mediastinum behind sternum; in early life is necessary for proper development of immune system; by puberty it has begun to shrink (see again Figure 9.1)

9.7 Thymus gland

> **TERMINOLOGY TIDBIT**
> The Greek term *thymos,* meaning "warty," was used to describe the bumpy appearance of the thymus gland.

    a. pertaining to the thymus gland   _____ / _____
                                                r   *s*

    b. surgical removal of the thymus gland   _____ / _____
                                                r   *s*

    c. thymus gland tumor   _____ / _____
                                              r   *s*

---

10. tonsill/o–combining form meaning **tonsils**

Three sets of tonsils are located in throat: palatine, pharyngeal, and lingual; contain lymphatic tissue that protects body from pathogens in air breathed and food eaten (see again Figure 9.1)

a. pertaining to the tonsils

_____/_____
                            r   *s*

b. surgical removal of the tonsils

_____/_____
                            r   *s*

c. inflammation of the tonsils

_____/_____
                            r   *s*

Immunology Vocabulary

The immunology terms presented in this section include eponyms, modern English words, and those that contain Latin or Greek word parts but are not constructed solely from these word parts. When you recognize word parts within a term, they will give you a hint about the word's meaning. In these instances, look for the word parts to follow the term.

Term	Explanation
AIDS-related complex (ARC)	Early stage of human immunodeficiency virus (HIV) infection in which mild symptoms of infection are present, including lymphadenopathy, fatigue, fever, night sweats, weight loss, and diarrhea
acquired immunodeficiency syndrome (AIDS) **immun/o** = protection	Later stage of human immunodeficiency virus (HIV) infection when the cells of the immune system lose their ability to fight off infection; patients become unable to resist opportunistic infections such as pneumocystis pneumonia (PCP) and Kaposi sarcoma (KS)
allergist **-ist** = specialist	Physician specializing in diagnosis and treatment of allergies
allergy	Hypersensitivity to a common substance in environment (such as pollen), to food, or to medication
anaphylactic shock	Life-threatening condition resulting from severe allergic reaction causing cardiovascular and respiratory problems; may be triggered by bee stings, medications, or certain foods; also called *anaphylaxis*
antihistamine **anti-** = against	Medication that blocks effects of histamine released by body during allergic reactions
antinuclear antibody titer (ANA) **anti-** = against	Blood test that determines number of antibodies against cell nuclei present in bloodstream; elevated in autoimmune conditions
autoimmune disease **auto-** = self	Disease resulting from body's immune system attacking its own cells as if they were pathogens; examples include systemic lupus erythematosus and sarcoidosis
corticosteroids **cortic/o** = cortex	Hormones produced by adrenal cortex; used as medication to treat autoimmune diseases due to their very strong anti-inflammatory properties
cytotoxic cells **cyt/o** = cell **-toxic** = poison	Cells capable of physically attacking and killing pathogens or diseased cells

Term	Explanation
elephantiasis **-iasis** = abnormal condition	Results from blockage of lymphatic vessels that causes extreme tissue edema

Blocked lymphatic vessel

Swollen lymphatic vessel

9.8 Elephantiasis; note how a blocked lymphatic vessel causes fluid to collect in the leg

TERMINOLOGY TIDBIT
Elephantiasis causes so much swelling in the leg that the knee and ankle disappear, making it look like an elephant's leg.

Term	Explanation
enzyme-linked immuno-sorbent assay (ELISA) **immun/o** = protection	Blood test for antibody to acquired immunodeficiency syndrome (AIDS) virus; positive result means the person has been exposed to virus
hives	Common name for appearance of wheals during allergic reaction
Hodgkin disease (HD)	Cancer of lymphatic cells found in lymph nodes; also called *Hodgkin lymphoma*
immunodeficiency **immun/o** = protection	Having an immune system that is unable to respond properly to pathogens; also called *immunocompromised*
immunosuppressant **immun/o** = protection	Medication to block certain actions of immune system; used to prevent rejection of transplanted organ
inflammation	Tissue response to injury; characterized by redness, pain, swelling, and feeling hot to touch

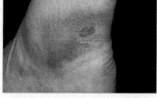

9.9 Inflammation associated with skin trauma to the ankle; note that the area is red and swollen; it is also painful and hot to touch
Source: Baciu/Shutterstock

Term	Explanation
Kaposi sarcoma (KS) **-oma** = tumor	Type of skin cancer often seen in patients with AIDS; consists of brownish-purple papules that begin in skin and spread to internal organs **9.10** Skin lesions characteristic of Kaposi sarcoma Source: National Cancer Institute (NCI Visuals Online) visualsonline.cancer.gov
mononucleosis (mono) **mono-** = one **-osis** = abnormal condition	Acute viral infection of lymphoid tissue with large number of abnormal white blood cells circulating in bloodstream
non-Hodgkin lymphoma (NHL) **lymph/o** = lymph **-oma** = tumor	Cancer of the lymphatic tissues other than Hodgkin lymphoma
opportunistic infections	Infections seen in patients with compromised immune systems
pneumocystis pneumonia (PCP)	Opportunistic infection common in immunodeficient persons; caused by fungus *Pneumocystis jiroveci*
sarcoidosis **-osis** = abnormal condition	Autoimmune disease with fibrous lesions forming in lymph nodes, liver, skin, lungs, spleen, eyes, and small bones of hands and feet
scratch test	Type of allergy testing in which body is exposed to allergens through a light scratch in skin
severe combined immu-nodeficiency syndrome (SCIDS) **immun/o** = protection	Genetic condition of children born with nonfunctioning immune system who are often forced to live in sealed sterile rooms
systemic lupus erythema-tosus (SLE) **system/o** = system **-ic** = pertaining to	Autoimmune disease in which immune system attacks connective tissue throughout body such as in joints and skin
urticaria	Severe itching associated with hives, usually seen in allergic reactions to food, stress, or medications
vaccination	Exposure to weakened pathogen to stimulate immune response and antibody production to give future protection against full-blown disease; also called *immunization*
Western blot test	Blood test to detect various antibodies in bloodstream such as HIV antibodies; considered more precise than ELISA

TERMINOLOGY TIDBIT
The first vaccine provided protection against smallpox; it was made from the drainage from cowpox sores, a condition closely related to smallpox. The term *vaccination* comes from the Latin word *vaccinus* meaning "relating to a cow."

Immunology Abbreviations

The following list presents common immunology abbreviations.

AIDS	acquired immunodeficiency syndrome	**KS**	Kaposi sarcoma
		mono	mononucleosis
ANA	antinuclear antibody titer	**NHL**	non-Hodgkin lymphoma
ARC	AIDS-related complex	**PCP**	pneumocystis pneumonia
ELISA	enzyme-linked immunosorbent assay	**SCIDS**	severe combined immunodeficiency syndrome
HD	Hodgkin disease		
HIV	human immunodeficiency virus	**SLE**	systemic lupus erythematosus
Ig	immunoglobulins (IgA, IgD, IgE, IgG, IgM)	**T&A**	tonsillectomy and adenoidectomy

CASE STUDY

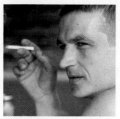

Source: Chubykin Arkady/ Shutterstock

History of Present Illness
Patient is a 39-year-old male referred to the AIDS Clinic by the family physician. Patient was seen three weeks ago by family physician when white spots on his tongue and throat were noted and patient had difficulty swallowing. Review of his physician's chart noted that this patient has had a 30-lb weight loss and several episodes of sinusitis and bronchitis over the past two years. When questioned, patient admitted that he was having regular bouts of diarrhea, night sweats, extreme fatigue, and unexplained fevers. Because of patient's past drug abuse history and current symptoms, he was referred to this clinic for evaluation.

Past Medical History
Patient is a recovering heroin abuser currently receiving treatment with methadone. Patient is on no other medication.

Family and Social History
Patient was a house painter but is becoming physically unable to perform the duties of his job. He is not married. Patient's parents are both alive and well.

Physical Examination
Patient appears older than his stated age, lethargic, and with muscular wasting. Temperature is 102°F, and the cervical and inguinal lymph nodes are enlarged.

Diagnostic Tests
ELISA was positive for HIV.

Diagnosis
AIDS-related complex

Plan of Treatment

1. Oral antifungal medication for treatment of thrush
2. Started on HIV drug regimen of Zidovudine (AZT), Epivir, and Viracept
3. Order Western blot to verify HIV infection
4. Monitor CD4 count

Critical Thinking Questions

Answer the following questions regarding this case study. Do not just copy words out of the case study but translate all medical terms. In order to answer some of these questions, you may need to look up information from another chapter of this text, in a medical dictionary, or online. Answers are found at the back of the book.

1. How was this patient probably infected by HIV? List two other ways in which persons may become exposed to HIV.

2. The white spots in the mouth of this patient are thrush. What causes this infection?

3. Read the entire case study carefully and list all of this patient's symptoms.

4. What is the first test used to diagnosis HIV infection, and why was a follow-up test ordered?

5. At this point, the patient is diagnosed with AIDS-related complex. What is the difference between ARC and AIDS?

6. What is an opportunistic infection? Name two that are commonly seen in AIDS patients.

7. This patient was started on an HIV drug regimen of three different medications. Use a website such as www.drugs.com or www.webmd.com to look up these drugs and briefly describe how they work.

8. A CD4 count was ordered for this patient. This is a count of a specific type of white blood cell targeted by HIV. Why do you think this piece of information is important for following this patient's progress?

Sound It Out

The following are some of the key terms from this chapter written as their phonetic spelling. Sound out each term and write it in the blank. Pronunciations for all terms are included in the audio glossary at www.mymedicalterminologylab.com.

1. lim-FOH-mah _____

2. AL-er-jee _____

3. path-OL-oh-gee _____

4. IM-yoo-noh-thair-ah-pee _____

5. in-flah-MAY-shun _____

6. splen-oh-MEG-ah-lee _____

7. lim-fad-eh-NEK-toh-mee _____

8. an-tih-HIST-ah-meen _____

9. lim-fad-en-EYE-tis _____

10. lim-fad-eh-NOG-rah-fee _____

11. LIM-fan-jee-EYE-tis _____

12. lim-FAN-jee-oh-gram _____

13. lim-fan-jee-OH-mah _____

14. sar-koyd-OH-sis _____

15. lim-foh-STAY-sis _____

16. mon-oh-nook-lee-OH-sis _____

17. path-oh-JEN-ik _____

18. lim-foh-sigh-TOE-mah _____

19. splen-EK-toh-mee _____

20. ton-sih-LEK-toh-mee _____

21. SPLEN-oh-PEKS-ee _____

22. thigh-MEK-toh-mee _____

23. vak-sih-NAY-shun _____

24. thigh-MOH-mah _____

25. ADD-eh-noy-DYE-tis _____

MyMedicalTerminologyLab™

MyMedicalTerminologyLab is a premium online homework management system that includes a host of features to help you study. Registered users will find:

- A multitude of activities and assignments built within the MyLab platform
- Powerful tools that track and analyze your results—allowing you to create a personalized learning experience
- Videos and audio pronunciations to help enrich your progress
- Streaming lesson presentations and self-paced learning modules
- A space where you and your instructors can view and manage your assignments

Transcription Practice

Each of the following sentences is written in common English. Underline any words or phrases that can be replaced by a medical term. Then rewrite the entire sentence using medical terms. Answers can be found at the back of the book.

1. Marcie's repeated bouts of tonsil inflammation required her to have the tonsils and adenoids surgically removed.

   _____

   _____

2. The lymph vessel record revealed a lymph vessel tumor.

   _____

   _____

3. The one who studies immunity is a physician who treats diseases in which the body's immune system attacks itself.

   _____

   _____

4. Jamar had a history of a life-threatening allergic reaction in response to a bee sting.

   _____

   _____

5. Mykos had to take medication to prevent transplant rejection after his kidney transplant.

   _____

   _____

6. Joyce's hypersensitivity to pollen was treated with medication that blocks the effects of histamine.

   _____

   _____

7. The patient in the late stages of HIV infection developed an opportunistic type of pneumonia.

   _____

   _____

8. Jennifer's allergic reactions consisted of wheals appearing and severe itching.

   _____

   _____

9. Shona's hand pain turned out to be caused by an autoimmune disease in which the immune system attacks connective tissue of her joints.

   _____

   _____

10. Carlos's lymph node disease turned out to be cancer of the lymphatic cells in the lymph nodes.

   _____

   _____

Build Medical Terms

Use each of the following word parts to build the indicated medical terms.

The combining form *lymphaden/o* means lymph node.

1. surgical removal of lymph node _____

2. lymph node record _____

3. lymph node disease _____

The combining form *immun/o* means protection or immunity.

4. protection protein _____

5. one who studies immunity _____

The combining form *splen/o* means spleen.

6. enlarged spleen _____

7. resembling a spleen _____

8. pertaining to the spleen _____

The combining form *tonsill/o* means tonsils.

9. tonsil inflammation _____

10. surgical removal of tonsil _____

11. pertaining to tonsils _____

The combining form *lymphangi/o* means lymph vessel.

12. lymph vessel inflammation _____

13. surgical repair of lymph vessel _____

14. process of recording lymph vessel _____

15. lymph vessel tumor _____

Labeling Exercise

Write the name of each structure on the numbered line. Also use this space to write the combining form where appropriate.

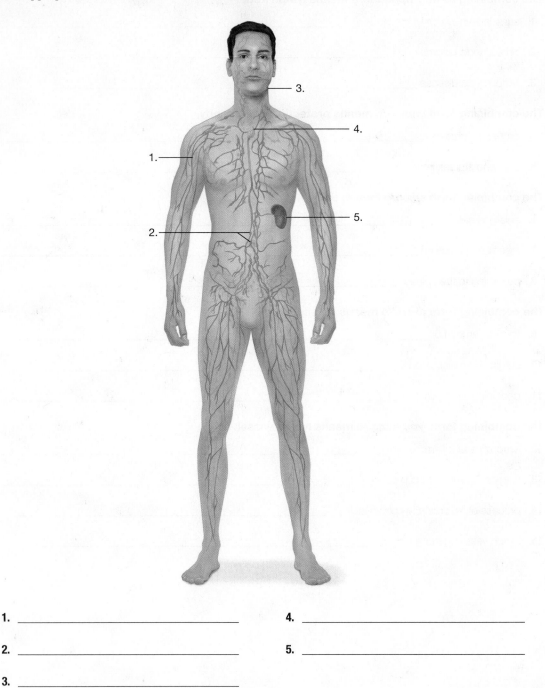

1. _____

2. _____

3. _____

4. _____

5. _____

Spelling

Some of the following terms are misspelled. Identify the incorrect terms and spell them correctly in the blank provided.

1. urticoria _____

2. sarcoidosis _____

3. corticosteroids _____

4. anaphylactic _____

5. lymphadanosis _____

6. immunosuppressents _____

7. splenomalasia _____

8. tonsilitis _____

9. mononucleosis _____

10. antihistamine _____

Fill in the Blank

Fill in the blank to complete each of the following sentences.

1. The _____ is a physician specializing in treating allergies.

2. A(n) _____ disease results when the body's own immune system attacks itself.

3. Elephantiasis occurs when _____ become blocked causing extreme tissue _____.

4. Hives are the common name for _____ that appear during an allergic reaction.

5. _____ are hormones that can be used to treat autoimmune diseases.

6. The early stage of an HIV infection with mild symptoms is called _____.

7. Vaccinations may also be called _____.

8. Kaposi sarcoma is a type of _____ cancer seen in AIDS patients.

9. _____ is a life-threatening severe allergic reaction.

10. The _____ is considered more sensitive than an ELISA.

Abbreviation Matching

Match each abbreviation with its definition.

_____ **1.** T&A   **A.** severe combined immunodeficiency syndrome

_____ **2.** PCP   **B.** acquired immunodeficiency syndrome

_____ **3.** HD   **C.** pneumocystis pneumonia

_____ **4.** Ig   **D.** mononucleosis

_____ **5.** mono   **E.** non-Hodgkin lymphoma

_____ **6.** SCIDS   **F.** enzyme-linked immunosorbent assay

_____ **7.** NHL   **G.** tonsillectomy and adenoidectomy

_____ **8.** KS   **H.** immunoglobulin

_____ **9.** AIDS   **I.** Kaposi sarcoma

_____**10.** ELISA   **J.** Hodgkin disease

Medical Term Analysis

Examine each of the following terms. Begin by dividing it into its word parts and writing them in the indicated blanks (*P = prefix*; *WR = word root*; *CF = combining form*; *S = suffix*). Follow with the definition of each word part and then finally the meaning of the full term.

1. adenoiditis

WR _____

means _____

S _____

means _____

Term meaning: _____

_____

2. lymphogenic

CF _____

means _____

S _____

means _____

Term meaning: _____

_____

3. immunotherapy

CF _____

means _____

S _____

means _____

Term meaning: _____

_____

4. **lymphocytoma**

   CF _____

   means _____

   WR _____

   means _____

   S _____

   means _____

   Term meaning: _____

   _____

5. **phagocytic**

   CF _____

   means _____

   WR _____

   means _____

   S _____

   means _____

   Term meaning: _____

   _____

6. **lymphadenopathy**

   CF _____

   means _____

   S _____

   means _____

   Term meaning: _____

   _____

7. **pathology**

   CF _____

   means _____

   S _____

   means _____

   Term meaning: _____

   _____

8. **lymphangiectasis**

   WR _____

   means _____

   S _____

   means _____

   Term meaning: _____

   _____

9. **thymectomy**

   WR _____

   means _____

   S _____

   means _____

   Term meaning: _____

   _____

10. **lymphedema**

    WR _____

    means _____

    S _____

    means _____

    Term meaning: _____

    _____

Photomatch Challenge

The following figure illustrates what happens when inflammation occurs. The letters represent the order of events. The events listed are out of order. Your challenge is to match each letter on the figure with its description.

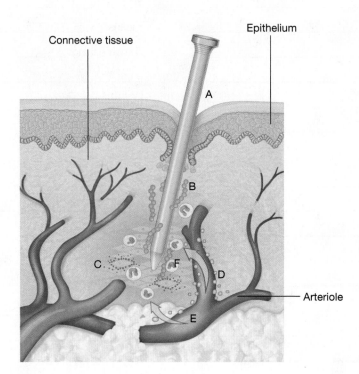

_____ **1.** Bacteria enter and multiply

_____ **2.** Arterioles dilate and become leaky

_____ **3.** Dirty nail punctures skin

_____ **4.** Injured cells release chemicals

_____ **5.** Materials are released into damaged tissue to begin repairs

_____ **6.** White blood cells destroy the bacteria

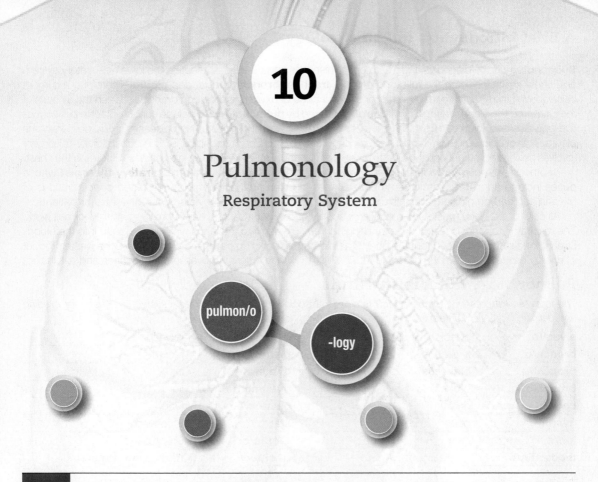

10

Pulmonology

Respiratory System

pulmon/o

-logy

⌄ Learning Objectives

Upon completion of this chapter, you will be able to:

10-1 Describe the medical specialty of pulmonology.

10-2 Understand the functions of the respiratory system.

10-3 Define pulmonology-related combining forms, prefixes, and suffixes.

10-4 Identify the organs treated in pulmonology.

10-5 Build pulmonology medical terms from word parts.

10-6 Explain pulmonology medical terms.

10-7 Use pulmonology abbreviations.

A Brief Introduction to Pulmonology

Pulmonology is the diagnosis and treatment of diseases and conditions affecting the lower respiratory system and chest cavity including the following organs: **trachea**, **bronchi**, **lungs**, and **pleura**. Therefore, it is most involved with the structures responsible for the exchange of oxygen and carbon dioxide between the air sacs of the lungs and the bloodstream. Conditions often treated by **pulmonologists** include cancer, infections, obstructive lung diseases, injuries, respiratory failure, environmental and occupational lung diseases, and disorders of the pleura. A **thoracic surgeon** surgically treats lung and thoracic cavity conditions. This subspecialty of surgery involves performing surgery on the lungs, trachea, esophagus, chest wall, heart, and other structures in the chest.

Another health care provider intimately involved in respiratory care is the **respiratory therapist** whose duties include administering oxygen therapy, measuring lung capacity, monitoring blood concentrations of oxygen and carbon dioxide, administering breathing treatments, and providing care for ventilator patients.

All cells of the body must have a constant supply of **oxygen** (O_2) in order to produce energy for cell work. The respiratory system is responsible for bringing fresh oxygen into the lungs where it is loaded into the bloodstream for distribution throughout the body. The blood then picks up **carbon dioxide** (CO_2), the waste product of energy production, from the cells and returns it to the lungs where it moves into the air sacs and is exhaled.

Pulmonology Combining Forms

The following list presents combining forms closely associated with the respiratory system and used for building and defining pulmonology terms.

alveol/o	alveolus (air sac)		**ox/i**	oxygen
bronch/o	bronchus		**pleur/o**	pleura
bronchi/o	bronchus		**pneum/o**	lung, air
bronchiol/o	bronchiole		**pneumon/o**	lung
coni/o	dust		**pulmon/o**	lung
cyan/o	blue		**spir/o**	breathing
lob/o	lobe		**thorac/o**	chest
mediastin/o	mediastinum		**trache/o**	trachea (windpipe)

The following list presents combining forms that are not specific to the respiratory system but are also used for building and defining pulmonology terms.

angi/o	vessel		**embol/o**	plug
arteri/o	artery		**fibr/o**	fibrous
atel/o	incomplete		**hem/o**	blood
carcin/o	cancer		**orth/o**	straight
cardi/o	heart		**py/o**	pus
cyt/o	cell			

Suffix Review

These suffixes introduced in Chapter 2 are being reviewed in this chapter because they are especially important for building pulmonology terms.

-al	pertaining to		**-genic**	producing
-algia	pain		**-gram**	record
-ar	pertaining to		**-graph**	instrument for recording
-ary	pertaining to		**-graphy**	process of recording
-centesis	puncture to withdraw fluid		**-ia**	state of
-dynia	pain		**-ic**	pertaining to
-ectasis	dilated		**-itis**	inflammation
-ectomy	surgical removal		**-logist**	one who studies

-logy	study of	**-oxia**	oxygen
-meter	instrument for measuring	**-plasty**	surgical repair
-metry	process of measuring	**-pnea**	breathing
-ole	small	**-ptysis**	spitting
-oma	tumor, mass	**-scope**	instrument for viewing
-osis	abnormal condition	**-scopy**	process of visually examining
-ostomy	surgically create an opening	**-spasm**	involuntary muscle contraction
-otomy	cutting into	**-thorax**	chest

Prefix Review

These prefixes introduced in Chapter 3 are being reviewed here because they are especially important for building pulmonology terms.

a-	without	**eu-**	normal, good
an-	without	**hyper-**	excessive
brady-	slow	**hypo-**	below, insufficient
dys-	painful, difficult, abnormal	**tachy-**	fast
endo-	within, inner		

Organs Commonly Treated in Pulmonary Disease

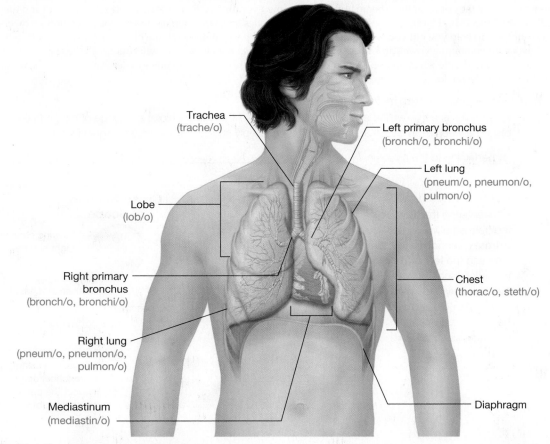

Trachea
(trache/o)

Left primary bronchus
(bronch/o, bronchi/o)

Left lung
(pneum/o, pneumon/o,
pulmon/o)

Lobe
(lob/o)

Right primary
bronchus
(bronch/o, bronchi/o)

Chest
(thorac/o, steth/o)

Right lung
(pneum/o, pneumon/o,
pulmon/o)

Mediastinum
(mediastin/o)

Diaphragm

10.1 Respiratory organs in the thoracic cavity

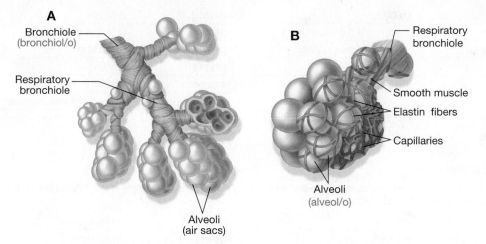

A

Bronchiole
(bronchiol/o)

Respiratory
bronchiole

Alveoli
(air sacs)

B

Respiratory
bronchiole

Smooth muscle

Elastin fibers

Capillaries

Alveoli
(alveol/o)

10.2 Microscopic lung structure: (A) Alveoli clustered at end of respiratory bronchioles
(B) Arrangement of capillaries and elastin fibers around cluster of alveoli

Building Pulmonology Terms

This section presents word parts most often used to build pulmonology terms. Following the explanation of the term, you have the opportunity to begin building your own vocabulary. Read the meaning for each term and then fill in the blanks to build a single medical term. Use the slashes to divide prefixes, word roots, combining vowels, and suffixes. To help you out you will find a key to the word parts underneath the blanks: **r** for word roots, **p** for prefix, **cv** for combining vowel, and **s** for suffix. Remember that not every term will contain all these word parts; it's up to you to decide which to use. As you gain experience, this process becomes easier. Answers can be found at the back of the book.

1. **alveol/o**–combining form meaning **alveolus**

    An alveolus is a thin-walled air sac at the end of respiratory bronchiole; exchange of oxygen takes place between air in alveoli and capillary blood supply surrounding them (see again Figure 10.2)

    a. pertaining to the alveolus

    _____ / _____
                                  r   *s*

---

2. **bronch/o**–combining form meaning **bronchus**

    After entering the thoracic cavity, the trachea divides into the **right primary bronchus** to the right lung and the **left primary bronchus** to the left lung; they subdivide into more narrow secondary and tertiary bronchi and eventually become the narrowest bronchioles (see again Figure 10.1)

Cross-Section of Scope

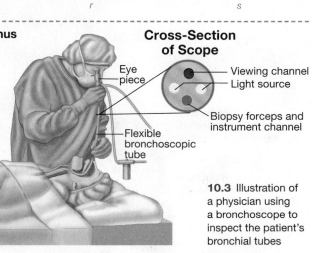

Eye piece

Viewing channel

Light source

Biopsy forceps and instrument channel

Flexible bronchoscopic tube

10.3 Illustration of a physician using a bronchoscope to inspect the patient's bronchial tubes

a. record of the bronchus   _____/_____/_____

r   CV   S

b. process of recording the bronchus   _____/_____/_____

r   CV   S

c. bronchus inflammation   _____/_____

r   S

d. instrument for viewing the bronchus   _____/_____/_____

r   CV   S

e. process of visually examining the bronchus   _____/_____/_____

r   CV   S

f. involuntary muscle contraction of the bronchus   _____/_____/_____

r   CV   S

g. bronchus producing   _____/_____/_____

r   CV   S

---

3. bronchi/o–combining form meaning **bronchus**

10.4 Bronchial tree

a. pertaining to the bronchus   _____/_____

r   S

b. small bronchus   _____/_____

r   S

c. dilated bronchus   _____/_____

r   S

---

4. bronchiol/o–combining form meaning **bronchiole**

A bronchiole is the narrowest airway tube; carries air from bronchi to alveoli; as a bronchiole approaches a group of alveoli, it becomes a respiratory bronchiole that terminates in the alveoli (see again Figure 10.2)

a. pertaining to a bronchiole   _____/_____

r   S

---

5. coni/o–combining form meaning **dust**

Used to refer to particles inhaled into lungs

a. abnormal condition of dust in the lung   _____/_____/_____/_____

r   CV   r   S

---

6. cyan/o–combining form meaning **blue**

Blood that is low in oxygen is a deep, dark red color that gives skin a blue tint

a. abnormal condition of being blue   _____/_____

r   S

---

7. **lob/o**–combining form meaning **lobe**

Each lung is subdivided into **lobes;** right lung has three lobes, left lung has two (see again Figure 10.1)

a. pertaining to a lobe   _____ / _____
                                                             r   *s*

b. surgical removal of a lobe   _____ / _____
                                                             r   *s*

8. **mediastin/o**–combining form meaning **mediastinum**

The mediastinum is the central region of the thoracic cavity between the lungs; contains trachea, heart, aorta, esophagus, lymph nodes, and thymus gland (see again Figure 10.1)

a. pertaining to the mediastinum   _____ / _____
                                                             r   *s*

b. cutting into the mediastinum   _____ / _____
                                                             r   *s*

9. **orth/o**–combining form meaning **straight**

Primarily used to refer to bone or skeleton terms; in pulmonology, is used to indicate sitting straight up; people who have difficulty breathing often feel they can breathe easier if they are sitting up rather than lying down

a. breathing (sitting up) straight   _____ / _____ / _____
                                                             r   *cv*   *s*

10. **-oxia**–suffix meaning **oxygen**

Oxygen is a gas required by every cell of body for cell metabolism; main function of lungs is to inhale oxygen and load it into the bloodstream

a. without oxygen   _____ / _____
                                                             p   *s*

11. **ox/i**–combining form meaning **oxygen**

a. instrument for measuring oxygen   _____ / _____ / _____
                                                             r   *cv*   *s*

b. process of measuring oxygen   _____ / _____ / _____
                                                             r   *cv*   *s*

12. **pleur/o**–combining form meaning **pleura**

The pleura is a double-layered membrane that forms protective sac around lungs; outer layer called **parietal pleura** and lines thoracic cavity; inner layer called **visceral pleura** and covers lungs; space formed by folded pleura is called **pleural cavity**

a. pertaining to the pleura   _____ / _____
                                                             r   *s*

b. puncture pleura to withdraw fluid   _____ / _____ / _____
                                                             r   *cv*   *s*

c. pleura pain   _____ / _____ / _____
                                                             r   *cv*   *s*

d. pleura pain   _____ / _____
                                                               r   *s*

e. pleura inflammation   _____ / _____
                                                              r   *s*

13. **-pnea**–suffix meaning **breathing**

A prefix is placed before this suffix to indicate what is happening with person's breathing pattern

a. without breathing

_____/_____
p   s

b. difficult breathing

_____/_____
p   s

c. normal breathing

_____/_____
p   s

d. excessive (deep) breathing

_____/_____
p   s

e. insufficient (shallow) breathing

_____/_____
p   s

f. slow breathing

_____/_____
p   s

g. fast breathing

_____/_____
p   s

14. **pneum/o**–combining form meaning **lung** or **air**

Lungs are paired organs found in thoracic cavity; each consists of tubelike airways that carry air to and from alveoli, or air sacs; gas exchange between outside air and bloodstream takes place in alveoli (see again Figure 10.1)

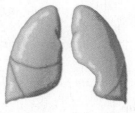

10.5 Lungs

a. record of a lung

_____/_____/_____
r   cv   s

b. instrument to record the lung

_____/_____/_____
r   cv   s

c. process of recording the lung

_____/_____/_____
r   cv   s

d. air in the chest

_____/_____/_____
r   cv   s

15. **pneumon/o**–combining form meaning **lung**

a. pertaining to the lung

_____/_____
r   s

b. lung puncture to withdraw fluid

_____/_____/_____
r   cv   s

c. surgical removal of the lung

_____/_____
r   s

d. cutting into the lung

_____/_____
r   s

16. pulmon/o–combining form meaning **lung**

    a. pertaining to a lung

        _____ / _____
                      r   s

    b. study of the lung

        _____ / _____ / _____
                      r   cv   s

    c. one who studies lungs

        _____ / _____ / _____
                      r   cv   s

- -

17. -ptysis–suffix meaning **spitting**

    The main medical term built using this suffix means coughing up and spitting out of blood coming from lungs or bronchi

    a. spitting (up) blood

        _____ / _____ / _____
                      r   cv   s

- -

18. spir/o–combining form meaning **breathing**

    a. record of breathing

        _____ / _____ / _____
                      r   cv   s

    b. instrument to measure breathing

        _____ / _____ / _____
                      r   cv   s

    c. process of measuring breathing

        _____ / _____ / _____
                      r   cv   s

- -

19. thorac/o–combining form meaning **chest**

10.6 Thoracocentesis: a needle is inserted between the ribs to withdraw fluid from the pleural sac at the base of the left lung; also known as thoracentesis or pleurocentesis

Needle inserted into pleural space to withdraw fluid

    a. chest pain

        _____ / _____
                      r   s

    b. chest pain

        _____ / _____ / _____
                      r   cv   s

    c. pertaining to the chest

        _____ / _____
                      r   s

    d. cutting into the chest

        _____ / _____
                      r   s

    e. puncture chest to withdraw fluid

        _____ / _____ / _____
                      r   cv   s

    f. surgically create an opening in the chest

        _____ / _____
                      r   s

- -

20. -thorax–suffix meaning **chest**

Used to indicate presence of substance in chest

a. blood in the chest

_____ / _____ / _____
r   cv   s

b. pus in the chest

_____ / _____ / _____
r   cv   s

c. air in the chest

_____ / _____ / _____
r   cv   s

---

21. trache/o–combining form meaning **trachea**

Trachea is the tube that carries air from throat down into chest cavity; splits into two main bronchi; commonly called *windpipe* (see again Figure 10.1)

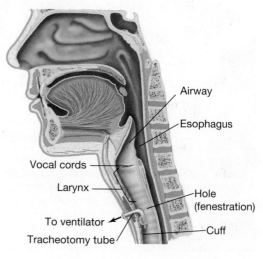

10.7 Trachea

a. pertaining to the trachea

_____ / _____
r   s

b. surgical repair of trachea

_____ / _____ / _____
r   cv   s

c. surgically create an opening in trachea

_____ / _____
r   s

d. cutting into the trachea

_____ / _____
r   s

e. trachea inflammation

_____ / _____
r   s

f. pertaining to within the trachea

_____ / _____ / _____
p   r   s

Airway

Esophagus

Vocal cords

Larynx

Hole (fenestration)

To ventilator

Tracheotomy tube

Cuff

10.8 A tracheotomy tube in place, inserted through an opening in the front of the neck and anchored within the trachea

Pulmonology Vocabulary

The pulmonology terms presented in this section include eponyms, modern English words, and those that contain Latin or Greek word parts but are not constructed solely from these word parts. When you recognize word parts within a term, they will give you a hint about the word's meaning. In these instances, look for the word parts to follow the term.

Term	Explanation
adult respiratory distress syndrome (ARDS)	Acute respiratory failure in adults characterized by tachypnea, dyspnea, cyanosis, tachycardia, and hypoxia
arterial blood gases (ABGs) **arteri/o** = artery **-al** = pertaining to	Laboratory test for levels of oxygen and carbon dioxide present in blood
asphyxia, asphyxiation	Lack of oxygen that can lead to unconsciousness and death if not corrected immediately; some common causes are drowning, foreign body in respiratory tract, poisoning, and electric shock; also called *suffocation*
aspirate	Inhaling fluid or foreign object into airways
asthma	Disease caused by various conditions, such as allergies, and resulting in broncho-spasm, excessive mucus production, inflammation, airway constriction, wheezing, and coughing

> **TERMINOLOGY TIDBIT**
> The term *aspirate* is built from the Latin prefix *a-* meaning "without" and *spiro* meaning "breathing." A person who has inhaled an object that blocks the airways is not able to breathe.

Normal bronchiole

Constricted bronchiole

Asthma attack

Contracted smooth muscle

Mucous membrane

Smooth muscle

Swollen mucous membrane

Excessive mucus secretion

A

B

10.9 (A) Normal bronchiole tube; (B) Bronchospasms and excessive mucus production associated with an asthma attack

atelectasis **atel/o** = incomplete **-ectasis** = dilated	Condition in which lung tissue collapses, preventing respiratory exchange of oxygen and carbon dioxide

> **TERMINOLOGY TIDBIT**
> The term *atelectasis* is built from the Greek terms *atelos* meaning "incomplete" and *ektasis* meaning "expansion." When *incomplete* modifies expansion, the term means *unexpanded* or, in other words, *collapsed*.

Term	Explanation
bronchodilator **bronch/o** = bronchus	Any medication that causes bronchi to dilate
bronchogenic carcinoma **bronch/o** = bronchus **-genic** = producing **carcin/o** = cancer **-oma** = tumor	Malignant lung tumor that originates in bronchi; often associated with a history of cigarette smoking Bronchial tumor Primary tumor **10.10** Illustration of a lung with two tumors growing out of the bronchial wall **TERMINOLOGY TIDBIT** The best known meaning of the Greek term *karkinos* is "cancer," as in the zodiac sign. However, the term also means a sore that won't heal, which is one of the warning signs of cancer.
cardiopulmonary resuscitation (CPR) **cardi/o** = heart **pulmon/o** = lung **-ary** = pertaining to	Combination of external compressions to sternum and rescue breathing to maintain blood flow and air movement in and out of lungs during cardiac and respiratory arrest
chronic obstructive pulmonary disease (COPD) **pulmon/o** = lung **-ary** = pertaining to	Progressive, chronic, and usually irreversible condition in which airflow to and from lungs is decreased; patient can have severe dyspnea with exertion and cough; also called *chronic obstructive lung disease (COLD)*
crackles	Abnormal rattling or crackling sound made during inhalation; caused by mucus or fluid in airways; also called *rales* **TERMINOLOGY TIDBIT** The term *rales* is a French word meaning "rattle."
croup	Acute viral infection in infants and children; symptoms include dyspnea and a characteristic barking cough **TERMINOLOGY TIDBIT** This term is unusual because its origin is not Latin or Greek. *Croup* comes from the Anglo-Saxon word *kropan*, which means to "cry aloud" or "croak."
cystic fibrosis (CF) **fibr/o** = fibrous **-osis** = abnormal condition	Genetic condition that causes patient to produce very thick mucus resulting in severe congestion within lungs and digestive system

Term	Explanation
emphysema	Pulmonary condition resulting from destruction of alveolar walls leading to overinflated alveoli; can occur as result of long-term heavy smoking or exposure to air pollution; characterized by dyspnea on exertion

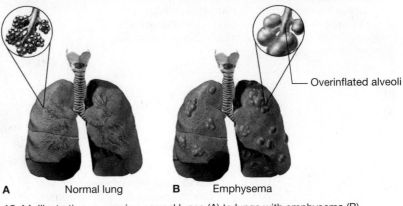

A   Normal lung   **B**   Emphysema

10.11 Illustration comparing normal lungs (A) to lungs with emphysema (B)

Term	Explanation
endotracheal (ET) **intubation** **endo-** = within **trache/o** = trachea **-al** = pertaining to	Placing tube through mouth and into trachea to maintain open airway and facilitate artificial ventilation

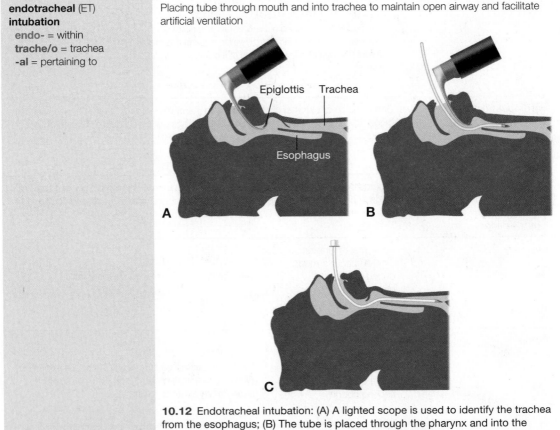

10.12 Endotracheal intubation: (A) A lighted scope is used to identify the trachea from the esophagus; (B) The tube is placed through the pharynx and into the trachea; (C) The scope is removed, leaving the tube in place

Term	Explanation
hyperventilation hyper- = excessive	To breathe too quickly (tachypnea) and too deeply (hyperpnea)
hypoventilation hypo- = insufficient	To breathe too slowly (bradypnea) and too shallowly (hypopnea)
hypoxia hypo- = insufficient -oxia = oxygen	Having insufficient amount of oxygen in body
infant respiratory distress syndrome (IRDS)	Condition seen in premature infants whose lungs have not had time to fully develop; lungs are not able to expand fully, causing extreme difficulty in breathing and can result in death; also known as *hyaline membrane disease (HMD)*
influenza (flu)	Acute viral infection of airways; usually highly contagious; symptoms include chills, fever, body aches, and dry cough
intermittent positive pressure breathing (IPPB)	Method of artificial ventilation using mask connected to machine that produces pressure to assist air to fill lungs **10.13** Patient receiving assistance to breathe with an intermittent positive pressure breathing machine Source: Ron May/Pearson Education
phlegm	Thick mucus secreted by mucous membranes lining respiratory tract; phlegm that is coughed out through mouth is called *sputum*
pleural effusion pleur/o = pleura -al = pertaining to	Abnormal presence of fluid or gas in pleural cavity; presence of this fluid can be detected by tapping chest (percussion) or listening with stethoscope (auscultation)
pleurisy pleur/o = pleura	Inflammation of pleura
pneumonia pneumon/o = lung -ia = state of	Acute inflammatory condition of lung, which can be caused by bacterial and viral infections, diseases, and chemicals; severe dyspnea and death can result when alveoli fill with fluid (pulmonary infiltrate)
pneumothorax pneum/o = air -thorax = chest	Collection of air or gas in pleural cavity, which can result in collapse of lung **10.14** Illustration showing how outside air entering pleural cavity results in collapsed lung of pneumothorax

Term	Explanation
postural drainage	Drainage of secretions from bronchi by placing patient in position that uses gravity to promote drainage; used for treatment of cystic fibrosis and bronchiectasis
pulmonary angiography **pulmon/o** = lung **-ary** = pertaining to **angi/o** = vessel **-graphy** = process of recording	Injecting dye into blood vessel for purpose of taking X-ray of arteries and veins of lungs; test for pulmonary embolism
pulmonary edema **pulmon/o** = lung **-ary** = pertaining to	Condition in which lung tissue retains excessive amount of fluid; results in dyspnea
pulmonary embolism (PE) **pulmon/o** = lung **-ary** = pertaining to **embol/o** = plug	Blood clot or air bubble in pulmonary artery or one of its branches; results in infarct of lung tissue
pulmonary function test (PFT) **pulmon/o** = lung **-ary** = pertaining to	Diagnostic procedure to assess respiratory function by using spirometer to measure airflow and lung volumes; often performed by respiratory therapists **10.15** Patient breathing into a spirometer during a pulmonary function test
purulent	Containing pus, as in purulent sputum
respiratory rate (RR)	Number of breaths per minute; one of vital signs (respiratory rate, heart rate, temperature, blood pressure)
rhonchi	Whistling sound that can be heard during either inhalation or exhalation; caused by narrowing of bronchi as in asthma or infection; also called *wheezing*
severe acute respiratory syndrome (SARS)	Severe and highly contagious viral lung infection with high fever; threatened worldwide epidemic in 2003
sputum	Mucus or phlegm coughed up and spit out from respiratory tract
sputum culture and sensitivity (C&S)	Testing sputum by placing it on culture medium and observing any bacterial growth; specimen tested to determine selection of effective antibiotic
sputum cytology **cyt/o** = cell **-logy** = study of	Examination of sputum for malignant cells

> **TERMINOLOGY TIDBIT**
> The term *rhonchi* comes from the Greek word *rhenchos* meaning "snoring."

Term	Explanation
sudden infant death syndrome (SIDS)	Unexpected and unexplained death of apparently well infant; sleep apnea, airway spasms, and failure of nerves to stimulate diaphragm have been studied as possible causes
sweat test	Diagnostic test for cystic fibrosis; children with this disease lose excessive amount of salt in their sweat
tuberculin skin tests (TB test)	Diagnostic test for exposure to tuberculosis bacteria by applying chemical agent (Tine or Mantoux tests) under surface of skin and evaluating site for reaction

0.1 ml tuberculin injected just under skin surface of forearm. Pale elevation results. Needle bevel directed upward to prevent too deep penetration.

Test read in 48 to 72 hours. Extent of induration determined by direct observation and palpation; limits marked. Area of erythema has no significance.

Diameter of marked indurated area measured in transverse plane. Reactions over 9 mm in diameter are regarded as positive; those 5 to 9 mm are questionable, and test may be repeated after 7 or more days to obtain booster effect. Less than 5 mm of induration is regarded as negative.

10.16 Steps of a TB skin test

Term	Explanation
tuberculosis (TB)	Infectious disease caused by tubercle bacillus, *Mycobacterium tuberculosis;* most commonly affects respiratory system and causes inflammation and calcification in lungs
ventilation-perfusion scan	Nuclear medicine image particularly useful in diagnosing pulmonary emboli; involves inhalation of radioactive tagged air to evaluate air movement (ventilation) and injection of radioactive tagged dye into bloodstream to evaluate blood flow (perfusion) to lungs
ventilator	Mechanical device to assist patient to breathe; also called *respirator*

10.17 Male patient breathing with the assistance of a ventilator attached to an endotracheal tube.
Source: Tyler Olson/Shutterstock

Pulmonology Abbreviations

The following list presents common pulmonology abbreviations.

ABGs	arterial blood gases	**IRDS**	infant respiratory distress syndrome
ARF	acute respiratory failure		
AP view	anteroposterior view (in radiology)	**LLL**	left lower lobe
		LUL	left upper lobe
ARD	acute respiratory disease	**O$_2$**	oxygen
ARDS	adult respiratory distress syndrome	**PA view**	posteroanterior view (in radiology)
Broncho	bronchoscopy	**PE**	pulmonary embolism
BS	breath sounds	**PFT**	pulmonary function test
CF	cystic fibrosis	**PPD**	purified protein derivative (tuberculin test)
CO$_2$	carbon dioxide		
COLD	chronic obstructive lung disease	**R**	respirations
		RD	respiratory disease
COPD	chronic obstructive pulmonary disease	**RDS**	respiratory distress syndrome
CPR	cardiopulmonary resuscitation	**RLL**	right lower lobe
		RML	right middle lobe
C&S	(sputum) culture and sensitivity	**RR**	respiratory rate
		RUL	right upper lobe
CTA	clear to auscultation	**SARS**	severe acute respiratory syndrome
CXR	chest X-ray		
DOE	dyspnea on exertion	**SIDS**	sudden infant death syndrome
ET	endotracheal		
flu	influenza	**SOB**	shortness of breath
HMD	hyaline membrane disease	**TB**	tuberculosis
IPPB	intermittent positive pressure breathing	**TPR**	temperature, pulse, and respiration

CASE STUDY

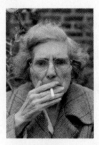

Source: Image Source/ Getty Images

History of Present Illness
Female who is 72 years old complaining of increasing level of dyspnea with activity over the past six months. She now has a frequent harsh cough producing thick sputum and occasional hemoptysis.

Past Medical History
Patient has had hysterectomy for endometriosis at age 45, cholecystectomy for cholelithiasis at age 62, and recent compression fracture of lumbar spine secondary to osteoporosis. Patient takes only calcium supplement for osteoporosis.

Family and Social History
Patient began smoking at age 15 and currently smokes two packs a day. Denies use of alcohol. She is a retired school teacher who lives at home with her husband. She continues to drive a car, do light house-work, and shop. Children are alive and well. She has one brother with hypertension. Mother died at age 60 from cerebrovascular accident. Father died at age 82 from complications of diabetes mellitus. There is no family history of asthma or emphysema.

Physical Examination
Patient is thin and short of stature. She has mild kyphosis. She is alert and answers all questions appro-priately. She is not SOB sitting in examination room. Auscultation of chest reveals marked crackles but no rhonchi. She has a persistent cough, and sputum was collected for a sputum culture and sensitivity and a sputum cytology.

Radiology Findings
Chest radiograph, AP view, revealed a suspicious cloudy area in right lung. Follow-up with CT scan of the bronchial tree confirmed the presence of a mass in the right lung.

Laboratory Findings
Sputum C&S was negative for the presence of bacteria. Sputum cytology contained malignant cells, indicating presence of cancerous tumor in the lungs.

Diagnosis
Bronchogenic carcinoma

Plan of Treatment
1. Refer patient to thoracic surgeon for consultation regarding thoracotomy and lobectomy
2. Following surgery, she will be referred to oncologist for chemotherapy and to determine whether the tumor has metastasized

Critical Thinking Questions
Answer the following questions regarding this case study. Do not just copy words out of the case study but translate all medical terms. To answer some of these questions, you may need to look up information from another chapter of this text, in a medical dictionary, or online. Answers are found at the back of the book.

1. Which of the following is NOT a feature of this patient's history of the present illness?
   a. spitting up blood
   b. difficulty getting her breath when she is active
   c. coughing up mucus
   d. pain in the chest region

2. This patient's history is significant for three previous health problems. List and describe each health problem and the surgical treatment she received for two of them.
   _____
   _____

3. Is this patient's family history important to her current illness? Justify your answer.
   _____
   _____

4. What did the physician hear when listening to this patient's chest?
   _____
   _____

5. Two laboratory tests were performed. Explain the difference between the two tests. What were the results of each test?

_____

_____

6. List and describe the difference in the two types of X-ray procedures this patient underwent.

_____

_____

7. Explain why this patient was referred to two different physicians.

_____

_____

PRACTICE

Sound It Out

The following are some of the key terms from this chapter written as their phonetic spelling. Sound out each term and write it in the blank. Pronunciations for all terms are included in the audio glossary at www.mymedicalterminologylab.com.

1. tray-kee-OTT-oh-mee _____
2. AP-nee-ah _____
3. AZ-mah _____
4. brong-KIGH-tis _____
5. hee-moh-THOH-raks _____
6. brong-koh-JEN-ik _____
7. noo-mon-EK-toe-mee _____
8. BRONG-koh-spazm _____
9. sigh-ah-NO-sis _____
10. em-fih-SEE-mah _____
11. at-eh-LEK-tah-sis _____
12. HYE-per-vent-ill-a-shun _____
13. in-floo-EN-za _____
14. low-BEK-toh-mee _____
15. ox-IM-eh-ter _____
16. brong-KOG-rah-fee _____
17. PLOOR-ih-see _____
18. noo-moe-sen-TEE-sis _____
19. noo-moh-koh-nee-OH-sis _____
20. too-ber-kyoo-LOH-sis _____
21. pye-oh-THOH-raks _____
22. spy-ROM-eh-tree _____
23. ah-NOK-see-ah _____
24. thor-ah-KOT-oh-mee _____
25. TRAY-kee-oh-plas-tee _____

Transcription Practice

Each of the following sentences is written in common English. Underline any words or phrases that can be replaced by a medical term. Then rewrite the entire sentence using medical terms. Answers can be found at the back of the book.

1. During the process of listening to sounds within the body, the physician heard abnormal crackling sounds when the patient breathed in.

   _____

   _____

2. It was unclear from the chest X-ray whether the patient had blood in the chest cavity or pus in the chest cavity.

   _____

   _____

3. The results of the lab test for the levels of oxygen and carbon dioxide present in the blood revealed an insufficient amount of oxygen in the body.

   _____

   _____

4. The patient underwent a surgical removal of a lung lobe after the discovery of a malignant lung tumor originating in the bronchi.

   _____

   _____

5. Mr. Scott's slow breathing was so severe that he had a blue color to his skin.

   _____

   _____

6. Carlyn went to the one who studies the lung when she noticed spitting up of blood several mornings in a row.

   _____

   _____

7. The physician ordered a test to grow and observe bacteria from sputum because Lars was coughing up phlegm with pus in it.

   _____

   _____

8. The patient underwent diagnostic procedures to assess respiratory function using an instrument to measure breathing and an instrument to measure oxygen.

   _____

   _____

9. The patient had a long-term irreversible condition in which airflow to and from the lungs is decreased and as a result had developed hypertrophy of the right ventricle of the heart.

_____

_____

10. An X-ray with dye injected into the blood vessels of the lungs was ordered to determine whether a blood clot was in a pulmonary artery.

_____

_____

Spelling

Some of the following terms are misspelled. Identify the incorrect terms and spell them correctly in the blank provided.

1. pneumoconeosis _____

2. pneumonia _____

3. phlegm _____

4. ventilater _____

5. prurulent _____

6. influenza _____

7. asphyxia _____

8. hyperopnea _____

9. mediastinal _____

10. alveololar _____

Labeling Exercise

Write the name of each structure on the numbered line. Also use this space to write the combining form where appropriate.

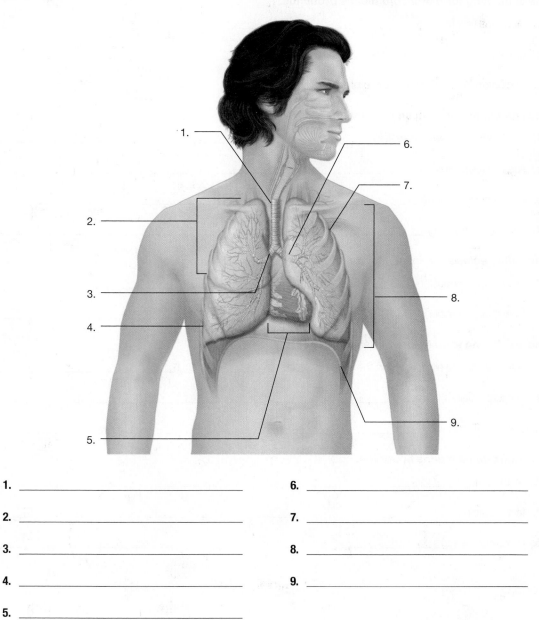

1. _____

2. _____

3. _____

4. _____

5. _____

6. _____

7. _____

8. _____

9. _____

Build Medical Terms

Use each of the following word parts to build the indicated medical terms.

The combining form *bronch/o* means bronchus.

1. bronchus record _____

2. process of visually examining bronchus _____

3. involuntary muscle contraction in bronchus _____

The combining form *pneumon/o* means lung.

4. lung puncture to withdraw fluid _____

5. surgical removal of lung _____

6. pertaining to the lung _____

7. cutting into the lung _____

The suffix *-ectasis* means dilated or expanded.

8. incomplete expansion _____

9. bronchus expansion _____

The combining form *trache/o* means trachea.

10. surgically create an opening in the trachea _____

11. surgical repair of trachea _____

12. trachea inflammation _____

The suffix *-pnea* means breathing.

13. no breathing _____

14. fast breathing _____

15. difficult breathing _____

Fill in the Blank

Fill in the blank to complete each of the following sentences.

1. Jenny's _____ attacks were brought on by her allergies and always involved broncho-spasms and coughing.

2. Mr. Wu had a(n) _____ to examine the inside of his bronchial tubes for possible cancer.

3. Mr. Michael's many years of smoking destroyed his alveolar walls; he has developed _____.

4. A sweat test confirmed that the new infant has _____.

5. The _____ is commonly called the *windpipe*.

6. The respiratory therapist used a(n) _____ to conduct a pulmonary function test.

7. Breathing too fast and too deep results in _____.

8. Hyaline membrane disease is also known as _____.

9. When air collects in the pleural cavity, causing the lung to collapse, it is referred to as a(n) _____.

10. The patient had a pulmonary angiography to determine whether she had a(n) _____.

Abbreviation Matching

Match each abbreviation with its definition.

_____ **1.** CXR   **A.** pulmonary embolism

_____ **2.** SOB   **B.** temperature, pulse, respiration

_____ **3.** TB   **C.** adult respiratory distress syndrome

_____ **4.** PE   **D.** chest X-ray

_____ **5.** LLL   **E.** arterial blood gases

_____ **6.** TPR   **F.** tuberculosis

_____ **7.** ET   **G.** chronic obstructive pulmonary disease

_____ **8.** ABGs   **H.** shortness of breath

_____ **9.** COPD   **I.** endotracheal

_____ **10.** ARDS   **J.** left lower lobe

Medical Term Analysis

Examine each of the following terms. Begin by dividing it into its word parts and writing them in the indicated blanks *(P = prefix; WR = word root; CF = combining form; S = suffix)*. Follow with the definition of each word part and then finally the meaning of the full term.

1. **thoracocentesis**

   CF _____

   means _____

   S _____

   means _____

   Term meaning: _____

   _____

2. **cyanosis**

   WR _____

   means _____

   S _____

   means _____

   Term meaning: _____

   _____

3. **pneumothorax**

   CF _____

   means _____

   S _____

   means _____

   Term meaning: _____

   _____

4. **endotracheal**

   P _____

   means _____

   WR _____

   means _____

   S _____

   means _____

   Term meaning: _____

   _____

5. **pneumoconiosis**

   CF _____

   means _____

   WR _____

   means _____

   S _____

   means _____

   Term meaning: _____

   _____

6. **oximeter**

   CF _____

   means _____

   S _____

   means _____

   Term meaning: _____

   _____

7. orthopnea

CF _____

means _____

S _____

means _____

Term meaning: _____

_____

8. pleurodynia

CF _____

means _____

S _____

means _____

Term meaning: _____

_____

9. bronchiectasis

WR _____

means _____

S _____

means _____

Term meaning: _____

_____

10. lobectomy

WR _____

means _____

S _____

means _____

Term meaning: _____

_____

MyMedicalTerminologyLab™

MyMedicalTerminologyLab is a premium online homework management system that includes a host of features to help you study. Registered users will find:

- A multitude of activities and assignments built within the MyLab platform
- Powerful tools that track and analyze your results—allowing you to create a personalized learning experience
- Videos and audio pronunciations to help enrich your progress
- Streaming lesson presentations and self-paced learning modules
- A space where you and your instructors can view and manage your assignments

Photomatch Challenge

Match each pulmonary condition with its name in the Word Bank.

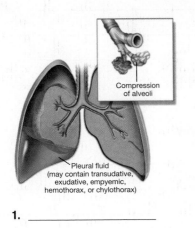

Pleural fluid
(may contain transudative,
exudative, empyemic,
hemothorax, or chylothorax)

Compression
of alveoli

1. _____

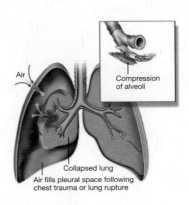

Air

Compression
of alveoli

Collapsed lung

Air fills pleural space following
chest trauma or lung rupture

2. _____

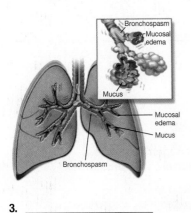

Bronchospasm

Mucosal
edema

Mucus

Mucosal
edema

Mucus

Bronchospasm

3. _____

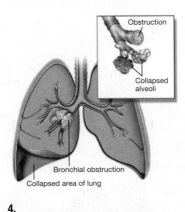

Obstruction

Collapsed
alveoli

Bronchial obstruction

Collapsed area of lung

4. _____

Word Bank:

asthma

atelectasis

emphysema

pleural effusion

pneumonia

pneumothorax

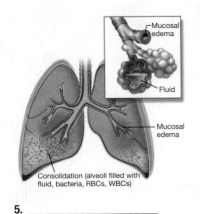

Mucosal
edema

Fluid

Mucosal
edema

Consolidation (alveoli filled with
fluid, bacteria, RBCs, WBCs)

5. _____

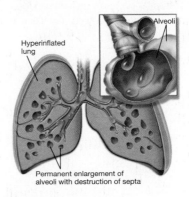

Hyperinflated
lung

Alveoli

Permanent enlargement of
alveoli with destruction of septa

6. _____

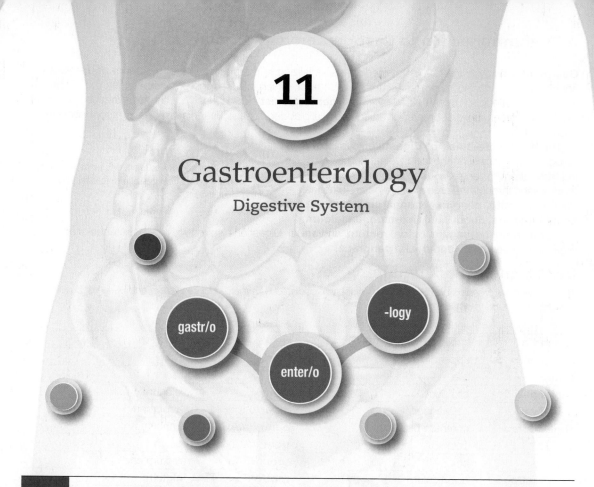

11

Gastroenterology

Digestive System

gastr/o

enter/o

-logy

Learning Objectives

Upon completion of this chapter, you will be able to:

11-1   Describe the medical specialty of gastroenterology.

11-2   Understand the functions of the digestive system.

11-3   Define gastroenterology-related combining forms, prefixes, and suffixes.

11-4   Identify the organs treated in gastroenterology.

11-5   Build gastroenterology medical terms from word parts.

11-6   Explain gastroenterology medical terms.

11-7   Use gastroenterology abbreviations.

A Brief Introduction to Gastroenterology

Gastroenterology is the branch of medicine specializing in the diagnosis and treatment of diseases and conditions affecting the lower gastrointestinal (GI) tract, which includes the organs between the esophagus and rectum. Conditions often treated by a **gastroenterologist** include bleeding, cancer, infections, nutritional disorders, inflammatory disorders, diverticulosis, gallbladder disease, liver disease, gastroesophageal reflux, and ulcers.

The **gastrointestinal**, or **digestive**, **system** is responsible for digesting the food we eat and absorbing the nutrient molecules. These processes occur as food passes through the organs of the gastrointestinal tract: the **mouth, pharynx, esophagus, stomach, small intestine** (**duodenum, jejunum,** and **ileum**)

> **TERMINOLOGY TIDBIT**
> The gastrointestinal tract is also referred to as the *alimentary canal.* This name comes from the Latin word *alimentum* meaning "nourishment."

and **large intestine** (**cecum, colon, rectum,** and **anus**). Digestion also requires the assistance of accessory organs: the **liver, gallbladder,** and **pancreas.**

Gastroenterology Combining Forms

The following list presents combining forms closely associated with the digestive system and used for building and defining gastroenterology terms.

an/o	anus		**esophag/o**	esophagus
append/o	appendix		**gastr/o**	stomach
appendic/o	appendix		**hepat/o**	liver
chol/e	bile		**ile/o**	ileum
cholangi/o	bile duct		**jejun/o**	jejunum
cholecyst/o	gallbladder		**lapar/o**	abdomen
choledoch/o	common bile duct		**pancreat/o**	pancreas
col/o	colon		**polyp/o**	polyp
colon/o	colon		**proct/o**	rectum and anus
diverticul/o	diverticulum		**rect/o**	rectum
duoden/o	duodenum		**sigmoid/o**	sigmoid colon
enter/o	intestine			

The following list presents combining forms that are not specific to the digestive system but are also used for building and defining gastroenterology terms.

hemat/o	blood
lith/o	stone

Suffix Review

These suffixes introduced in Chapter 2 are being reviewed in this chapter because they are especially important for building gastroenterology terms.

-al	pertaining to		**-gram**	record
-algia	pain		**-graphy**	process of recording
-cele	protrusion		**-iasis**	abnormal condition
-dynia	pain		**-ic**	pertaining to
-eal	pertaining to		**-itis**	inflammation
-ectomy	surgical removal		**-logist**	one who studies
-emesis	vomiting		**-logy**	study of

-oma	tumor, mass		-plasty	surgical repair
-osis	abnormal condition		-ptosis	drooping
-ostomy	surgically create an opening		-scope	instrument for viewing
-otomy	cutting into		-scopy	process of visually examining
-pepsia	digestion		-tripsy	surgical crushing
-phagia	eating, swallowing			

Prefix Review

These prefixes introduced in Chapter 3 are being reviewed here because they are especially important for building gastroenterology terms.

a-	without		hyper-	excessive
brady-	slow		poly-	many
dys-	painful, difficult, abnormal			

Organs Commonly Treated in Gastroenterology

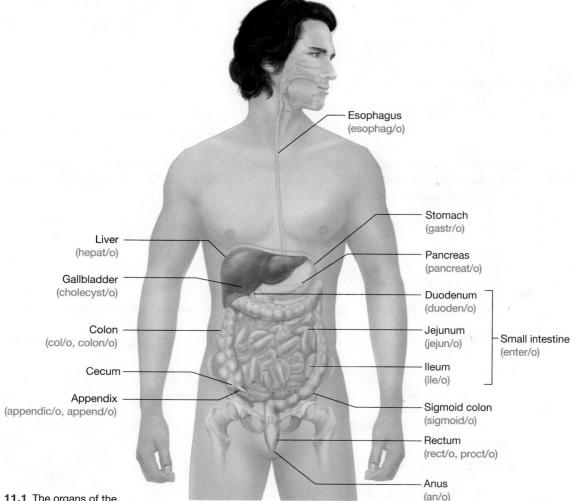

11.1 The organs of the gastrointestinal system

Building Gastroenterology Terms

This section presents word parts most often used to build gastroenterology terms. Following the explanation of the term, you have the opportunity to begin building your own vocabulary. Read the meaning for each term and then fill in the blanks to build a single medical term. Use the slashes to divide prefixes, word roots, combining vowels, and suffixes. To help you out you will find a key to the word parts underneath the blanks: **r** for word roots, **p** for prefix, **cv** for combining vowel, and **s** for suffix. Remember that not every term will contain all these word parts; it's up to you to decide which to use. As you gain experience, this process becomes easier. Answers can be found at the back of the book.

1. **an/o**—combining form meaning **anus**

   The anus is the distal opening of the digestive tract to the outside of the body; opening and closing is controlled by two rings of muscles, the **internal anal sphincter** (involuntary smooth muscle) and **external anal sphincter** (voluntary skeletal muscle) (see again Figure 11.1)

   a. pertaining to anus   _____/_____
                                                   r   *s*

2. **append/o**—combining form meaning **appendix**

   The appendix is a small pouch attached to the cecum; contains lymphatic tissue, but function is unclear (see again Figure 11.1)

   a. surgical removal of appendix   _____/_____
                                                 r   *s*

3. **appendic/o**—combining form meaning **appendix**

   a. appendix inflammation   _____/_____
                                                 r   *s*

4. **chol/e**—combining form meaning **bile**

   Bile is a substance produced by the liver and stored in the gallbladder; transported to duodenum by the **common bile duct**; aids fat digestion by breaking up large fat globules into smaller fat particles (a process called *emulsification*); also called *gall*

   a. condition of having bile stones (gallstones)   _____/_____/_____/_____
                                             r   *cv*   *r*   *s*

   b. surgical crushing of bile stones (gallstones)   _____/_____/_____/_____/_____
                                             r   *cv*   *r*   *cv*   *s*

5. **cholangi/o**—combining form meaning **bile duct**

   The bile duct is part of a series of tubes that transport bile between liver, gallbladder, and duodenum

   a. record of bile duct   _____/_____/_____
                                             r   *cv*   *s*

   b. process of recording bile duct   _____/_____/_____
                                           r   *cv*   *s*

6. **cholecyst/o**—combining form meaning **gallbladder**

   This organ stores bile produced by liver; releases bile into duodenum via common bile duct as needed (see again Figure 11.1)

   a. gallbladder inflammation   _____/_____
                                                 r   *s*

b. surgical removal of gallbladder

_____/_____
r   s

c. record of gallbladder

_____/_____/_____
r   cv   s

d. process of recording gallbladder

_____/_____/_____
r   cv   s

---

7. **choledoch/o**–combining form meaning **common bile duct**

The common bile duct is the main duct that transports bile from liver or gallbladder to duodenum

a. condition of stone in common bile duct

_____/_____/_____/_____
r   cv   r   s

b. surgical crushing of stone in common bile duct

_____/_____/_____/_____/_____
r   cv   r   cv   s

---

8. **col/o**–combining form meaning **colon**

The colon receives undigested food from small intestine; allows for water to be reabsorbed into body; what remains are called _feces;_ colon is divided into **ascending colon**, **transverse colon**, **descending colon**, and **sigmoid colon**; term _large intestine_ includes **cecum**, appendix, colon, rectum, and anus (see again Figure 11.1)

11.2 Colon

a. surgically create an opening in colon

_____/_____
r   s

b. colon inflammation

_____/_____
r   s

c. pertaining to colon and rectum

_____/_____/_____/_____
r   cv   r   s

---

9. **colon/o**–combining form meaning **colon**

a. instrument for viewing colon

_____/_____/_____
r   cv   s

b. process of visually examining colon

_____/_____/_____
r   cv   s

c. pertaining to colon

_____/_____
r   s

---

10. **diverticul/o**–combining form meaning **diverticulum**

Diverticula (singular is _diverticulum_) are small, abnormal, blind pouches that form off intestinal or colon wall; can become inflamed and infected

a. diverticulum inflammation

_____/_____
r   s

b. abnormal condition of having diverticula

_____/_____
r   s

c. surgical removal of diverticulum

_____/_____
r   s

---

11. **duoden/o**–combining form meaning **duodenum**

The duodenum is the first section of small intestine; receives food from the stomach, digestive enzymes from the pancreas, and bile from the liver; final digestion of food and absorption of nutrients begins in duodenum (see again Figure 11.1)

a. pertaining to duodenum

_____/_____
                     r   s

b. surgically create an opening in duodenum

_____/_____
                     r   s

12. **-emesis**–suffix meaning **vomiting**

a. vomiting blood

_____/_____
                     r   s

b. excessive vomiting

_____/_____
                     p   s

13. **enter/o**–combining form meaning **intestine**

May refer to either the small or large intestine; small intestine receives food from the stomach, digestive enzymes from the pancreas, and bile from the liver; digestion of food into nutrient molecules and absorption of these molecules occurs in the small intestine; fluid that remains after digestion and absorption enters the large intestine where water is reabsorbed and the remaining material is compacted into **feces** (see again Figure 11.1)

11.3 Small and large intestines

a. intestine inflammation

_____/_____
                     r   s

b. pertaining to intestine

_____/_____
                     r   s

14. **esophag/o**–combining form meaning **esophagus**

The esophagus is a muscular tube that carries food from throat to stomach (see again Figure 11.1)

11.4 Esophagus

a. pertaining to esophagus

_____/_____
                     r   s

b. surgical repair of esophagus

_____/_____/_____
                     r   cv   s

c. esophagus inflammation

_____/_____
                     r   s

d. instrument for viewing esophagus

_____/_____/_____
                     r   cv   s

e. process of visually examining esophagus

_____/_____/_____
                     r   cv   s

15. gastr/o–combining form meaning **stomach**

The stomach is a muscular sac producing hydrochloric acid and digestive enzymes for protein; begins digestive process by mixing food received from esophagus with acid and enzymes; watery mixture, called **chyme**, leaves stomach and enters duodenum (see again Figure 11.1)

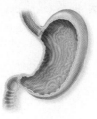

11.5 Stomach

a. pertaining to stomach

_____ / _____
                     r   s

b. stomach inflammation

_____ / _____
                     r   s

c. stomach and intestine inflammation

_____ / _____ / _____ / _____
        r   cv   r   s

d. surgical removal of stomach

_____ / _____
                     r   s

e. surgically create an opening in stomach

_____ / _____
                     r   s

f. instrument for viewing stomach

_____ / _____ / _____
        r   cv   s

g. process of visually examining stomach

_____ / _____ / _____
        r   cv   s

h. stomach pain

_____ / _____ / _____
        r   cv   s

i. stomach pain

_____ / _____
                     r   s

j. one who studies stomach and intestine

_____ / _____ / _____ / _____ / ____
     r   cv   r   cv   s

k. study of stomach and intestine

_____ / _____ / _____ / _____ / ____
     r   cv   r   cv   s

- -

16. hepat/o–combining form meaning **liver**

The liver is a complex abdominal organ; in gastroenterology, plays role in digestion by producing **bile** to aid in fat digestion (see again Figure 11.1)

11.6 Liver

a. liver inflammation

_____ / _____
                     r   s

b. pertaining to liver

_____ / _____
                     r   s

c. liver tumor

_____ / _____
                     r   s

- -

17. **ile/o**–combining form meaning **ileum**

The ileum is the third section of small intestine; receives digested food from jejunum and completes process of digestion and nutrient absorption (see again Figure 11.1)

a. pertaining to ileum

_____/_____
r   s

b. surgically create an opening in ileum

_____/_____
r   s

18. **jejun/o**–combining form meaning **jejunum**

The jejunum is the second portion of small intestine; receives digested food from duodenum and continues process of digestion and nutrient absorption (see again Figure 11.1)

a. pertaining to jejunum

_____/_____
r   s

b. surgically create an opening in jejunum

_____/_____
r   s

19. **lapar/o**–combining form meaning **abdomen**

The abdomen is a body cavity that houses organs of digestion, reproduction, and excretion

a. cutting into abdomen

_____/_____
r   s

b. instrument for viewing abdomen

_____/_____/_____
r   cv   s

c. process of visually examining abdomen

_____/_____/_____
r   cv   s

20. **pancreat/o**–combining form meaning **pancreas**

This organ produces digestive enzymes and buffers to neutralize acidic chyme entering duodenum from stomach; pancreatic duct carries these enzymes and buffers to duodenum where they aid in food digestion (see again Figure 11.1)

11.7 Pancreas

a. pertaining to pancreas

_____/_____
r   s

b. pancreas inflammation

_____/_____
r   s

21. **-pepsia**–suffix meaning **digestion**

a. without digestion

_____/_____
p   s

b. painful digestion

_____/_____
p   s

c. slow digestion

_____/_____
p   s

22. **-phagia**–suffix meaning **eating** or **swallowing**

    a. without swallowing

             _____ / _____
                           p   *s*

    b. difficult swallowing

             _____ / _____
                           p   *s*

    c. many (or excessive) eating

             _____ / _____
                           p   *s*

---

23. **polyp/o**–combining form meaning **polyp**

    A polyp is a small mushroom-shaped tumor that grows on mucous membranes of colon and extends into lumen of colon; can become cancerous

    a. abnormal condition of having polyps

             _____ / _____
                           r   *s*

    b. surgical removal of polyp

             _____ / _____
                           r   *s*

---

24. **proct/o**–combining form meaning **rectum** and **anus**

    Refers to both the rectum and anus (see again Figure 11.1)

    a. drooping of rectum and anus

             _____ / _____ / _____
                     r   *cv*   *s*

    b. instrument for viewing rectum and anus

             _____ / _____ / _____
                     r   *cv*   *s*

    c. process of visually examining rectum and anus

             _____ / _____ / _____
                     r   *cv*   *s*

    d. one who studies rectum and anus

             _____ / _____ / _____
                     r   *cv*   *s*

    e. study of rectum and anus

             _____ / _____ / _____
                     r   *cv*   *s*

---

25. **rect/o**–combining form meaning **rectum**

    Rectum is the final segment of large intestine; receives feces from the sigmoid colon and stores it prior to elimination (see again Figure 11.1)

    a. protrusion of rectum

             _____ / _____ / _____
                     r   *cv*   *s*

    b. pertaining to rectum

             _____ / _____
                     r   *s*

---

26. **sigmoid/o**–combining form meaning **sigmoid colon**

    The sigmoid colon is the final S-shaped section of the colon; feces pass out of sigmoid colon and into rectum (see again Figure 11.1)

    a. instrument for viewing sigmoid colon

             _____ / _____ / _____
                     r   *cv*   *s*

    b. process of visually examining sigmoid colon

             _____ / _____ / _____
                     r   *cv*   *s*

Gastroenterology Vocabulary

The gastroenterology terms presented in this section include eponyms, modern English words, and those that contain Latin or Greek word parts but are not constructed solely from these word parts. When you recognize word parts within a term, they will give you a hint about the word's meaning. In these instances, look for the word parts to follow the term.

Term	Explanation
ascites	Accumulation of fluid in abdominal cavity

> **TERMINOLOGY TIDBIT**
> The term *ascites* comes from the Latin word *askos* meaning "a bag." This describes the swollen appearance of the abdomen in a person with ascites.

Umbilicus may be protuberant

11.8 Patient with swollen abdomen and protruding umbilicus characteristic of ascites

Bulging flank with fluid

Term	Explanation
barium enema (BE)	X-ray examination of large intestine using barium as contrast medium; also known as *lower GI series*
cirrhosis **-osis** = abnormal condition	Chronic liver disease

11.9 Chronic destruction and scarring of liver due to cirrhosis
Source: Pearson Education

Term	Explanation
Crohn disease	Chronic inflammatory bowel disease (IBD) with mucous membrane ulcers; most often found in ileum
dysentery **dys-** = abnormal **enter/o** = intestine	Acute intestinal condition with pain, diarrhea, and blood and mucus in stool; usually caused by bacterial or parasitic infection
esophageal atresia **esophag/o** = esophagus **-eal** = pertaining to	Congenital lack of the connection between esophagus and stomach; food cannot enter stomach

> **TERMINOLOGY TIDBIT**
> The term *atresia* is formed by combining the Greek prefix *a-* meaning "without" and the word *tresis* meaning "a hole."

Term	Explanation
esophageal varices **esophag/o** = esophagus **-eal** = pertaining to	Varicose veins in esophagus; result in massive bleeding if rupture **11.10** Blood clots forming from ruptured esophageal varices at point where esophagus meets the stomach Source: Pearson Education
fecal occult blood test (FOBT) **-al** = pertaining to	Clinical lab test for presence of small amounts of blood in feces; also called *hemoccult test* or *stool guaiac test* **TERMINOLOGY TIDBIT** The term *occult* comes from the Latin word *occulere* meaning "hidden." This is a test for amounts of blood that are too small to see, even with a microscope.
gastric bypass **gastr/o** = stomach **-ic** = pertaining to	Surgical treatment for obesity; portion of stomach is stapled off and bypassed so that it holds less food; also called *stomach stapling* **TERMINOLOGY TIDBIT** The combining form for stomach, *gastr/o,* comes from the Greek word *gaster* meaning "stomach." Flow of food Esophagus Small pouch of stomach that still receives food Duodenum attached to small stomach pouch that receives food Bypassed portion of stomach Bypassed section of duodenum **11.11** Gastric bypass surgery
gastroesophageal **reflux disease** (GERD) **gastr/o** = stomach **esophag/o** = esophagus **-eal** = pertaining to	Occurs when stomach acid backs up into esophagus
Helicobacter pylori **antibody test**	Clinical lab test for presence of bacteria known to cause gastric ulcers
hemorrhoids	Varicose veins in rectum
ileus	Obstruction of intestine that occurs when muscular movements stop moving food or blockage prevents food from moving through digestive tract

Term	Explanation
intussusception	Occurs when one section of intestine slips or telescopes into another section of intestine **11.12** Intussusception: a short length of small intestine has telescoped into itself
irritable bowel syndrome (IBS)	Disturbance in normal functioning of bowel characterized by abdominal pain and diarrhea; often associated with stress; also called *spastic colon*
jaundice	Yellow-colored skin and whites of eyes associated with liver disease **11.13** Yellow eyeballs of person with jaundice Source: Dr. Thomas F. Sellers/Emory University/Centers for Disease Control and Prevention
melena	Very dark, tarry stool due to presence of blood
nausea	Feeling the urge to vomit
ova and parasites (O&P)	Clinical lab test for presence of parasites or their eggs in feces **11.14** Hookworms attached to the intestinal lining; eggs released by these parasites would be detected by an O&P Source: Centers for Disease Control and Prevention

> **TERMINOLOGY TIDBIT**
> The term *nausea* comes from the Latin word *nausia* meaning "seasickness."

Term	Explanation
peptic ulcer disease (PUD)	Craterlike erosion occurring on mucous membrane of lower esophagus, stomach, and/or duodenum; more dangerous if ulcer eats into blood vessel and becomes *bleeding ulcer,* or if ulcer eats through wall of stomach and becomes a *perforated ulcer* allowing stomach acids to escape into abdominal cavity **Gastric juices are released into the stomach** • **Duodenal ulcer** • **Gastric juices (acidic)** • **Acid secretions further break down the lining of the stomach, forming an ulcer** • **Gastric ulcer** **11.15** Figure illustrating the location and appearance of peptic ulcers in both the stomach and the duodenum
total parenteral nutrition (TPN)	Nutrient-complete solution given directly into bloodstream when person cannot eat by mouth
ulcerative colitis col/o = colon -itis = inflammation	Chronic inflammatory bowel disease (IBD) characterized by formation of ulcers on mucous membrane of colon
upper gastrointestinal series (UGI) gastr/o = stomach -al = pertaining to	X-ray examination of esophagus and stomach using barium as contrast medium; also known as *barium swallow* **Barium** **11.16** Patient drinks liquid barium solution in order to outline her stomach for an upper GI series
volvulus	Length of bowel that becomes twisted around itself **Colon** • **Small intestine** • **Twisted portion of small intestine** **11.17** Volvulus: a length of small intestine has twisted around itself, cutting off blood circulation to the twisted loop
vomit	Forceful return of stomach contents out of mouth

Gastroenterology Abbreviations

The following list presents common gastroenterology abbreviations.

Ba	barium	**GB**	gallbladder
BE	barium enema	**GERD**	gastroesophageal reflux disease
BM	bowel movement	**GI**	gastrointestinal
BS	bowel sounds	**IBD**	inflammatory bowel disease
CBD	common bile duct	**IBS**	irritable bowel syndrome
CUC	chronic ulcerative colitis	**N&V**	nausea and vomiting
EGD	esophagogastroduodenoscopy	**O&P**	ova and parasites
ERCP	endoscopic retrograde cholangiopancreatography	**PUD**	peptic ulcer disease
		TPN	total parenteral nutrition
FOBT	fecal occult blood test	**UGI**	upper gastrointestinal series

CASE STUDY

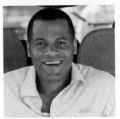

Source: Monkey Business Images/Shutterstock

History of the Present Illness

The patient is a 35-year-old man who has had a gradual increase in upper abdominal pain for the past eight months. He has no prior history of upper abdominal pain. He now reports a sharp pain in the epigastric area about 30 minutes after meals, which has been somewhat relieved by Tums or Rolaids or over-the-counter Zantac. Spicy foods make the pain more frequent and severe. Milk and ice cream relieve the pain sometimes. The pain is a deep aching feeling that does not radiate. The pain does not interfere with normal activities including work and sleep. On a scale from 1 (barely perceptible) to 10 (worst imaginable) he rates it a 3–4. It occurs almost daily and lasts about one hour. His appetite is good, and he has not lost weight. The patient denies dysphagia, substernal burning, N&V, lower abdominal pain, hematemesis, melena, and diarrhea. He has had intermittent constipation since his early 20s that he treats with Milk of Magnesia once every 2–3 months. Ten years ago he had some rectal bleeding from hemorrhoids. Other than that episode, he denies other GI problems.

Past Medical History

Hemorrhoids at age 25 requiring hemorrhoidectomy. He takes no regular prescriptions; does use over-the-counter antacids and Milk of Magnesia.

Family and Social History

Married with two children. College graduate. Works in accounting firm as a computer programmer. Smoked from ages 16 to 23. Social drinker. No illegal substance use. No travel or unusual exposures. Mother had colon cancer. Father had prostate cancer. Brother had hepatitis.

Physical Examination

No evidence of ascites, jaundice, hepatomegaly, abdominal mass.

Laboratory Findings

Test for *Helicobacter pylori* was positive.

Endoscopic Findings

EGD revealed gastritis without hemorrhage or ulcer.

Diagnosis

Dyspepsia without evidence of gastric or duodenal ulcer.

Plan of Treatment

1. Patient will be placed on medication to block release of acidic stomach secretions for the gastritis and an antibiotic to treat the *Helicobacter pylori* infection
2. Repeat EGD in three months if symptoms do not resolve

Critical Thinking Questions

Answer the following questions regarding this case study. Do not just copy words out of the case study, but translate all medical terms. To answer some of these questions, you may need to look up information from another chapter of this text, in a medical dictionary, or online. Answers are found at the back of the book.

1. What complaint brought this patient to the doctor?

   _____

   _____

2. What foods make the pain better? What foods make it worse? What is the main thing this patient has done to treat the problem on his own?

   _____

   _____

3. Two diagnostic tests/procedures were performed. Name them, describe them, and explain the findings.

   _____

   _____

4. The history states the pain is in the epigastric region and does not radiate. Where is the epigastric region? This chapter does not explain what *radiating pain* means. What do you think it means?

   _____

   _____

5. Describe the symptoms the patient denies having.

   _____

   _____

6. Why is this patient's family history important to this episode?

   _____

   _____

7. Which of the following is NOT one of the symptoms denied by the patient in the history?
   a. vomiting blood
   b. difficulty swallowing
   c. yellow-colored skin
   d. dark, tarry stool

8. Explain the physician's plan of treatment.

   _____

   _____

Sound It Out

The following are some of the key terms from this chapter written as their phonetic spelling. Sound out each term and write it in the blank. Pronunciations for all terms are included in the audio glossary at www.mymedicalterminologylab.com.

1. sig-MOYD-oh-scope _____

2. RECK-toh-seal _____

3. gas-TRY-tis _____

4. koh-LAN-jee-oh-gram _____

5. sih-ROH-sis _____

6. koh-LYE-tis _____

7. koh-lon-OSS-koh-pee _____

8. koh-lee-sis-TEK-toh-mee _____

9. dis-PEP-see-ah _____

10. eh-soff-ah-go-PLAS-tee _____

11. gas-troh-en-ter-EYE-tis _____

12. GAS-troh-scope _____

13. ah-pen-dih-SIGH-tis _____

14. HEM-oh-roydz _____

15. dis-in-TARE-ee _____

16. high-per-EM-eh-sis _____

17. brad-ee-PEP-see-ah _____

18. ill-ee-OSS-toh-mee _____

19. lap-ar-OSS-koh-pee _____

20. lap-ah-ROT-oh-mee _____

21. dis-FAY-jee-ah _____

22. gas-TREK-toh-mee _____

23. VOL-vyoo-lus _____

24. sig-moid-OS-koh-pee _____

25. ah-PEN-diks _____

Transcription Practice

Each of the following sentences is written in common English. Underline any words or phrases that can be replaced by a medical term. Then rewrite the entire sentence using medical terms. Answers can be found at the back of the book.

1. Mr. Mercado was noted to have yellow skin color, leading to a diagnosis of liver inflammation.

_____

_____

2. Mrs. Mendez underwent a visual examination of her esophagus, stomach, and duodenum that revealed a craterlike erosion in her stomach.

_____

_____

3. Mr. Brown's severe inflamed pouch extending off his colon resulted in his having the pouch surgically removed.

_____

_____

4. The patient presented in the emergency room with a severe urge to vomit and vomiting blood.

_____

_____

5. The physician ordered an X-ray of the colon using barium as a contrast medium because of concern that the patient could have an abnormal condition of mushroom-shaped tumors.

_____

_____

6. Because of her abnormal condition of gallstones, Ms. Katopolis had a cutting into her abdomen and gallbladder removal.

_____

_____

7. Common symptoms of stomach acid backing up into the esophagus include difficulty swallowing and stomach pain.

_____

_____

8. The patient was found to have an obstruction in the intestine due to the loss of muscular movements and required a surgical creation of an opening into the second section of intestine.

_____

_____

9. The bowel movement was tested for the presence of small amounts of blood in the feces and the presence of parasites or their eggs in the feces.

_____

_____

10. To evaluate Mr. Habib's very dark, tarry stool, his stomach and intestine specialist performed a visual exam of the rectum and anus, a visual exam of the S-shaped region of the colon, and a visual exam of the colon.

_____

_____

Labeling Exercise

Write the name of each organ on the numbered line. Also use this space to write the combining form where appropriate.

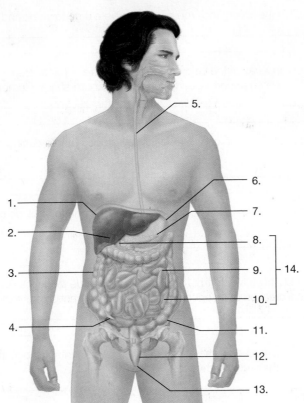

1. _____

2. _____

3. _____

4. _____

5. _____

6. _____

7. _____

8. _____

9. _____

10. _____

11. _____

12. _____

13. _____

14. _____

Build Medical Terms

Use each of the following word parts to build the indicated medical terms.

The combining form *gastr/o* means stomach.

1. stomach inflammation _____

2. surgical removal of stomach _____

3. instrument for viewing the stomach _____

4. one term that means stomach pain _____

5. a different term that means stomach pain _____

The combining forms *proct/o* and *rect/o* both refer to the rectum.

6. Use *proct/o* to build rectum drooping. _____

7. Use *rect/o* to build rectum protrusion. _____

The combining form *cholecyst/o* means gallbladder.

8. gallbladder inflammation _____

9. surgical removal of gallbladder _____

The suffix *-ostomy* means to surgically create an opening.

10. artificial opening in the duodenum _____

11. artificial opening in the colon _____

12. artificial opening in the stomach _____

The suffix *-pepsia* means digestion.

13. without digestion _____

14. difficult digestion _____

15. slow digestion _____

Abbreviation Matching

Match each abbreviation with its definition.

_____	**1.** ERCP	**A.**	gastroesophageal reflux disease
_____	**2.** GI	**B.**	barium
_____	**3.** BE	**C.**	total parenteral nutrition
_____	**4.** IBD	**D.**	gastrointestinal
_____	**5.** TPN	**E.**	nausea and vomiting
_____	**6.** GERD	**F.**	irritable bowel syndrome
_____	**7.** Ba	**G.**	barium enema
_____	**8.** IBS	**H.**	endoscopic retrograde cholangiopancreatography
_____	**9.** EGD	**I.**	inflammatory bowel disease
_____	**10.** N&V	**J.**	esophagogastroduodenoscopy

Fill in the Blank

Fill in the blank to complete each of the following sentences.

1. The patient had a nutrient-complete solution given directly into her bloodstream. The medical term for this is called _____.

2. In peptic ulcer disease, the ulcers may be found in the _____, _____, or _____.

3. The forceful return of stomach contents out of the mouth is to _____.

4. Another term for an upper GI series is _____.

5. Bile is produced by the _____ and stored in the _____.

6. The nurse's notes indicated that the patient's abdomen was swollen by fluid accumulating in the abdominal cavity. This accumulation is called _____.

7. The term that describes an intestinal blockage that occurs when the colon muscles stop pushing food through the colon is _____.

8. After finding ulcers on the mucous membrane of Mr. Fong's colon during a colonoscopy, the physician was able to tell him that he had a chronic condition called _____.

9. Miss Matthews did not recognize what condition she had when her doctor told her she had irritable bowel syndrome. She was more familiar with the name _____.

10. _____ is a surgical treatment for obesity.

Spelling

Some of the following terms are misspelled. Identify the incorrect terms and spell them correctly in the blank provided.

1. cholecystogram _____

2. esophogal _____

3. pancreasitis _____

4. duodenum _____

5. gastroitis _____

6. intussusception _____

7. *Helicobacter pylori* _____

8. cirhosis _____

9. volvolus _____

10. jaundice _____

Medical Term Analysis

Examine each of the following terms. Begin by dividing it into its word parts and writing them in the indicated blanks (*P = prefix*; *WR = word root*; *CF = combining form*; *S = suffix*). Follow with the definition of each word part and then finally the meaning of the full term.

1. **esophagoplasty**

   CF _____

   means _____

   S _____

   means _____

   Term meaning: _____

   _____

2. **appendectomy**

   WR _____

   means _____

   S _____

   means _____

   Term meaning: _____

   _____

3. **choledocholithotripsy**

CF _____

means _____

CF _____

means _____

S _____

means _____

Term meaning: _____

_____

4. **hyperemesis**

P _____

means _____

S _____

means _____

Term meaning: _____

_____

5. **gastroenteritis**

CF _____

means _____

WR _____

means _____

S _____

means _____

Term meaning: _____

_____

6. **hepatoma**

WR _____

means _____

S _____

means _____

Term meaning: _____

_____

7. **diverticulosis**

WR _____

means _____

S _____

means _____

Term meaning: _____

_____

8. **ileostomy**

WR _____

means _____

S _____

means _____

Term meaning: _____

_____

9. laparoscope

CF _____

means _____

S _____

means _____

Term meaning: _____

_____

10. polyphagia

P _____

means _____

S _____

means _____

Term meaning: _____

_____

MyMedicalTerminologyLab™

MyMedicalTerminologyLab is a premium online homework management system that includes a host of features to help you study. Registered users will find:

- A multitude of activities and assignments built within the MyLab platform
- Powerful tools that track and analyze your results—allowing you to create a personalized learning experience
- Videos and audio pronunciations to help enrich your progress
- Streaming lesson presentations and self-paced learning modules
- A space where you and your instructors can view and manage your assignments

Photomatch Challenge

Use the Word Bank below to build a term for each figure.

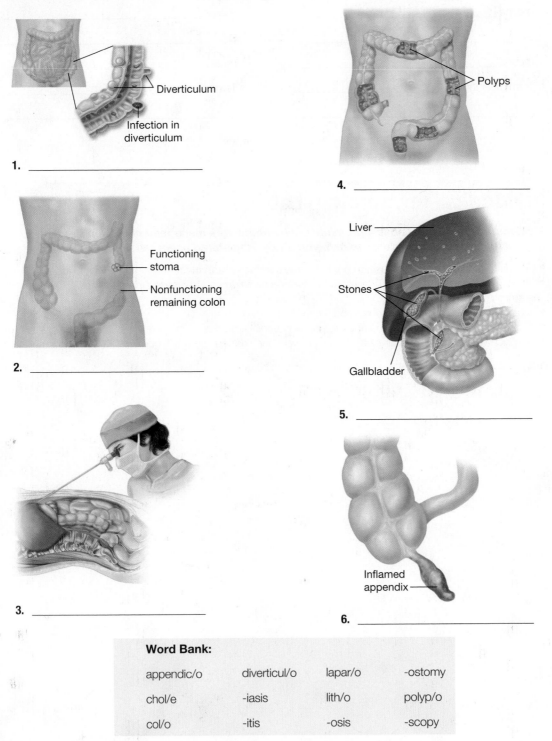

Diverticulum

Infection in diverticulum

1. _____

Polyps

4. _____

Functioning stoma

Nonfunctioning remaining colon

2. _____

Liver

Stones

Gallbladder

5. _____

3. _____

Inflamed appendix

6. _____

Word Bank:

appendic/o	diverticul/o	lapar/o	-ostomy
chol/e	-iasis	lith/o	polyp/o
col/o	-itis	-osis	-scopy

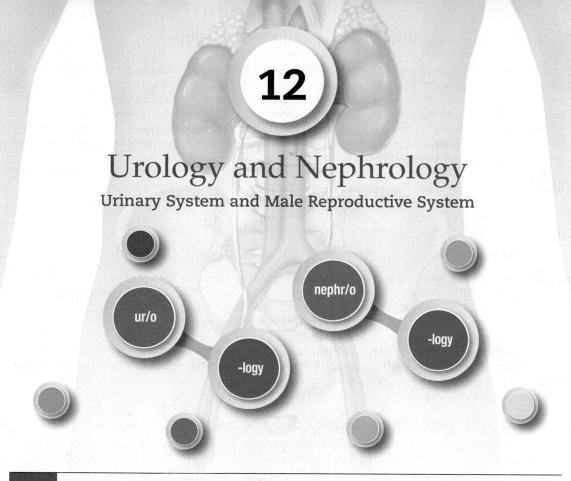

12

Urology and Nephrology

Urinary System and Male Reproductive System

ur/o

nephr/o

-logy

-logy

Learning Objectives

Upon completion of this chapter, you will be able to:

12-1 Describe the medical specialties of urology and nephrology.

12-2 Understand the functions of the urinary and male reproductive systems.

12-3 Define urology- and nephrology-related combining forms, prefixes, and suffixes.

12-4 Identify the organs treated in urology and nephrology.

12-5 Build urology and nephrology medical terms from word parts.

12-6 Explain urology and nephrology medical terms.

12-7 Use urology and nephrology abbreviations.

A Brief Introduction to Urology and Nephrology

Two medical specialty areas are involved in the diagnosis and treatment of conditions affecting the urinary system: **urology** and **nephrology. Urologists** treat conditions of the female and male urinary tract. In addition, because of the overlap between organs of the urinary tract and male reproductive system, urologists also treat conditions affecting the testes, epididymis, vas deferens, prostate gland, seminal vesicles, bulbourethral glands, and penis. Nephrology is more specifically involved with treating kidney disease. Conditions commonly treated by **nephrologists** include renal failure, problems with fluid and electrolyte balance, kidney transplants, and kidney disease in dialysis patients.

The urinary system is responsible for several very important processes necessary to maintain **homeostasis**, a stable internal environment. These processes include:

- Removing waste products
- Adjusting water and electrolyte levels in the body
- Maintaining normal pH

Beginning in the two **kidneys**, unneeded and unwanted substances are removed from the body along with excess water to produce **urine**. Urine then flows from each kidney through a **ureter** to the **urinary bladder** where it is stored. When urine is released from the body, it flows out through the **urethra**.

In males, the reproductive system is closely associated with the urinary system because both share the urethra. For this reason, these two systems are sometimes referred to as the **genitourinary system**. The testes are responsible for producing **sperm** and secreting **testosterone**, the male sex hormone. The remaining organs of this system include the **epididymis**, **vas deferens**, **seminal vesicles**, **prostate gland**, **bulbourethral glands**, **urethra**, and **penis**. These organs store and transport sperm or secrete seminal fluids to nourish the sperm.

Urology and Nephrology Combining Forms

The following list presents combining forms closely associated with the urinary and male reproductive systems and used for building and defining urology and nephrology terms.

balan/o	glans penis	**ren/o**	kidney
cyst/o	urinary bladder, sac	**semin/i**	semen
epididym/o	epididymis	**sperm/o**	sperm
glomerul/o	glomerulus	**spermat/o**	sperm
lith/o	stone	**testicul/o**	testes
nephr/o	kidney	**ur/o**	urine
orch/o	testes	**ureter/o**	ureter
orchi/o	testes	**urethr/o**	urethra
orchid/o	testes	**urin/o**	urine
prostat/o	prostate gland	**vas/o**	vas deferens
pyel/o	renal pelvis	**vesicul/o**	seminal vesicle

The following list presents combining forms that are not specific to the urinary or male reproductive systems but are also used for building and defining urology and nephrology terms.

albumin/o	albumin	**crypt/o**	hidden
azot/o	nitrogen waste	**genit/o**	genitals
bacteri/o	bacteria	**glycos/o**	sugar, glucose
corpor/o	body	**hem/o**	blood

hemat/o	blood		py/o	pus
hydr/o	water		rect/o	rectum
noct/i	night		ven/o	vein
olig/o	scanty			

Suffix Review

These suffixes introduced in Chapter 2 are being reviewed in this chapter because they are especially important for building urology and nephrology terms.

-al	pertaining to		-megaly	enlarged
-algia	pain		-meter	instrument for measuring
-ar	pertaining to		-oma	tumor, mass
-ary	pertaining to		-osis	abnormal condition
-cele	protrusion		-ostomy	surgically create an opening
-cyte	cell		-otomy	cutting into
-eal	pertaining to		-ous	pertaining to
-ectomy	surgical removal		-pathy	disease
-emia	blood condition		-pexy	surgical fixation
-genesis	produces, generates		-plasia	formation of cells
-gram	record, picture		-plasty	surgical repair
-graphy	process of recording		-ptosis	drooping
-ia	state		-rrhaphy	suture
-iasis	abnormal condition		-rrhea	discharge, flow
-ic	pertaining to		-sclerosis	hardening
-ism	state of		-scope	instrument for viewing
-itis	inflammation		-scopy	process of visually examining
-lith	stone		-stenosis	narrowing
-logist	one who studies		-tripsy	surgical crushing
-logy	study of		-uria	urine condition
-lysis	to destroy			

Prefix Review

These prefixes introduced in Chapter 3 are being reviewed here because they are especially important for building urology and nephrology terms.

a-	without		hyper-	excessive
an-	without		intra-	within
dys-	abnormal, difficult, painful		poly-	many
extra-	outside of		trans-	across

Organs Commonly Treated in Urology and Nephrology

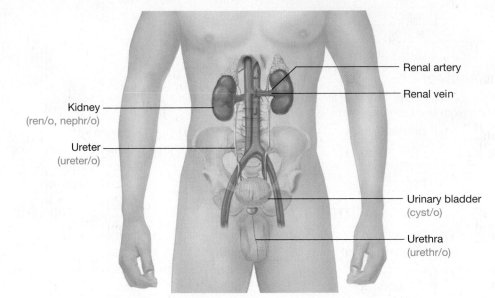

Renal artery

Renal vein

Kidney
(ren/o, nephr/o)

Ureter
(ureter/o)

Urinary bladder
(cyst/o)

Urethra
(urethr/o)

12.1 The urinary system

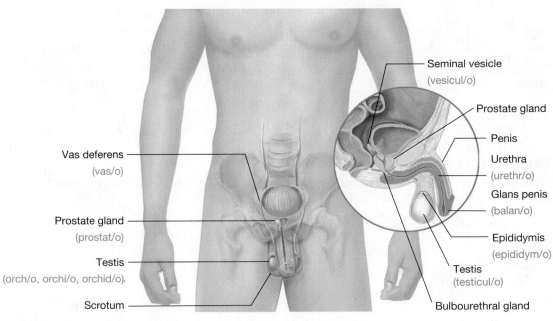

Seminal vesicle
(vesicul/o)

Prostate gland

Penis

Vas deferens
(vas/o)

Urethra
(urethr/o)

Glans penis
(balan/o)

Prostate gland
(prostat/o)

Epididymis
(epididym/o)

Testis
(orch/o, orchi/o, orchid/o)

Testis
(testicul/o)

Scrotum

Bulbourethral gland

12.2 The male reproductive system

Building Urology and Nephrology Terms

This section presents word parts most often used to build urology and nephrology terms. Following the explanation of the term, you have the opportunity to begin building your own vocabulary. Read the meaning for each term and then fill in the blanks to build a single medical term. Use the slashes to divide prefixes, word roots, combining vowels, and suffixes. To help you out you will find a key to the word parts underneath the blanks: **r** for word roots, **p** for prefix, **cv** for combining vowel, and **s** for suffix. Remember that not every term will contain all these word parts; it's up to you to decide which to use. As you gain experience, this process becomes easier. Answers can be found at the back of the book.

1. **balan/o**–combining form meaning **glans penis**

    The glans penis is the enlarged tip of the penis; glans is covered by the **prepuce** (or **foreskin**) (see again Figure 12.2)

    a. glans penis inflammation _____/_____
                                                      r   *s*

    b. discharge from the glans penis _____/_____/_____
                                                      r   *cv*   *s*

2. **cyst/o**–combining form meaning **urinary bladder, sac**

    The urinary bladder is an elastic muscular organ that stores urine produced by the kidneys; urine drains into bladder from ureters and exits bladder in urethra (see again Figure 12.1)

    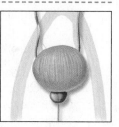

    12.3 Urinary bladder

    a. bladder pain _____/_____
                     r   *s*

    b. protrusion of the bladder _____/_____/_____
                     r   *cv*   *s*

    c. surgical removal of the bladder _____/_____
                     r   *s*

    d. bladder inflammation _____/_____
                     r   *s*

    e. process of visually examining the bladder _____/_____/_____
                     r   *cv*   *s*

    f. record of the bladder _____/_____/_____
                     r   *cv*   *s*

    g. process of recording the bladder _____/_____/_____
                     r   *cv*   *s*

    h. instrument for viewing the bladder _____/_____/_____
                     r   *cv*   *s*

    i. pertaining to the bladder _____/_____
                     r   *s*

    j. stone in the bladder _____/_____/_____
                     r   *cv*   *s*

3. **epididym/o**–combining form meaning **epididymis**

The epididymis sits on surface of each testis; receives sperm produced by testes; location of sperm maturation and storage until released during ejaculation (see again Figure 12.2)

a. epididymis inflammation

_____/_____
r   s

b. pertaining to the epididymis

_____/_____
r   s

- -

4. **lith/o**–combining form meaning **stone**

Stones form in many parts of body, usually formed from the accumulation of mineral salts within an organ; may form in kidney, renal pelvis, ureters, urinary bladder, or urethra; also called a *calculus* (plural is *calculi*)

a. surgical crushing of a stone

_____/_____/_____
r   cv   s

b. abnormal condition of stone in ureter

_____/_____/_____/_____
r   cv   r   s

c. abnormal condition of stone in kidney

_____/_____/_____/_____
r   cv   r   s

d. abnormal condition of stone in bladder

_____/_____/_____/_____
r   cv   r   s

- -

5. **nephr/o**–combining form meaning **kidney**

One kidney is located on either side of spine at level of lower ribs; each consists of thousands of **nephrons**; **glomerulus** portion of each nephron filters waste products and excess water and electrolytes out of blood to produce urine; urine collects in **renal pelvis** and drains out of kidney into ureter and on to urinary bladder for storage; blood is delivered to each kidney by renal arteries and carried away by renal veins (see again Figure 12.1)

12.4 Kidney

a. surgical removal of the kidney

_____/_____
r   s

b. kidney inflammation

_____/_____
r   s

c. enlarged kidney

_____/_____/_____
r   cv   s

d. kidney tumor

_____/_____
r   s

e. drooping kidney

_____/_____/_____
r   cv   s

f. cutting into the kidney

_____/_____
r   s

g. kidney disease

_____ / _____ / _____
r   cv   s

h. surgical fixation of the kidney

_____ / _____ / _____
r   cv   s

i. hardening of the kidney

_____ / _____ / _____
r   cv   s

j. glomerulus and kidney inflammation

_____ / _____ / _____ / _____
r   cv   r   s

k. kidney stone

_____ / _____ / _____
r   cv   s

l. abnormal condition of the kidney

_____ / _____
r   s

---

6. orch/o–combining form meaning **testes**

The testes (singular is _testis_) are the male reproductive organs that produce sperm and testosterone; the two testes are suspended outside body in the **scrotum**; as sperm are produced, they travel to epididymis for storage and maturation (see again Figure 12.2); another term for testes is **testicles** (singular is _testicle_)

12.5 Testis

a. state of being without testes

_____ / _____ / _____
p   r   s

b. testes inflammation

_____ / _____
r   s

c. state of hidden testes

_____ / _____ / _____
r   r   s

---

7. orchi/o–combining form meaning **testes**

a. surgical fixation of the testes

_____ / _____ / _____
r   cv   s

b. testes pain

_____ / _____
r   s

---

8. orchid/o–combining form meaning **testes**

a. surgical removal of testes

_____ / _____
r   s

---

9. -ostomy–suffix meaning **to surgically create an opening**

Describes the creation of new opening between two organs or between organ and external surface of body; new opening on surface of body is called **stoma**

a. surgically create an opening in the bladder

_____ / _____
r   s

b. surgically create an opening in the kidney

_____ / _____
r   s

c. surgically create an opening in the ureter

_____ / _____
r   s

d. surgically create an opening in the renal pelvis

_____ / _____
r   s

e. surgically create an opening in the urethra

_____ / _____
r   s

f. surgically create an opening between (one section of) vas deferens and (another section of) vas deferens

_____ / _____ / _____ / _____
r   cv   r   s

---

10. **prostat/o**–combining form meaning **prostate gland**

The prostate gland is one of the male reproductive glands; this single gland is located surrounding urethra at base of bladder; secretes milky fluid that makes up much of liquid portion of semen and serves to nourish sperm (see again Figure 12.2)

12.6 Prostate gland

a. surgical removal of prostate gland

_____ / _____
r   s

b. prostate gland inflammation

_____ / _____
r   s

c. pertaining to prostate gland

_____ / _____
r   s

---

11. **pyel/o**–combining form meaning **renal pelvis**

The renal pelvis is an area inside each kidney where urine collects as it is being made; each renal pelvis then drains into one of the ureters

12.7 Sectioned kidney

a. renal pelvis and kidney inflammation

_____ / _____ / _____ / _____
r   cv   r   s

b. record of the renal pelvis

_____ / _____ / _____
r   cv   s

c. process of recording the renal pelvis

_____ / _____ / _____
r   cv   s

---

12. **ren/o**–combining form meaning **kidney**

a. pertaining to kidney

_____ / _____
r   s

b. record of kidney

_____ / _____ / _____
r   cv   s

c. process of recording kidney

_____ / _____ / _____
r   cv   s

---

13. **semin/i**–combining form meaning **semen**

Semen is the fluid ejaculated from penis during intercourse; contains sperm and fluids secreted by reproductive glands: prostate gland, seminal vesicles, and bulbourethral glands

a. pertaining to semen

_____/_____

r   s

b. condition of semen in urine

_____/_____

r   s

14. **sperm/o**–combining form meaning **sperm**

Sperm are the male reproductive cells; produced in testes and ejaculated from body in semen; contain one-half of normal complement of chromosomes; when sperm fertilizes ovum (which also has one-half set of chromosomes from mother), new baby is created with full set of chromosomes

a. state of being without sperm

_____/_____/_____

p   r   s

b. state of having scanty sperm

_____/_____/_____/_____

r   cv   r   s

15. **spermat/o**–combining form meaning **sperm**

a. generates sperm

_____/_____/_____

r   cv   s

b. to destroy sperm

_____/_____/_____

r   cv   s

c. pertaining to sperm

_____/_____

r   s

d. sperm cell

_____/_____/_____

r   cv   s

16. **testicul/o**–combining form meaning **testes**

a. pertaining to a testis

_____/_____

r   s

17. **ur/o**–combining form meaning **urine**

a. study of urine

_____/_____/_____

r   cv   s

b. one who studies urine

_____/_____/_____

r   cv   s

c. condition of urine (components) [nitrogenous waste products] in blood

_____/_____

r   s

18. **ureter/o**–combining form meaning **ureter**

The ureter is a tube leading away from renal pelvis of each kidney; carries urine from kidney to urinary bladder (see again Figure 12.1)

12.8 Ureters

a. ureter inflammation

_____/_____

r   s

b. narrowing of ureter

_____/_____/_____
r   cv   s

c. pertaining to ureter

_____/_____
r   s

---

19. **urethr/o**–combining form meaning **urethra**

The single urethra leads out of bladder and carries urine to outside
of body; external opening is **meatus** (see again Figures 12.1 and 12.2)

12.9 Male urethra

a. surgical repair of urethra

_____/_____/_____
r   cv   s

b. urethra pain

_____/_____
r   s

c. urethra inflammation

_____/_____
r   s

d. instrument for viewing urethra

_____/_____/_____
r   cv   s

e. process of visually examining urethra

_____/_____/_____
r   cv   s

f. narrowing of urethra

_____/_____/_____
r   cv   s

g. cutting into urethra

_____/_____
r   s

h. pertaining to urethra

_____/_____
r   s

---

20. **-uria**–suffix meaning **urine condition**

Used with a prefix or combining form to indicate something found in urine or associated with
urination

a. sugar urine condition

_____/_____
r   s

b. night urine condition

_____/_____
r   s

c. scanty urine condition

_____/_____
r   s

d. pus urine condition

_____/_____
r   s

e. without urine condition

_____/_____
p   s

f. abnormal urine condition

_____/_____
p   s

g. blood urine condition

_____/_____
r   s

h. many (excessive) urine condition

_____/_____
p   s

i. albumin (protein) urine condition   _____ / _____
                                                              r   s

j. nitrogen waste urine condition   _____ / _____
                                                              r   s

k. bacteria urine condition   _____ / _____
                                                              r   s

---

21. **urin/o**–combining form meaning **urine**

    Urine is the fluid produced by nephrons of each kidney as they filter wastes, water, and dissolved substances from blood

    a. pertaining to urine   _____ / _____
                                                      r   s

    b. instrument to measure urine   _____ / _____ / _____
                                                                  r   cv   s

---

22. **vas/o**–combining form meaning **vas deferens**

    The vas deferens is a long tube that carries sperm from epididymis to urethra; reproductive glands connected to vas deferens add fluids to sperm as they pass by, making semen (see again Figure 12.2)

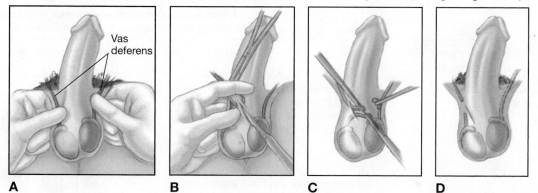

A   **B**   **C**   **D**

12.10 Steps in performing a vasectomy: (A) vas deferens are located; (B) small skin incision is made; (C) vas deferens are cut and ends are cauterized; (D) vas deferens are returned to scrotum and skin is sutured

    a. surgical removal of vas deferens   _____ / _____
                                                                        r   s

    b. suture vas deferens   _____ / _____ / _____
                                                    r   cv   s

---

23. **vesicul/o**–combining form meaning **seminal vesicles**

    The seminal vesicles are the male reproductive glands found behind bladder; add fluids to sperm as they pass by in vas deferens (see again Figure 12.2)

    a. seminal vesicle inflammation   _____ / _____
                                                                  r   s

    b. surgical removal of seminal vesicle   _____ / _____
                                                                            r   s

    c. pertaining to seminal vesicle   _____ / _____
                                                                r   s

Urology and Nephrology Vocabulary

The urology and nephrology terms presented in this section include eponyms, modern English words, and those that contain Latin or Greek word parts but are not constructed solely from these word parts. When you recognize word parts within a term, they will give you a hint about the word's meaning. In these instances, look for the word parts to follow the term.

Term	Explanation
benign prostatic hyperplasia (BPH) **prostat/o** = prostate gland **-ic** = pertaining to **hyper-** = excessive **-plasia** = formation of cells	Noncancerous enlargement of prostate gland; condition places pressure on urethra and narrows it, resulting in frequency, urgency, and nocturia; commonly seen in males over age 50

> **TERMINOLOGY TIDBIT**
> The word *benign* comes from the Latin word *benignus* meaning "kind." Benign growths are not cancerous.

Enlarged prostate gland
Narrowed urethra
Urinary bladder

12.11 Benign prostatic hyperplasia: the enlarged prostate gland pinches the urethra, making urination difficult

Term	Explanation
blood urea nitrogen (BUN)	Blood test to determine kidney function by measuring level of nitrogenous waste, or urea, in blood
calculus	Term for "stone formed within organ"; most are formed from mineral salts; commonly found in kidney, renal pelvis, ureters, bladder, or urethra; plural is *calculi*

> **TERMINOLOGY TIDBIT**
> The word *calculus* comes from the Latin word *calculus* meaning "pebble."

Kidney
Stone
Renal pelvis
Ureter
Stones
Bladder
Stone
Urethra

12.12 Common locations for calculi in the urinary system: kidney, renal pelvis, ureter, and bladder

Term	Explanation
chlamydia	Bacterial sexually transmitted disease; causes inflammation of urethra of males or cervix of females with purulent discharge
circumcision	Surgical removal of prepuce, or foreskin, from glans penis; commonly performed on newborn male at request of parents; primary reason is for ease of hygiene; also a ritual practiced in some religions

> **TERMINOLOGY TIDBIT**
> The word *circumcision* comes from the Latin word *circumcido* meaning "to cut around." This describes the incision required to remove the prepuce.

Term	Explanation
clean catch specimen (CC)	Procedure for obtaining urine sample after cleaning off urethral meatus and catching urine in midstream (halfway through urination process) to minimize contamination from skin
digital rectal exam (DRE) **rect/o** = rectum **-al** = pertaining to	Direct examination for presence of enlarged prostate gland performed by palpating (feeling) prostate gland with fingers (digital) through wall of rectum
erectile dysfunction (ED)	Inability to achieve erection of penis for coitus; also called *impotence*
extracorporeal shockwave lithotripsy (ESWL) **extra-** = outside of **corpor/o** = body **-eal** = pertaining to **lith/o** = stone **-tripsy** = surgical crushing	Treatment procedure for urinary system stones; utilizes ultrasound waves to break up stones; process is noninvasive, meaning it does not require surgery Beam focused on kidney stones Shockwave generator Reflector **12.13** Extracorporeal shockwave lithotripsy, a noninvasive procedure using high-frequency sound waves to shatter kidney stones
frequency	Condition of feeling urge to urinate more often than normal but without increase in total daily volume of urine; can indicate inflammation of bladder or urethra or benign prostatic hyperplasia
genital herpes **genit/o** = genitals **-al** = pertaining to	Highly infectious viral sexually transmitted disease; causes blisterlike lesions on penis of males or cervix and vagina of females
gonorrhea **-rrhea** = discharge	Bacterial sexually transmitted disease; infects mucous membranes and can spread throughout entire genitourinary system; often does not cause many symptoms until widespread
hemodialysis (HD) **hem/o** = blood	Treatment for renal failure using artificial kidney machine to filter waste from blood **12.14** Patient undergoing hemodialysis; patient's blood passes through the hemodialysis machine for cleansing and is then returned to the body Source: Gopixa/Shutterstock
hesitancy	State of difficulty initiating flow of urine; often symptom of blockage along urethra, such as caused by benign prostatic hyperplasia
hydrocele **hydr/o** = water **-cele** = protrusion	Accumulation of fluid within scrotum

Term	Explanation
intravenous pyelogram (IVP) **intra-** = within **ven/o** = vein **-ous** = pertaining to **pyel/o** = renal pelvis **-gram** = record	X-ray of kidney following injection of dye into vein to visualize renal pelvis as kidney filters dye out of bloodstream and puts it into urine
peritoneal dialysis **-al** = pertaining to	Artificial means to remove waste substances from body by placing warm, chemically balanced solutions into peritoneal cavity; treatment for renal failure **12.15** In peritoneal dialysis, a chemically balanced solution is placed into the abdominal cavity to draw impurities out of the bloodstream; it is removed after several hours
phimosis	Narrowing of prepuce over glans penis; can cause difficulty with urination and infection; treatment is circumcision **TERMINOLOGY TIDBIT** The word *phimosis* comes from the Greek word *phimos* meaning "to muzzle." This describes how the prepuce constricts the glans penis.
polycystic kidney disease (PKD) **poly-** = many **cyst/o** = sac **-ic** = pertaining to	Inherited kidney disease characterized by presence of multiple cysts throughout kidney tissue; eventually destroys kidneys and results in kidney failure
prostate-specific antigen (PSA)	Blood test to screen for prostate cancer
prostatic cancer **prostat/o** = prostate gland **-ic** = pertaining to	Common and slow-growing cancer of prostate gland occurring in males over age 50; prostate-specific antigen (PSA) test is used to assist in early detection of this disease
renal failure **ren/o** = kidney **-al** = pertaining to	Inability of kidneys to filter wastes from blood and/or produce urine; treatment of severe renal failure is dialysis or renal transplant
renal transplant **ren/o** = kidney **-al** = pertaining to	Replacement of diseased kidney by donor kidney **12.16** Figure illustrates the location of transplanted donor kidney

Term	Explanation
retrograde pyelogram (RP) **pyel/o** = renal pelvis **-gram** = record	X-ray of urinary bladder, ureters, and renal pelvis following insertion of dye through urethra
semen analysis	Evaluation of semen for fertility; sperm in semen analyzed for number, swimming strength, and shape; procedure is also used to determine whether vasectomy has been successful
sexually transmitted disease (STD)	Contagious disease acquired through sexual contact; formerly referred to as *venereal disease (VD)*
sterility	Inability to produce children; in males, usually due to problem with sperm production, such as aspermia or oligospermia; also called *infertility*
syphilis	Bacterial sexually transmitted disease; begins as localized ulcer at point of infection; chronic disease that spreads through lymph nodes to nervous system after years, causing death
testicular cancer **testicul/o** = testes **-ar** = pertaining to	Cancer of one or both testicles; more commonly seen in young men or boys
transurethral resection of the prostate (TURP) **trans-** = across **urethr/o** = urethra **-al** = pertaining to	Surgical removal of prostate gland tissue by inserting device called *resectoscope* through urethra and removing prostate tissue; may also be referred to simply as *transurethral resection* (TUR)
trichomoniasis **-iasis** = abnormal condition	Protozoan sexually transmitted disease; causes inflammation of genitourinary tract in both men and women
undescended testicle	Congenital anomaly involving failure of one or both of testes to descend into scrotal sac before birth; surgical procedure called *orchiopexy* may be required to bring testes down into scrotum permanently; also called *cryptorchism* **12.17** Undescended testicle or cryptorchism: in (A) both testes have failed to descend; in (B) one testis correctly descended while the other is partially descended
urgency	Feeling the need to urinate immediately

Term	Explanation
urinalysis (U/A, UA) **urin/o** = urine	Laboratory test that consists of physical, chemical, and microscopic examination of urine 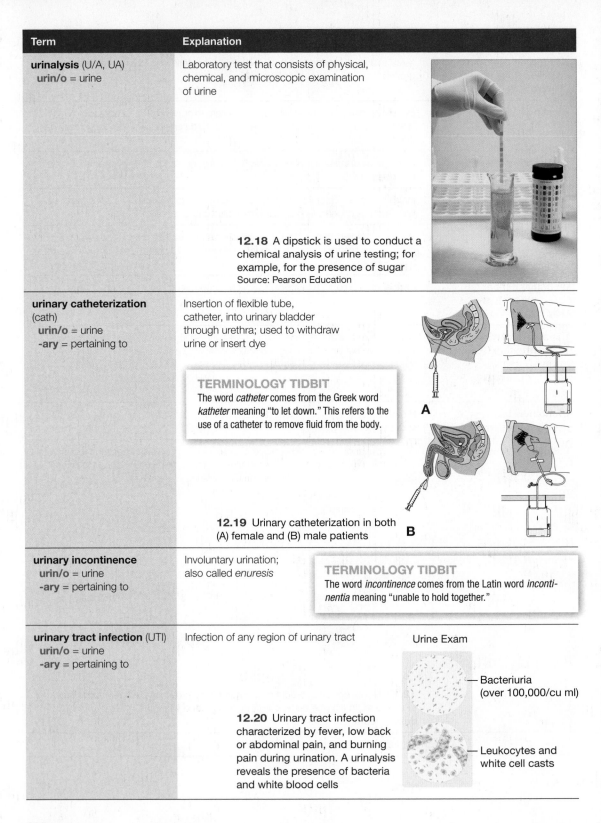 **12.18** A dipstick is used to conduct a chemical analysis of urine testing; for example, for the presence of sugar Source: Pearson Education
urinary catheterization (cath) **urin/o** = urine **-ary** = pertaining to	Insertion of flexible tube, catheter, into urinary bladder through urethra; used to withdraw urine or insert dye **TERMINOLOGY TIDBIT** The word *catheter* comes from the Greek word *katheter* meaning "to let down." This refers to the use of a catheter to remove fluid from the body. **12.19** Urinary catheterization in both (A) female and (B) male patients
urinary incontinence **urin/o** = urine **-ary** = pertaining to	Involuntary urination; also called *enuresis* **TERMINOLOGY TIDBIT** The word *incontinence* comes from the Latin word *incontinentia* meaning "unable to hold together."
urinary tract infection (UTI) **urin/o** = urine **-ary** = pertaining to	Infection of any region of urinary tract Urine Exam Bacteriuria (over 100,000/cu ml) Leukocytes and white cell casts **12.20** Urinary tract infection characterized by fever, low back or abdominal pain, and burning pain during urination. A urinalysis reveals the presence of bacteria and white blood cells

Term	Explanation
urine culture & sensitivity (C&S)	Diagnostic lab procedure that identifies bacterial infection of urinary system and determines best antibiotic to treat it; involves growing bacteria in culture medium and testing different antibiotics on it
varicocele **-cele** = protrusion	Development of varicose veins in the scrotal veins
voiding cystourethrography (VCUG) **cyst/o** = bladder **urethr/o** = urethra **-graphy** = process of recording	X-ray made while patient voids dye that has been placed in urinary bladder through urethra

Urology and Nephrology Abbreviations

The following list presents common urology and nephrology abbreviations.

ARF	acute renal failure	**I&O**	intake and output
BPH	benign prostatic hyperplasia	**IVP**	intravenous pyelogram
BUN	blood urea nitrogen	**KUB**	kidney, ureter, bladder
cath	catheterization	**PKD**	polycystic kidney disease
CC	clean-catch urine specimen	**PSA**	prostate-specific antigen
CRF	chronic renal failure	**RP**	retrograde pyelogram
C&S	culture and sensitivity	**STD**	sexually transmitted disease
cysto	cystoscopy	**TUR**	transurethral resection
DRE	digital rectal exam	**TURP**	transurethral resection of the prostate
ED	erectile dysfunction		
ESRD	end-stage renal disease	**U/A, UA**	urinalysis
ESWL	extracorporeal shockwave lithotripsy	**UC**	urine culture
		UTI	urinary tract infection
GU	genitourinary	**VCUG**	voiding cystourethrography
HD	hemodialysis	**VD**	venereal disease
HPV	human papilloma virus		

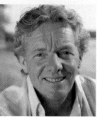

Source: Leifstiller/ Shutterstock

History of Present Illness

The patient is a 57-year-old male seen in the urologist's office to follow up an above normal prostate-specific antigen level found on his annual exam. His prostate-specific antigen values have been in the normal range but have gradually risen over the past three years. He reports nocturnal frequency and hesitancy but denies urinary incontinence or erectile dysfunction.

Past Medical History

Patient has a history of an acute myocardial infarction two years ago, which was treated by a percutaneous transluminal coronary angioplasty. He also had an inguinal herniorrhaphy 10 years ago. Patient has taken medication for hypertension for four years and for hyperlipidemia for two years.

Family and Social History

Patient is a professional golfer but has been unable to tolerate walking long distances for the past three years. He quit smoking following his myocardial infarction and denies using alcohol or illicit drugs. He is married and has three children. Family history is negative for cardiac problems. His father died of bone cancer at the age of 64 and his mother is alive but in poor health with metastatic breast cancer.

Physical Examination

Patient is an average size male, alert and oriented x3, does not appear in any distress. His vital signs are normal, his abdomen is soft to palpation without organomegaly or lymphadenopathy. Digital rectal exam reveals a uniformly enlarged prostate gland but no nodules.

Diagnostic Tests

Urinalysis was positive for red blood cells but negative for bacteria, and a urine culture and sensitivity was negative. Multiple prostatic biopsies were taken. One biopsy revealed prostatic cancer. A bone scan and computed tomography scan of the abdomen and pelvis failed to demonstrate any evidence of metastases.

Diagnosis

Localized prostatic cancer without apparent metastases.

Plan of Treatment

1. Patient elected to undergo a prostatectomy
2. Because the tumor was well localized in the prostate gland and all lymph nodes were clear of metastatic disease, oncology did not recommend radiation or chemotherapy at this time
3. He is to have a repeat prostate-specific antigen level every three months

Critical Thinking Questions

Answer the following questions regarding this case study. Do not just copy words out of the case study but translate all medical terms. To answer some of these questions, you may need to look up information from another chapter of this text, in a medical dictionary, or online. Answers are found at the back of the book.

1. Describe the two urinary tract symptoms this patient does have and the two of which he does not complain.

_____

_____

2. An elevated prostate-specific antigen level is often associated with:
   a. benign prostatic hyperplasia
   b. syphilis
   c. epispadias
   d. prostatic cancer

3. What are the vital signs?

_____

_____

4. Several terms in this case study can be replaced by an abbreviation. List five of them and their abbreviations.

_____

_____

5. What is a urinalysis? Describe the results of this patient's urinalysis.

_____

_____

6. What is an oncologist? Explain the oncologist's recommendations.

_____

_____

7. Two tests did not find any evidence of metastases. What were these tests, and what are _metastases_?

_____

_____

8. This patient has had a myocardial infarction that was treated with a percutaneous transluminal coronary angioplasty. Define these cardiology terms.

_____

_____

PRACTICE

Sound It Out

The following are some of the key terms from this chapter written as their phonetic spelling. Sound out each term and write it in the blank. Pronunciations for all terms are included in the audio glossary at www.mymedicalterminologylab.com.

1. yoo-ree-ter-oh-sten-OH-sis _____

2. bah-lah-noh-REE-ah _____

3. krip-TOR-kizm _____

4. yoo-rin-OH-meh-ter _____

5. ah-SPER-mee-ah _____

6. neh-FROH-ma _____

7. dis-YOO-ree-ah _____

8. ep-ih-did-ih-MYE-tis _____

9. veh-SIC-yoo-LYE-tis _____

10. hee-mah-TOO-ree-ah _____

11. hee-moh-dye-AL-ih-sis _____

12. gon-oh-REE-ah _____

13. pye-eh-loh-neh-FRYE-tis _____

14. neh-FROH-sis _____

15. LITH-oh-trip-see _____

16. nef-roh-skleh-ROH-sis _____

17. ol-ih-goh-SPER-mee-ah _____

18. or-kid-EK-toh-mee _____

19. pol-ee-YOO-ree-ah _____

20. pross-tah-TYE-tis _____

21. ree-NOG-rah-fee _____

22. vas-EK-toh-mee _____

23. yoo-rih-NAL-ih-sis _____

24. VAIR-ih-koh-seel _____

25. nef-roh-MEG-ah-lee _____

Transcription Practice

Each of the following sentences is written in common English. Underline any words or phrases that can be replaced by a medical term. Then rewrite the entire sentence using medical terms. Answers can be found at the back of the book.

1. A procedure to visually examine the bladder revealed the presence of a bladder stone, and the patient underwent a surgical procedure to crush the stone.

   _____

   _____

2. When noting the discharge from the glans penis and the inflammation of the glans penis, the physician knew she needed to determine whether the patient had developed a disease following sexual activity.

   _____

   _____

3. An X-ray record of the renal pelvis made after the insertion of a dye through the urethra confirmed the diagnosis of inflammation of the renal pelvis and kidney.

   _____

   _____

4. An evaluation of the semen for fertility performed six weeks after the surgical removal of the vas deferens confirmed the lack of sperm.

   _____

   _____

5. The patient's kidneys forming many small cysts resulted in the inability of his kidneys to filter waste from the blood, necessitating the use of a machine to filter the blood.

   _____

   _____

6. The results of the physical examination of the urine showed that there was pus in the urine, bacteria in the urine, and sugar in the urine.

   _____

   _____

7. After the patient developed an absence of urine, a kidney record revealed that the patient had developed hardening of the kidney.

   _____

   _____

8. The elderly gentleman required the surgical removal of the prepuce for narrowing of the prepuce.

   _____

   _____

9. The patient required a creation of an opening to the ureter following the removal of the bladder for bladder cancer.

_____

_____

10. The patient developed the abnormal condition of stones in the kidneys and underwent a procedure utilizing ultrasound waves to break up the stones.

_____

_____

Abbreviation Matching

Match each abbreviation with its definition.

_____ **1.** ARF   **A.** blood urea nitrogen

_____ **2.** UTI   **B.** hemodialysis

_____ **3.** PSA   **C.** genitourinary

_____ **4.** HD   **D.** digital rectal exam

_____ **5.** BUN   **E.** intravenous pyelogram

_____ **6.** IVP   **F.** prostate-specific antigen

_____ **7.** TURP   **G.** urinary tract infection

_____ **8.** UA   **H.** urinalysis

_____ **9.** DRE   **I.** transurethral resection of the prostate

_____ **10.** GU   **J.** acute renal failure

Labeling Exercise

Write the name of each structure on the numbered line. Also use this space to write the combining form where appropriate.

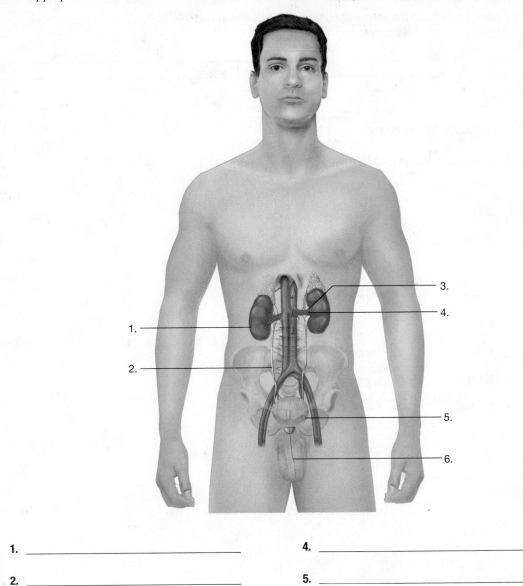

1. _____

2. _____

3. _____

4. _____

5. _____

6. _____

Build Medical Terms

Use each of the word parts below to build the indicated medical terms.

The combining form *nephr/o* means kidney.

1. study of the kidney _____

2. enlarged kidney _____

3. kidney disease _____

4. drooping kidney _____

5. surgical fixation of kidney _____

The combining form *spermat/o* means sperm.

6. to destroy sperm _____

7. pertaining to sperm _____

The combining form *cyst/o* means bladder.

8. record of bladder _____

9. procedure to view bladder _____

The combining form *prostat/o* means prostate gland.

10. prostate gland inflammation _____

11. surgical removal of prostate gland _____

The suffix *-uria* means urine condition.

12. blood urine condition _____

13. night urine condition _____

14. abnormal urine condition _____

15. sugar urine condition _____

Fill in the Blank

Fill in the blank to complete each of the following sentences.

1. The development of varicose veins leading to the testes is called _____.

2. _____ is the noncancerous enlargement of the prostate gland.

3. The male sex hormone is _____.

4. In a semen analysis, the sperm are checked for _____, _____, and
   _____.

5. An X-ray made while the person voids dye that has been placed in the bladder is called a(n)
   _____.

6. The treatment for phimosis is _____.

7. _____ is difficulty initiating the flow of urine.

8. _____ is a blood test used to screen for prostate cancer.

9. A _____ is a blood test to determine kidney function by measuring the level of nitrogenous
   waste in the blood.

10. The term for a stone formed within an organ is a(n) _____.

Spelling

Some of the following terms are misspelled. Identify the incorrect terms and spell them correctly in the blank provided.

1. epidydimitis _____

2. nefrolithiasis _____

3. orchidectomy _____

4. pylography _____

5. ureterostenosis _____

6. catheterization _____

7. hidrocele _____

8. tricomoniasis _____

9. urinalysis _____

10. varicocele _____

Medical Term Analysis

Examine each term of the following terms. Begin by dividing it into its word parts and writing them in the indicated blanks (*P = prefix*; *WR = word root*; *CF = combining form*; *S = suffix*). Follow with the definition of each word part and then finally the meaning of the full term.

1. balanitis

WR _____

means _____

S _____

means _____

Term meaning: _____

_____

2. vasectomy

WR _____

means _____

S _____

means _____

Term meaning: _____

_____

3. pyuria

WR _____

means _____

S _____

means _____

Term meaning: _____

_____

4. ureterostomy

WR _____

means _____

S _____

means _____

Term meaning: _____

_____

5. nephrolithiasis

CF _____

means _____

WR _____

means _____

S _____

means _____

Term meaning: _____

_____

6. urology

CF _____

means _____

S _____

means _____

Term meaning: _____

_____

7. testicular

WR _____

means _____

S _____

means _____

Term meaning: _____

_____

8. cryptorchism

WR _____

means _____

WR _____

means _____

S _____

means _____

Term meaning: _____

_____

9. prostatectomy

WR _____

means _____

S _____

means _____

Term meaning: _____

_____

10. cystoscope

CF _____

means _____

S _____

means _____

Term meaning: _____

_____

MyMedicalTerminologyLab™

MyMedicalTerminologyLab is a premium online homework management system that includes a host of features to help you study. Registered users will find:

- A multitude of activities and assignments built within the MyLab platform
- Powerful tools that track and analyze your results—allowing you to create a personalized learning experience
- Videos and audio pronunciations to help enrich your progress
- Streaming lesson presentations and self-paced learning modules
- A space where you and your instructors can view and manage your assignments

Photomatch Challenge

Match each scrotal condition with its name in the Word Bank.

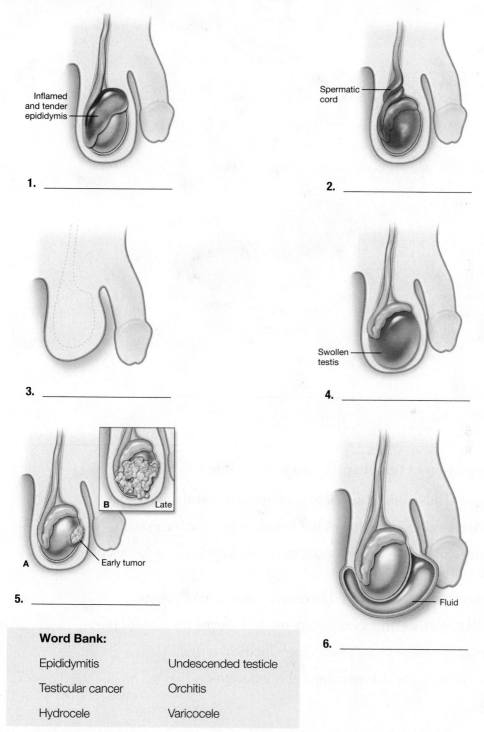

Inflamed and tender epididymis

1. _____

Spermatic cord

2. _____

3. _____

Swollen testis

4. _____

B   Late

A

Early tumor

5. _____

Fluid

6. _____

Word Bank:

Epididymitis	Undescended testicle
Testicular cancer	Orchitis
Hydrocele	Varicocele

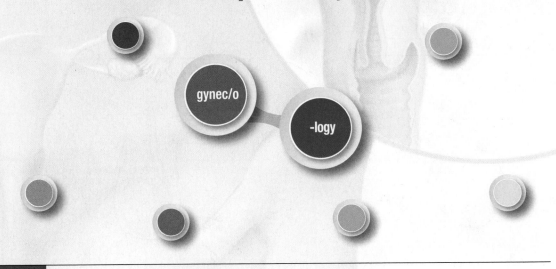

13

Obstetrics and Gynecology

Female Reproductive System

gynec/o

-logy

Learning Objectives

Upon completion of this chapter, you will be able to:

13-1 Describe the medical specialties of obstetrics and gynecology.

13-2 Understand the function of the female reproductive system.

13-3 Define obstetrics- and gynecology-related combining forms, prefixes, and suffixes.

13-4 Identify the organs treated in obstetrics and gynecology.

13-5 Build obstetrics and gynecology medical terms from word parts.

13-6 Explain obstetrics and gynecology medical terms.

13-7 Use obstetrics and gynecology abbreviations.

A Brief Introduction to Obstetrics and Gynecology

Gynecology is the branch of medicine that diagnoses and treats conditions of the female reproductive organs as well as provides general medical care for women. **Obstetrics** is the specialty concerned with childbirth and the care of pregnant women. Most physicians in this field train as both **gynecologists** and **obstetricians** at the same time. However, they can choose to further specialize in only one of the two areas.

The female reproductive system is vital to the continuation of the human race. **Ovaries** begin the process by producing egg cells called **ova** (singular is *ovum*). **Fertilization**, the joining of ovum and sperm, typically occurs in the **uterine** (or **fallopian**) **tubes**. The fertilized ovum then implants in the lining of the **uterus** where the new embryo develops. During birth, the baby passes through the **vagina** as it enters the world. The newborn is then nourished by milk made by the mother's **breasts**. In addition, the ovaries secrete the female sex hormones **estrogen** and **progesterone**, which regulate the reproductive cycle and produce the female secondary sexual characteristics.

Obstetrics and Gynecology Combining Forms

The following list presents combining forms closely associated with the female reproductive system and used for building and defining obstetrics and gynecology terms.

amni/o	amnion		**mast/o**	breast
cervic/o	neck, cervix		**men/o**	menses, menstruation
chori/o	chorion		**metr/o**	uterus
colp/o	vagina		**nat/o**	birth
embry/o	embryo		**o/o**	egg
episi/o	vulva		**oophor/o**	ovary
fet/o	fetus		**ovari/o**	ovary
gynec/o	woman, female		**salping/o**	uterine (fallopian) tube
hyster/o	uterus		**uter/o**	uterus
lapar/o	abdomen		**vagin/o**	vagina
mamm/o	breast			

The following list presents combining forms that are not specific to the female reproductive system but are also used for building and defining obstetrics and gynecology terms.

carcin/o	cancer		**olig/o**	scanty
cyst/o	urinary bladder, sac		**pelv/o**	pelvis
fibr/o	fibrous		**rect/o**	rectum
hem/o	blood			

Suffix Review

These suffixes introduced in Chapter 2 are being reviewed in this chapter because they are especially important for building obstetrics and gynecology terms.

-al	pertaining to		**-lytic**	destruction
-algia	pain		**-metry**	process of measuring
-an	pertaining to		**-nic**	pertaining to
-ary	pertaining to		**-oid**	resembling
-cele	protrusion		**-oma**	tumor, mass
-centesis	puncture to withdraw fluid		**-osis**	abnormal condition
-cyesis	pregnancy		**-otomy**	cutting into
-cyte	cell		**-para**	to bear (offspring)
-ectomy	surgical removal		**-partum**	childbirth
-genesis	produces, generates		**-pexy**	surgical fixation
-genic	producing		**-plasty**	surgical repair
-gram	record		**-rrhagia**	abnormal flow condition
-graphy	process of recording		**-rrhaphy**	suture
-gravida	pregnancy		**-rrhea**	flow, discharge
-ic	pertaining to		**-rrhexis**	rupture
-ine	pertaining to		**-scope**	instrument for viewing
-itis	inflammation		**-scopy**	process of visually examining
-logist	one who studies		**-tic**	pertaining to
-logy	study of			

Prefix Review

These prefixes introduced in Chapter 3 are being reviewed here because they are especially important for building obstetrics and gynecology terms.

a-	without		**multi-**	many
ante-	before		**neo-**	new
dys-	painful, difficult, abnormal		**post-**	after
endo-	within, inner		**pre-**	before
intra-	within		**primi-**	first
nulli-	none		**trans-**	across

Organs Commonly Treated in Obstetrics and Gynecology

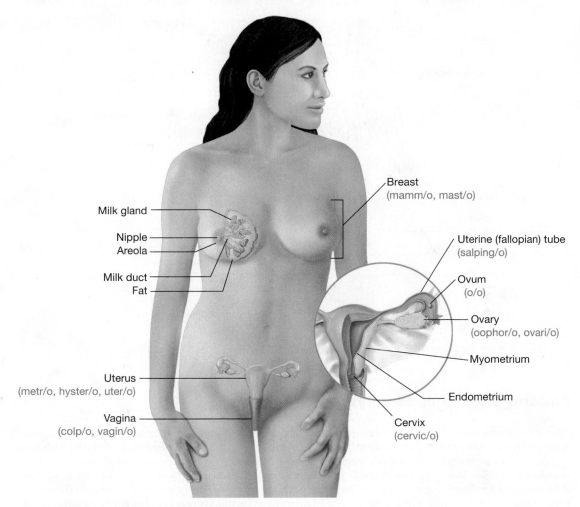

Milk gland

Nipple

Areola

Milk duct

Fat

Breast
(mamm/o, mast/o)

Uterine (fallopian) tube
(salping/o)

Ovum
(o/o)

Ovary
(oophor/o, ovari/o)

Myometrium

Endometrium

Uterus
(metr/o, hyster/o, uter/o)

Vagina
(colp/o, vagin/o)

Cervix
(cervic/o)

13.1 Female reproductive system, anterior view

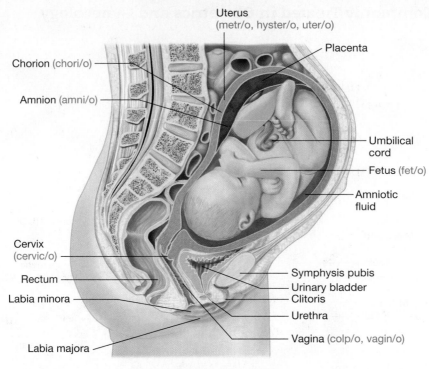

13.2 Full-term pregnancy, internal structures, lateral view

Building Obstetrics and Gynecology Terms

This section presents word parts most often used to build obstetrics and gynecology terms. Following the explanation of the term, you have the opportunity to begin building your own vocabulary. Read the meaning for each term and then fill in the blanks to build a single medical term. Use the slashes to divide prefixes, word roots, combining vowels, and suffixes. To help you out you will find a key to the word parts underneath the blanks: **r** for word roots, **p** for prefix, **cv** for combining vowel, and **s** for suffix. Remember that not every term will contain all these word parts; it's up to you to decide which to use. As you gain experience, this process becomes easier. Answers can be found at the back of the book.

1. **amni/o**–combining form meaning **amnion**

    Amnion is the inner sac surrounding the fetus; contains **amniotic fluid** in which fetus floats (see again Figure 13.2)

    a. pertaining to amnion _____/_____/_____
                                                       _r_   _cv_   _s_

    b. cutting into amnion _____/_____
                                                  _r_   _s_

    c. flow of amniotic (fluid) _____/_____/_____
                                                  _r_   _cv_   _s_

    d. puncture of amnion to withdraw fluid _____/_____/_____
                                                  _r_   _cv_   _s_

    e. rupture of amnion _____/_____/_____
                                                  _r_   _cv_   _s_

2. cervic/o–combining form meaning **cervix**

The cervix is the narrow, lower portion of uterus; opens into vagina to allow passage of menstrual fluids; dilates during labor to allow birth of baby; also called *neck of the uterus* (see again Figures 13.1 and 13.2)

a. pertaining to cervix

_____/_____
r   s

b. surgical removal of cervix

_____/_____
r   s

c. cervix inflammation

_____/_____
r   s

d. inflammation within cervix

_____/_____/_____
p   r   s

e. surgical repair of cervix

_____/_____/_____
r   cv   s

---

3. chori/o–combining form meaning **chorion**

Chorion is the outer sac surrounding and protecting fetus; forms part of **placenta**; placenta is formed from both maternal and fetal tissue; it lies along inner wall of uterus; fetus is connected to placenta by **umbilical cord**; point of exchange between maternal and fetal circulations (oxygen and nutrients are delivered to fetus and carbon dioxide and wastes are removed) (see again Figure 13.2)

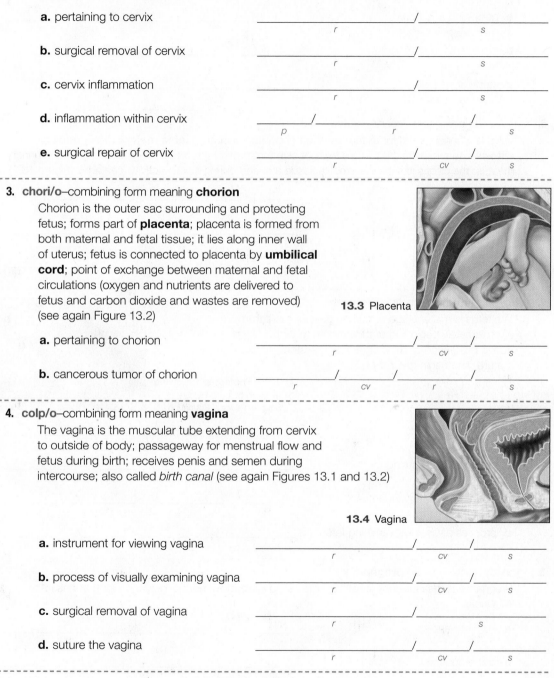

13.3 Placenta

a. pertaining to chorion

_____/_____/_____
r   cv   s

b. cancerous tumor of chorion

_____/_____/_____/_____
r   cv   r   s

---

4. colp/o–combining form meaning **vagina**

The vagina is the muscular tube extending from cervix to outside of body; passageway for menstrual flow and fetus during birth; receives penis and semen during intercourse; also called *birth canal* (see again Figures 13.1 and 13.2)

13.4 Vagina

a. instrument for viewing vagina

_____/_____/_____
r   cv   s

b. process of visually examining vagina

_____/_____/_____
r   cv   s

c. surgical removal of vagina

_____/_____
r   s

d. suture the vagina

_____/_____/_____
r   cv   s

---

5. embry/o–combining form meaning **embryo**

The embryo is an early stage of human development from time of fertilization until approximately end of second month of pregnancy; during this time period, all the major organs and body systems are formed

a. pertaining to embryo

_____/_____/_____
                 r   *cv*   *s*

b. producing an embryo

_____/_____/_____
                 r   *cv*   *s*

c. study of embryo

_____/_____/_____
                 r   *cv*   *s*

6. episi/o–combining form meaning **vulva**

Vulva is a general term for all female external genitalia including **labia majora**, **labia minora**, and **clitoris**; the two pairs of labia are folds of skin that protect the clitoris, vaginal opening, and urinary meatus; the clitoris is sensitive erectile tissue aroused during sexual activity (see again Figure 13.2)

a. suture of vulva

_____/_____/_____
                 r   *cv*   *s*

b. surgical repair of vulva

_____/_____/_____
                 r   *cv*   *s*

c. cutting into vulva

_____/_____
                 r   *s*

7. fet/o–combining form meaning **fetus**

The fetus is a later stage of human development from approximately beginning of third month to birth; during this period of time, organs and systems grow, mature, and begin to function

13.5 Photograph showing fetus in the uterus
Source: Pearson Education

a. pertaining to fetus

_____/_____
                 r   *s*

b. process of measuring fetus

_____/_____/_____
                 r   *cv*   *s*

c. instrument for viewing fetus

_____/_____/_____
                 r   *cv*   *s*

d. process of visually examining fetus

_____/_____/_____
                 r   *cv*   *s*

8. -gravida–suffix meaning **pregnancy**

Pregnancy is measured by length of time called **gestation**; normal gestation for humans is 40 weeks

a. no pregnancies

_____/_____
                 p   *s*

b. first pregnancy

_____/_____
                 p   *s*

c. many pregnancies

_____/_____
                 p   *s*

9. gynec/o–combining form meaning **female**

    a. study of female

                                         _____ / _____ / _____
                                                 r   cv   s

    b. one who studies female

                                         _____ / _____ / _____
                                                 r   cv   s

---

10. hyster/o–combining form meaning **uterus**

The uterus is the hollow pear-shaped organ in lower pelvic cavity between urinary bladder and rectum; **fundus** is upper portion between where uterine tubes enter; **body** of uterus is largest central region; **cervix** is narrow lowest region that opens into vagina; **endometrium** is inner lining that thickens during the month and is sloughed off during **menstrual period**; **myometrium** is thick muscular wall that contracts to push fetus through birth canal (see again Figures 13.1 and 13.2)

13.6 Uterus

    a. surgical fixation of uterus

                        _____ / _____ / _____
                                r   cv   s

    b. ruptured uterus

                        _____ / _____ / _____
                                r   cv   s

    c. surgical removal of uterus

                        _____ / _____
                                r   s

    d. process of recording uterus

                        _____ / _____ / _____
                                r   cv   s

    e. record of uterus

                        _____ / _____ / _____
                                r   cv   s

---

11. lapar/o–combining form meaning **abdomen**

    a. cutting into abdomen

                      _____ / _____
                              r   s

    b. instrument for viewing abdomen

                      _____ / _____ / _____
                              r   cv   s

    c. process of visually examining abdomen

                      _____ / _____ / _____
                              r   cv   s

---

12. mamm/o–combining form meaning **breast**

The breast is a collection of glands to produce milk to nourish infant; pigmented area around the **nipple** is the **areola**; also called *mammary glands* (see again Figure 13.1)

13.7 Breast

    a. pertaining to breast

                      _____ / _____
                              r   s

    b. record of breast

                      _____ / _____ / _____
                              r   cv   s

c. process of recording breast   _____/_____/_____

                                                           r   *cv*   *s*

d. surgical repair of breast   _____/_____/_____

                                                            r   *cv*   *s*

- -

13. mast/o–combining form meaning **breast**

    a. breast pain   _____/_____

                                     r   *s*

    b. breast inflammation   _____/_____

                                     r   *s*

    c. surgical removal of breast   _____/_____

                                     r   *s*

- -

14. men/o–combining form meaning **menstruation**

Menstruation occurs when endometrial lining of uterus is shed each month; this process stops during pregnancy; appears as bloody flow through cervix and vagina

    a. without menstrual flow   _____/_____/_____/_____

                                   p   *r*   *cv*   *s*

    b. painful menstrual flow   _____/_____/_____/_____

                                   p   *r*   *cv*   *s*

    c. scanty menstrual flow   _____/_____/_____/_____/_____

                                   r   *cv*   *r*   *cv*   *s*

    d. abnormal flow condition (of excessive)   _____/_____/_____

    menstruation   *r*   *cv*   *s*

- -

15. metr/o–combining form meaning **uterus**

    a. inner uterus inflammation   _____/_____/_____

                                     p   *r*   *s*

    b. flow from uterus   _____/_____/_____

                                     r   *cv*   *s*

    c. abnormal flow condition from uterus   _____/_____/_____

                                     r   *cv*   *s*

- -

16. nat/o–combining form meaning **birth**

    a. pertaining to birth   _____/_____

                                     r   *s*

    b. pertaining to a newborn   _____/_____/_____

                                   p   *r*   *s*

    c. study of newborn   _____/_____/_____/_____

                                   p   *r*   *cv*   *s*

    d. one who studies newborn   _____/_____/_____/_____

                                   p   *r*   *cv*   *s*

- -

17. **o/o**–combining form meaning **egg**

The ovum is the egg cell that carries the mother's half of chromosomes; combines with sperm to form new human

a. egg cell

_____/_____/_____
 r   cv   s

b. produces an egg

_____/_____/_____
 r   cv   s

18. **oophor/o**–combining form meaning **ovary**

The ovary is an almond-shaped organ located on either side of uterus; connected to uterus by uterine (fallopian) tube; produces ova; release of ovum from ovary is called **ovulation**; secretes female hormones: estrogen and progesterone (see again Figure 13.1)

13.8 Ovary

a. ovary inflammation

_____/_____
 r   s

b. surgical removal of ovary

_____/_____
 r   s

c. surgical fixation of ovary

_____/_____/_____
 r   cv   s

19. **ovari/o**–combining form meaning **ovary**

a. pertaining to ovary

_____/_____
 r   s

b. ovary and uterine tube inflammation

_____/_____/_____/_____
 r   cv   r   s

20. **-para**–suffix meaning **to bear (offspring)**

Refers to the number of times a pregnancy has successfully ended with birth of infant

a. no births

_____/_____
 p   s

b. first birth

_____/_____
 p   s

c. many births

_____/_____
 p   s

21. **-partum**–suffix meaning **childbirth**

a. before childbirth

_____/_____
 p   s

b. after childbirth

_____/_____
 p   s

22. **salping/o**–combining form meaning **uterine (fallopian) tube**

The uterine tube is a narrow duct that runs from the area around each ovary to upper uterus; ova travel from ovary to uterus through uterine tube; normal location for **fertilization**; also called **fallopian tube** (see again Figure 13.1)

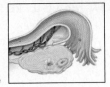

13.9 Uterine tube

a. surgical removal of uterine tube

_____/_____
　　　　　　　　　　r　　　　　　　　　　　s

b. uterine tube inflammation

_____/_____
　　　　　　　　　　r　　　　　　　　　　　s

c. process of recording uterine tube

_____/_____/_____
　　　　　　　r　　　　　cv　　　　　s

d. record of uterine tube

_____/_____/_____
　　　　　　　r　　　　　cv　　　　　s

e. pregnancy in uterine tube

_____/_____/_____
　　　　　　　r　　　　　cv　　　　　s

---

23. **uter/o**–combining form meaning **uterus**

a. pertaining to uterus

_____/_____
　　　　　　　r　　　　　　　　　s

b. surgical repair of uterus

_____/_____/_____
　　　　　　　r　　　　　cv　　　　　s

c. instrument for viewing uterus

_____/_____/_____
　　　　　　　r　　　　　cv　　　　　s

d. process of visually examining uterus

_____/_____/_____
　　　　　　　r　　　　　cv　　　　　s

e. pertaining to within uterus

_____/_____/_____
　　p　　　　　　r　　　　　　　s

---

24. **vagin/o**–combining form meaning **vagina**

a. pertaining to vagina

_____/_____
　　　　　　　　　　r　　　　　　　　　　　s

b. vagina inflammation

_____/_____
　　　　　　　　　　r　　　　　　　　　　　s

c. pertaining to across vagina

_____/_____/_____
　　p　　　　　　r　　　　　　　s

Obstetrics and Gynecology Vocabulary

The obstetrics and gynecology terms presented in this section include eponyms, modern English words, and those that contain Latin or Greek word parts but are not constructed solely from these word parts. When you recognize word parts within a term, they will give you a hint about the word's meaning. In these instances, look for the word parts to follow the term.

Term	Explanation
abortion (AB)	Discharge of embryo from uterus before about 20th week of gestation; *spontaneous abortion* (miscarriage) is unplanned and due to death of embryo; *elective abortion* is legal termination of pregnancy; *therapeutic abortion* is necessary for mother's health
abruptio placentae	Emergency condition occurring when placenta tears away from uterine wall prior to birth of fetus; requires immediate delivery of baby **13.10** Illustration showing the premature separation of the placenta in abruptio placentae **TERMINOLOGY TIDBIT** The term *abruptio* comes from the Latin word *abruptus* meaning "to break off." The term *placenta* comes from the Greek word *plakous* meaning "flat cake." This word was used to describe the appearance of the placenta.
atresia **a-** = without	Lack of normal body opening; for example, *hysteratresia* is closing of cervix, usually from scarring **TERMINOLOGY TIDBIT** The term *atresia* comes from combining the Greek prefix *a-* meaning "without" and the word *tresis* meaning "a hole." When combined, these form a term meaning the "lack of a normal body opening."
breast cancer	Malignant tumor of breast; usually forms in milk glands or lining of milk ducts Tumor — Lactiferous glands **13.11** Breast with a malignant tumor growing in the milk gland and duct

Term	Explanation
cervical cancer **cervic/o** = cervix **-al** = pertaining to	Malignant tumor of cervix; some cases caused by *human papilloma virus* (HPV), sexually transmitted virus for which there is now vaccine; regular Pap smear used for early detection
cesarean section (CS, C-section)	Surgical birth of baby through incision into abdominal and uterine walls; named for Roman emperor Julius Caesar, who is said to have been the first person born using this method **13.12** The head of a fetus emerges from the uterus during a cesarean section Source: Pearson Education
chorionic villus sampling (CVS) **chori/o** = chorion **-nic** = pertaining to	Removal of small piece of chorion for genetic analysis; can be done at earlier stage of pregnancy than amniocentesis
conization	Surgical removal of a core of cervical tissue for biopsy
cystocele **cyst/o** = bladder **-cele** = protrusion	Hernia or outpouching of bladder protrudes into vagina; can cause urinary frequency and urgency and block vagina
dilation and curettage (D&C)	Surgical procedure consisting of widening cervix and scraping or suctioning out endometrial lining of uterus; often performed after spontaneous abortion or to stop excessive bleeding from other causes **TERMINOLOGY TIDBIT** The term *curettage* comes from the French word *curer* meaning "to cleanse."
ectopic pregnancy **-ic** = pertaining to	Pregnancy occurring outside of uterus, usually in uterine tubes; growing fetus will rupture uterine tube requiring a salpingectomy; also called *salpingocyesis* **TERMINOLOGY TIDBIT** The term *ectopic* comes from the Greek word *ektopos* meaning "out of place." **13.13** Illustration of common sites for ectopic pregnancy Interstitial pregnancy Ovarian pregnancy

Term	Explanation
endometriosis **endo-** = inner **metr/o** = uterus **-osis** = abnormal condition	Condition when endometrial tissue appears throughout pelvic or abdominal cavity; causes recurring pain and scarring
endometrial cancer **endo-** = inner **metr/o** = uterus **-al** = pertaining to	Cancerous tumor forms in lining of uterus

A Stage I   **B** Stage II

C Stage III   **D** Stage IV

13.14 Illustration showing the stages of endometrial cancer: (A) Stage I–localized tumor forms in endometrial tissue; (B) Stage II–tumor grows larger within the uterus; (C) Stage III–tumor spreads to nearby organs; (D) Stage IV–cancerous tumors appear throughout the body

Term	Explanation
fetal monitoring **fet/o** = fetus **-al** = pertaining to	Use of electronic equipment placed on mother's abdomen or fetus' scalp to check fetal heart rate (FHR) and fetal heart tone (FHT) during labor; normal FHR ranges from 120 to 160 beats per minute; drop in fetal heart rate indicates fetal distress
fibrocystic breast disease **fibr/o** = fibrous **cyst/o** = sac **-ic** = pertaining to	Benign cysts in breast tissue; not precancerous

Adipose
Cysts
Lactiferous glands

13.15 Illustration showing the location of a fibrocystic lump in the adipose tissue of the breast

Term	Explanation
fibroid tumor **fibr/o** = fibrous **-oid** = resembling	Benign tumor of fiberlike tissue; the most common type of tumor in women

13.16 Common sites for the development of fibroid tumors

Term	Explanation
fistula	Abnormal passageway that develops between two structures; *vesicovaginal fistula* is between urinary bladder and vagina; *rectovaginal fistula* is between rectum and vagina

TERMINOLOGY TIDBIT
The term *fistula* comes directly from the Latin word *fistula* meaning "a pipe."

Term	Explanation
hemolytic disease of the newborn (HDN) **hem/o** = blood **-lytic** = destruction	Condition developing in fetus when mother's blood type is Rh-negative and baby's blood is Rh-positive; antibodies in mother's blood enter fetus' bloodstream through placenta and destroy fetus' red blood cells; causes anemia, jaundice, and enlargement of spleen; treated with intrauterine blood transfusion; also called *erythroblastosis fetalis*
***in vitro* fertilization** (IVF)	Infertility treatment; ova are removed from woman and fertilized by sperm externally; resulting embryos are returned to uterus for development; commonly called *test tube baby*
infertility	Inability to produce children; generally defined as no pregnancy after properly timed intercourse for one year
ovarian cancer **ovari/o** = ovary **-an** = pertaining to	Cancerous tumor formed within ovary
Papanicolaou (Pap) **smear**	Test for early detection of cervical cancer; named after developer George Papanicolaou, a Greek physician; cells are removed from cervix by simple scraping and examined under microscope
pelvic inflammatory disease (PID) **pelv/o** = pelvis **-ic** = pertaining to	Chronic or acute infection, usually bacterial, that ascends through female reproductive tract and out into pelvic cavity; can result in scarring that interferes with fertility

Term	Explanation
placenta previa	Placenta forms in lower portion of uterus and blocks birth canal; can require C-section for delivery Umbilical cord — Fetus — Placenta — Severe bleeding **13.17** Illustration of placenta previa showing the placenta growing over the opening of the cervix
premature birth pre- = before	Birth of fetus before 37 weeks of gestation **13.18** A premature infant Source: Courtesy of Lisa Smith-Pedersen, RN, MSN, NNP-BC/Pearson Education
premenstrual syndrome (PMS) pre- = before	Symptoms that develop just prior to onset of menstrual period; can include irritability, headache, tender breasts, and anxiety
prolapsed uterus	Fallen uterus that can cause cervix to protrude through vaginal opening TERMINOLOGY TIDBIT The term *prolapse* comes from the Latin word *prolapsus* meaning "falling." Prolapsed uterus Severely prolapsed uterus **13.19** Illustration of (A) mild and (B) severe prolapsed uterus **A** **B**
rectocele rect/o = rectum -cele = protrusion	Protrusion or herniation of rectum into vagina
stillbirth (SB)	Birth in which viable-aged fetus dies shortly before or at time of birth

Term	Explanation
tubal ligation **-al** = pertaining to	Surgical tying off of uterine tubes to prevent pregnancy

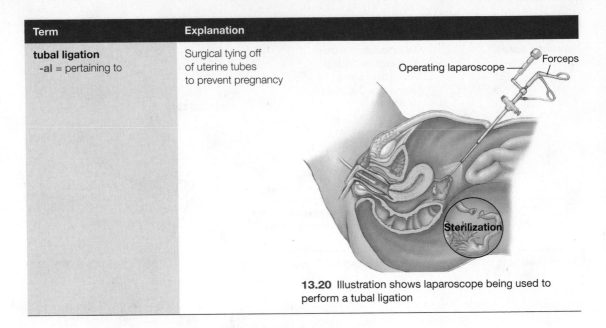

13.20 Illustration shows laparoscope being used to perform a tubal ligation

Obstetrics and Gynecology Abbreviations

The following list presents common obstetrics and gynecology abbreviations.

AB	abortion	**HRT**	hormone replacement therapy
BSE	breast self-examination	**HSG**	hysterosalpingography
CS, C-section	cesarean section	**IUD**	intrauterine device
CVS	chorionic villus sampling	**IVF**	*in vitro* fertilization
Cx	cervix	**LMP**	last menstrual period
D&C	dilation and curettage	**NB**	newborn
EMB	endometrial biopsy	**OB**	obstetrics
ERT	estrogen replacement therapy	**OCPs**	oral contraceptive pills
FHR	fetal heart rate	**Pap**	Papanicolaou test
FHT	fetal heart tone	**PI, para I**	first birth
FTND	full-term normal delivery	**PID**	pelvic inflammatory disease
GI, grav I	first pregnancy	**PMS**	premenstrual syndrome
GYN, gyn	gynecology	**SB**	stillbirth
HDN	hemolytic disease of the newborn	**TAH-BSO**	total abdominal hysterectomy–bilateral salpingo-oophorectomy
HPV	human papilloma virus		

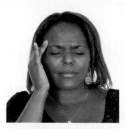

Source: Chris from Paris/
Shutterstock

History of Present Illness

The patient is a 52-year-old female who reports postmenopausal vaginal bleeding for the past two months. She states that her last known menstrual period was three years ago. She also reports mild to moderate uterine cramps, lower abdominal pain, and painful intercourse.

Past Medical History

Patient reports having migraine headaches about once every three months, asthma since her mid-20s, and hyperlipemia. She is grav2 para2. Patient currently uses pain medication prn for headaches and a bronchodilator to relieve asthma symptoms. She is not treating hyperlipemia.

Family and Social History

Patient is divorced. Her two living children are well.

Physical Examination

Patient appears her stated age and is in no distress. She is obese. Pelvic examination revealed normal-appearing cervix and vagina. A small amount of bright red blood was apparent, but no likely source of bleeding was identified.

Diagnostic Tests

An Hgb and HCT revealed anemia. Pap smear was negative. Pelvic ultrasound revealed no uterine fibroids or pelvic masses. A D&C was conducted and pathologist reports no abnormal findings. Finally, hysteroscopy was performed. During course of this procedure, a single small area of active bleeding was identified within the uterine cavity and EMB was completed. Results indicated endometrial cancer.

Diagnosis

Endometrial cancer, stage unknown

Plan of Treatment

1. Schedule patient for total abdominal hysterectomy with lymphadenectomy to stage the cancer
2. Begin iron supplement for anemia, can require transfusion prior to surgery
3. MRI to look for metastases
4. Referral to oncologist for evaluation for possible radiation therapy, hormone therapy, or chemotherapy

Critical Thinking Questions

Answer the following questions regarding this case study. Do not just copy words out of the case study but translate all medical terms. In order to answer some of these questions, you may need to look up information from another chapter of this text, in a medical dictionary, or online. Answers are found at the back of the book.

1. From the patient's history of present illness, explain why it was surprising and troublesome that she was experiencing vaginal bleeding. What are her additional symptoms?

   _____

   _____

2. Interpret the following abbreviations used in this case study: prn, grav2, para2, D&C, EMB.

   _____

   _____

3. List this patient's three previous medical conditions and the treatment she is using for each.

_____

_____

4. What is a Pap smear used to diagnose? Why was it not surprising that it was negative?

_____

_____

5. What are an Hgb and HCT? What is a possible explanation for why this patient is anemic?

_____

_____

6. Go to the following website, www.oncologychannel.com, under "All Topics," click on "Endometrial cancer" and then "Endometrial Cancer & Uterine Cancer Staging." Describe the four main Clinical Stages 1–4 (ignore the substages such as 1A and 1B), for endometrial cancer. If cancer cells are found in this patient's pelvic lymph nodes, what stage will her cancer be?

_____

_____

7. Carefully read the results of the D&C and hysteroscopy. Suggest why it might be possible that the D&C missed the cancer cells but the hysteroscopy found them.

_____

_____

8. What does lymphadenectomy mean and why is it helpful for determining this patient's diagnosis and treatment?

_____

_____

PRACTICE

Sound It Out

The following are some of the key terms from this chapter written as their phonetic spelling. Sound out each term and write it in the blank. Pronunciations for all terms are included in the audio glossary at www.mymedicalterminologylab.com.

1. am-nee-oh-sen-TEE-sis _____

2. SER-vih-koh-plas-tee _____

3. KOH-ree-oh-car-sih-no-mah _____

4. kol-POSS-koh-pee _____

5. SIS-toh-seel _____

6. dis-men-oh-REE-ah _____

7. en-doh-mee-tree-OH-sis _____

8. fee-TOM-eh-tree _____

9. hiss-ter-OG-rah-fee _____

10. IN-tra-YOU-ter-in _____

11. lap-ar-OSS-koh-pee _____

12. MAM-moh-gram _____

13. mass-TEK-toh-mee _____

14. mull-TIP-ah-rah _____

15. NEE-oh-NAY-tall _____

16. null-ih-GRAV-ih-dah _____

17. oh-off-oh-REK-toh-mee _____

18. oh-VAIR-ee-oh-sal-pin-JIH-tis _____

19. post-PAR-tum _____

20. prem-ih-GRAV-ih-dah _____

21. RECK-toh-seel _____

22. sal-ping-go-sigh-EE-sis _____

23. tranz-VAJ-ih-nal _____

24. YOU-ter-oh-plas-tee _____

25. vaj-ih-NIGH-tis _____

MyMedicalTerminologyLab™

MyMedicalTerminologyLab is a premium online homework management system that includes a host of features to help you study. Registered users will find:

- A multitude of activities and assignments built within the MyLab platform
- Powerful tools that track and analyze your results—allowing you to create a personalized learning experience
- Videos and audio pronunciations to help enrich your progress
- Streaming lesson presentations and self-paced learning modules
- A space where you and your instructors can view and manage your assignments

Transcription Practice

Each of the following sentences is written in common English. Underline any words or phrases that can be replaced by a medical term. Then rewrite the entire sentence using medical terms. Answers can be found at the back of the book.

1. Mrs. Scott's painful menstrual flow was treated with a surgical procedure to widen the cervix and scrape the endometrial lining.

   _____

   _____

2. Over time Mrs. Martinez had developed an abnormal passageway between her bladder and vagina.

   _____

   _____

3. The one who studies newborns assisted with the birth through an incision in the abdominal and uterine walls.

   _____

   _____

4. Jean's inability to produce children after properly timed intercourse for one year was the result of scarring caused by chronic bacterial infections ascending through the female reproductive tract.

_____

_____

5. A surgical removal of the uterus became necessary due to extensive endometrial tissue appearing outside the uterus in the pelvic cavity.

_____

_____

6. The new patient at the office of the one who studies women was in her first pregnancy and had no births.

_____

_____

7. Maria was happy to find out she had a benign breast tumor of fiberlike tissue, not a malignant tumor of the milk glands of the breast.

_____

_____

8. A surgical removal of a uterine tube was necessary following the discovery of a pregnancy occurring outside of the uterus in the uterine tubes.

_____

_____

9. Following abnormal test results in which cells were removed from the cervix by scraping, Tawanda's malignant tumor of the cervix was diagnosed by removal of a core of cervical tissue for biopsy.

_____

_____

10. A process of viewing the abdomen was conducted to examine the patient for a cancerous tumor forming within the ovary.

_____

_____

Build Medical Terms

Use each of the following word parts to build the indicated medical terms.

The combining form _hyster/o_ means uterus.

1. surgical fixation of uterus _____

2. surgical removal of uterus _____

3. ruptured uterus _____

4. record of the uterus _____

The combining form _fet/o_ means fetus.

5. pertaining to fetus _____

6. process of measuring the fetus _____

The suffix -*partum* means childbirth.

7. before childbirth _____

8. after childbirth _____

The combining form *men/o* means menstruation.

9. without menstrual flow _____

10. painful menstrual flow _____

11. scanty menstrual flow _____

12. abnormal flow condition (of excessive) menstruation _____

The combining form *mast/o* means breast.

13. breast pain _____

14. breast inflammation _____

15. surgical removal of breast _____

Spelling

Some of the following terms are misspelled. Identify the incorrect terms and spell them correctly in the blank provided.

1. histerectomy _____

2. laparoscopy _____

3. mammary _____

4. oogenesis _____

5. premenstral _____

6. antipartum _____

7. menorhagia _____

8. ovariosalpingitis _____

9. anmiotomy _____

10. endometriosis _____

Fill in the Blank

Fill in the blank to complete each of the following sentences.

1. Fertilization typically occurs in the _____ (or _____) tubes.

2. _____ is the branch of medicine that treats conditions of the female reproductive tract, and _____ is the branch that specializes in pregnancy.

3. The inner lining of the uterus is called the _____, and the muscular layer of the uterus is called the _____.

4. _____ is the removal of a small piece of chorion for genetic analysis.

5. Fetal monitoring uses equipment to check the _____ and _____.

6. Erythroblastosis fetalis is another name for _____.

7. An abnormal passageway that develops between two structures is called a(n) _____.

8. Tying off the uterine tubes to prevent pregnancy is called _____.

9. A prolapsed uterus can cause the _____ to protrude through the vaginal opening.

10. A(n) _____ occurs when the fetus dies shortly before or at time of birth.

Labeling Exercise

Write the name of each structure on the numbered line. Also use this space to write the combining form where appropriate.

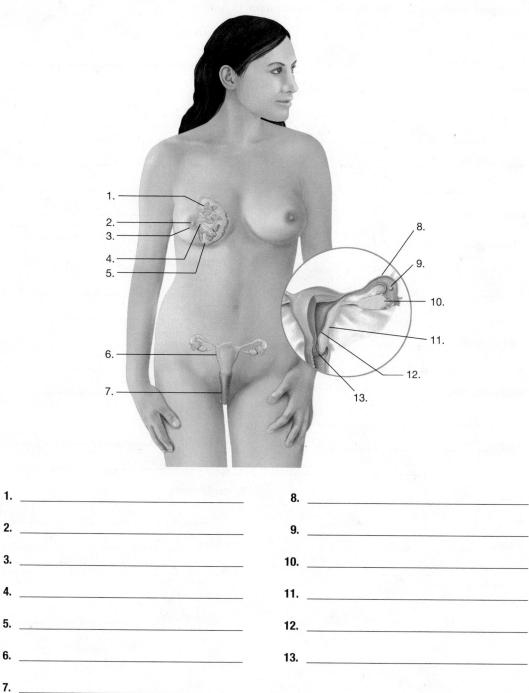

1. _____

2. _____

3. _____

4. _____

5. _____

6. _____

7. _____

8. _____

9. _____

10. _____

11. _____

12. _____

13. _____

Medical Term Analysis

Examine each of the following terms. Begin by dividing it into its word parts and writing them in the indicated blanks (*P = prefix*; *WR = word root*; *CF = combining form*; *S = suffix*). Follow with the definition of each word part and then finally the meaning of the full term.

1. **oophoropexy**

   CF _____

   means _____

   S _____

   means _____

   Term meaning: _____

   _____

2. **colposcope**

   CF _____

   means _____

   S _____

   means _____

   Term meaning: _____

   _____

3. **choriocarcinoma**

   CF _____

   means _____

   WR _____

   means _____

   S _____

   means _____

   Term meaning: _____

   _____

4. **intrauterine**

   P _____

   means _____

   WR _____

   means _____

   S _____

   means _____

   Term meaning: _____

   _____

5. **transvaginal**

   P _____

   means _____

   WR _____

   means _____

   S _____

   means _____

   Term meaning: _____

   _____

6. **embryonic**

   CF _____

   means _____

   S _____

   means _____

   Term meaning: _____

   _____

7. oocyte

CF _____

means _____

S _____

means _____

Term meaning: _____

_____

8. cervicoplasty

CF _____

means _____

S _____

means _____

Term meaning: _____

_____

9. ovariosalpingitis

CF _____

means _____

WR _____

means _____

S _____

means _____

Term meaning: _____

_____

10. episiotomy

WR _____

means _____

S _____

means _____

Term meaning: _____

_____

Abbreviation Matching

Match each abbreviation with its definition.

_____	**1.** NB	**A.**	hysterosalpingography
_____	**2.** Cx	**B.**	*in vitro* fertilization
_____	**3.** FHR	**C.**	cervix
_____	**4.** HSG	**D.**	estrogen replacement therapy
_____	**5.** HPV	**E.**	premenstrual syndrome
_____	**6.** IVF	**F.**	newborn
_____	**7.** grav I	**G.**	abortion
_____	**8.** ERT	**H.**	human papilloma virus
_____	**9.** AB	**I.**	fetal heart rate
_____	**10.** PMS	**J.**	first pregnancy

Photomatch Challenge

Match each procedure with its name in the Word Bank.

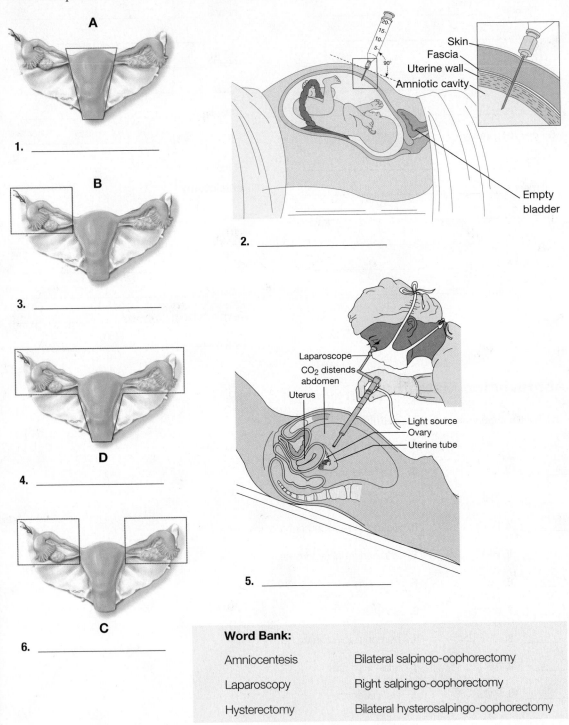

A

1. _____

B

3. _____

D

4. _____

C

6. _____

Skin
Fascia
Uterine wall
Amniotic cavity

Empty bladder

2. _____

Laparoscope
CO$_2$ distends abdomen
Uterus

Light source
Ovary
Uterine tube

5. _____

Word Bank:

Amniocentesis

Laparoscopy

Hysterectomy

Bilateral salpingo-oophorectomy

Right salpingo-oophorectomy

Bilateral hysterosalpingo-oophorectomy

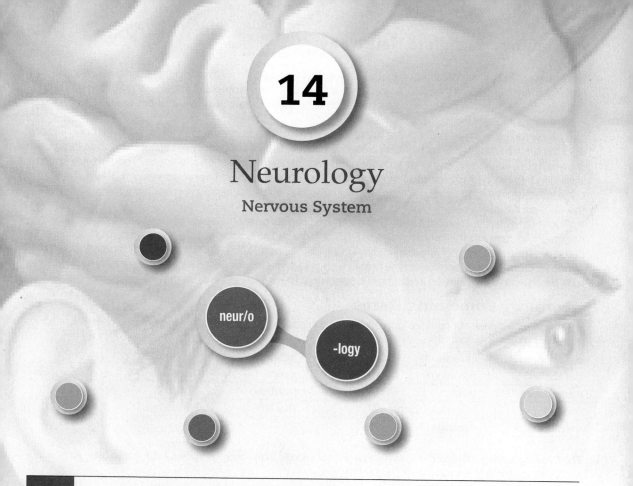

14

Neurology

Nervous System

neur/o — -logy

Learning Objectives

Upon completion of this chapter, you will be able to:

14-1   Describe the medical specialty of neurology.

14-2   Understand the function of the nervous system.

14-3   Define neurology-related combining forms, prefixes, and suffixes.

14-4   Identify the organs treated in neurology.

14-5   Build neurology medical terms from word parts.

14-6   Explain neurology medical terms.

14-7   Use neurology abbreviations.

A Brief Introduction to Neurology

Neurology is the branch of medicine that specializes in the diagnosis and treatment of conditions affecting the nervous system, including the brain, spinal cord, and nerves. A **neurologist** can also treat muscle conditions that are caused by nervous system problems. Another specialty, **neurosurgery**, includes surgical procedures in treating nervous system conditions.

The nervous system consists of the **brain**, **spinal cord**, and **nerves** and is responsible for coordinating all of the body's activity. This task involves receiving information from **sensory receptors** and then using that information to adjust the activity of **muscles** and **glands** to match the body's needs. The nervous system is divided into the **central nervous system (CNS)** and the **peripheral nervous system (PNS)**. The CNS consists of the brain and spinal cord; the PNS comprises all of the nerves carrying electrical impulses between the CNS and all of the body's organs.

The structures of the nervous system are composed of **neurons**. These cells conduct the electrical impulses necessary to carry information between the CNS and body. The point at which one neuron meets another is called a **synapse**. Electrical impulses cannot pass directly across the gap between two neurons, called the **synaptic cleft**. They instead require the help of a chemical messenger, called a **neurotransmitter**. Many neurons are covered by **myelin**, an insulating substance that helps neurons conduct their electrical impulses faster.

Neurology Combining Forms

The following list presents combining forms closely associated with the nervous system and used for building and defining neurology terms.

cerebell/o	cerebellum		**myel/o**	spinal cord
cerebr/o	cerebrum		**neur/o**	nerve
encephal/o	brain		**pont/o**	pons
medull/o	medulla oblongata		**thalam/o**	thalamus
mening/o	meninges			

The following list presents combining forms that are not specific to the nervous system but are also used for building and defining neurology terms.

cephal/o	head		**my/o**	muscle
electr/o	electricity		**scler/o**	hardening, sclera
hemat/o	blood		**spin/o**	spine
hydr/o	water		**tom/o**	to cut
lumb/o	low back		**vascul/o**	blood vessel

Suffix Review

These suffixes introduced in Chapter 2 are being reviewed in this chapter because they are especially important for building neurology terms.

-al	pertaining to		**-ic**	pertaining to
-algia	pain		**-ine**	pertaining to
-ar	pertaining to		**-itis**	inflammation
-ary	pertaining to		**-logist**	one who studies
-asthenia	weakness		**-logy**	study of
-cele	protrusion		**-malacia**	abnormal softening
-eal	pertaining to		**-oma**	tumor, mass
-ectomy	surgical removal		**-osis**	abnormal condition
-esthesia	feeling, sensation		**-otomy**	cutting into
-gram	record		**-pathy**	disease
-graphy	process of recording		**-phasia**	speech

-plasty	surgical repair		**-sclerosis**	hardening
-plegia	paralysis		**-trophic**	development
-rrhaphy	suture			

Prefix Review

These prefixes introduced in Chapter 3 are being reviewed here because they are especially important for building neurology terms.

a-	without		**hyper-**	excessive
an-	without		**mono-**	one
anti-	against		**para-**	two like parts of a pair, beside
di-	two		**poly-**	many
dys-	painful, difficult, abnormal		**quadri-**	four
hemi-	half		**sub-**	beneath, under

Organs Commonly Treated in Neurology

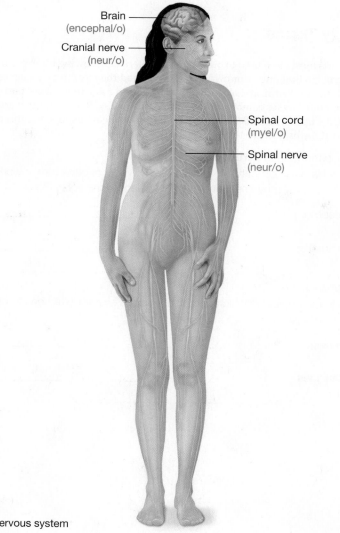

Brain — (encephal/o)

Cranial nerve — (neur/o)

Spinal cord (myel/o)

Spinal nerve (neur/o)

14.1 The nervous system

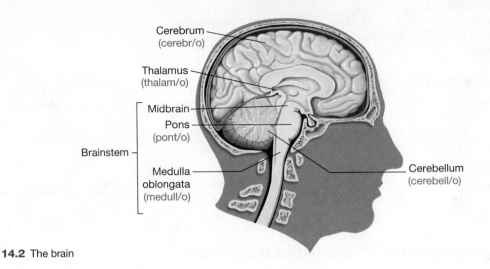

14.2 The brain

Building Neurology Terms

This section presents word parts most often used to build neurology terms. Following the explanation of the term, you have the opportunity to begin building your own vocabulary. Read the meaning for each term and then fill in the blanks to build a single medical term. To help you out you will find a key to the word parts underneath the blanks: **r** for word roots, **p** for prefix, **cv** for combining vowel, and **s** for suffix. Remember that not every term will contain all these word parts; it's up to you to decide which to use. As you gain experience, this process becomes easier. Answers can be found at the back of the book

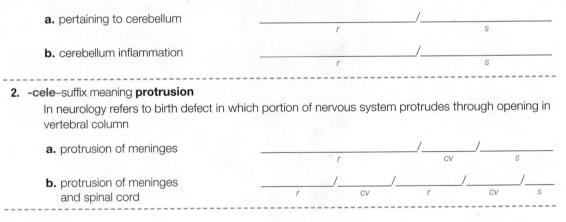

1. **cerebell/o**–combining form meaning **cerebellum**

    Cerebellum is second largest part of brain; located below posterior cerebrum; it works closely with cerebrum to coordinate body movement and maintain balance (see again Figure 14.2)

    a. pertaining to cerebellum
    _____/_____
                 r   s

    b. cerebellum inflammation
    _____/_____
                 r   s

2. **-cele**–suffix meaning **protrusion**

    In neurology refers to birth defect in which portion of nervous system protrudes through opening in vertebral column

    a. protrusion of meninges
    _____/_____/_____
             r   cv   s

    b. protrusion of meninges and spinal cord
    _____/_____/_____/_____/_____
       r   cv   r   cv   s

3. **cerebr/o**–combining form meaning **cerebrum**

Cerebrum is largest part of brain; located in upper portion of brain, its surface is highly convoluted (folded) gray matter called **cerebral cortex**; receives sensory information, integrates all incoming messages with memories, selects responses, and sends motor commands; also responsible for memory, problem solving, and language; divided into **frontal**, **parietal**, **temporal**, and **occipital lobes** (see again Figure 14.2)

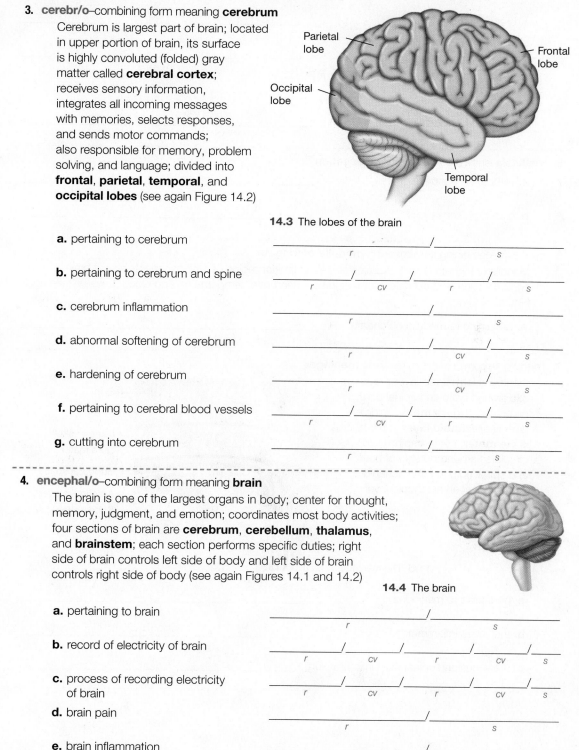

14.3 The lobes of the brain

a. pertaining to cerebrum

_____ / _____
r   s

b. pertaining to cerebrum and spine

_____ / _____ / _____ / _____
r   cv   r   s

c. cerebrum inflammation

_____ / _____
r   s

d. abnormal softening of cerebrum

_____ / _____ / _____
r   cv   s

e. hardening of cerebrum

_____ / _____ / _____
r   cv   s

f. pertaining to cerebral blood vessels

_____ / _____ / _____ / _____
r   cv   r   s

g. cutting into cerebrum

_____ / _____
r   s

- -

4. **encephal/o**–combining form meaning **brain**

The brain is one of the largest organs in body; center for thought, memory, judgment, and emotion; coordinates most body activities; four sections of brain are **cerebrum**, **cerebellum**, **thalamus**, and **brainstem**; each section performs specific duties; right side of brain controls left side of body and left side of brain controls right side of body (see again Figures 14.1 and 14.2)

14.4 The brain

a. pertaining to brain

_____ / _____
r   s

b. record of electricity of brain

_____ / _____ / _____ / _____ / _____
r   cv   r   cv   s

c. process of recording electricity of brain

_____ / _____ / _____ / _____ / _____
r   cv   r   cv   s

d. brain pain

_____ / _____
r   s

e. brain inflammation

_____ / _____
r   s

f. brain disease
　　　　　　/　　　　　　/　　　　　
　　　　　　r　　　　cv　　　　s

g. brain tumor
　　　　　　/　　　　　　　　　　
　　　　　　r　　　　　　　s

h. abnormal softening of brain
　　　　　　/　　　　　　/　　　　　
　　　　　　r　　　　cv　　　　s

i. hardening of brain
　　　　　　/　　　　　　/　　　　　
　　　　　　r　　　　cv　　　　s

---

5. **-esthesia**–suffix meaning **feeling, sensation**

   a. without sensation
　　　　　　/　　　　　　　　　　
　　　　　　p　　　　　　s

   b. excessive sensations
　　　　　　/　　　　　　　　　　
　　　　　　p　　　　　　s

---

6. **medull/o**–combining form meaning **medulla oblongata**
   Medulla oblongata is part of brainstem; most inferior region of brain; connects rest of brain to spinal cord; contains control centers for respiration, heart rate, temperature, and blood pressure (see again Figure 14.2)

   a. pertaining to medulla oblongata
　　　　　　/　　　　　　　　　　
　　　　　　r　　　　　　s

---

7. **mening/o**–combining form meaning **meninges**
   Meninges form three-layer protective sac around brain and spinal cord; outer layer is **dura mater**, middle layer is **arachnoid layer**, inner layer is **pia mater**; cerebrospinal fluid circulates around outside of brain and spinal cord in subarachnoid space (between arachnoid layer and pia mater)

   Skin
   Bone of skull
   Dura mater
   Subdural space
   Arachnoid layer
   Subarachnoid space
   Pia mater
   Brain

   14.5 The meninges

   a. pertaining to meninges
　　　　　　/　　　　　　　　　　
　　　　　　r　　　　　　s

   b. meninges inflammation
　　　　　　/　　　　　　　　　　
　　　　　　r　　　　　　s

   c. meninges and spinal cord inflammation
　　　　　　/　　　　　/　　　　　/　　　　
　　　　　r　　　cv　　　r　　　s

---

8. myel/o–combining form meaning **spinal cord**

Spinal cord is a column of nervous tissue; extends from medulla oblongata to approximately second lumbar vertebra; provides path for messages traveling to and from brain; incoming sensory information enters **gray matter** of spinal cord on dorsal side via **dorsal roots** and rises to brain within **ascending tracts**, which are located in the **white matter**; outgoing motor commands travel from brain by **descending tracts**, which are also located in the white matter, and exit spinal cord from ventral-side gray matter via **ventral roots** (see again Figure 14.1)

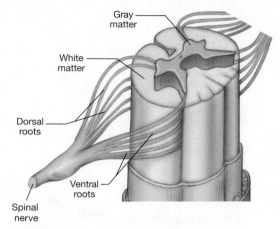

Gray matter

White matter

Dorsal roots

Ventral roots

Spinal nerve

14.6 Cross-section of spinal cord

a. record of spinal cord

_____ / _____ / _____
r   cv   s

b. process of recording spinal cord

_____ / _____ / _____
r   cv   s

c. spinal cord inflammation

_____ / _____
r   s

d. abnormal softening of spinal cord

_____ / _____ / _____
r   cv   s

e. spinal cord and nerve inflammation

_____ / _____ / _____ / _____
r   cv   r   s

f. spinal cord disease

_____ / _____ / _____
r   cv   s

g. hardening of spinal cord

_____ / _____ / _____
r   cv   s

h. cutting into spinal cord

_____ / _____
r   s

---

9. neur/o–combining form meaning **nerve**

A nerve is a cordlike bundle of neurons carrying messages between CNS and muscles and organs of body; **sensory nerves** carry information to CNS; **motor nerves** carry messages from CNS to muscles and organs; there are 12 pairs of **cranial nerves** attached to the brain and 31 pairs of **spinal nerves** attached to the spinal cord (see again Figure 14.1)

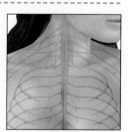

14.7 Nerves

a. pertaining to nerves

_____ / _____
r   s

b. nerve pain

_____ / _____
r   s

c. surgical removal of a nerve

_____ / _____
r   s

d. study of nerves

_____/_____/_____
                    r   cv   s

e. one who studies nerves

_____/_____/_____
                    r   cv   s

f. nerve tumor

_____/_____
                    r   s

g. nerve disease

_____/_____/_____
                    r   cv   s

h. surgical repair of nerve

_____/_____/_____
                    r   cv   s

i. inflammation of many nerves

_____/_____/_____
     p   r   s

j. suture a nerve

_____/_____/_____
                    r   cv   s

---

10. -phasia–suffix meaning **speech**

a. without speech

_____/_____
                    p   s

b. difficult, abnormal speech

_____/_____
                    p   s

---

11. -plegia–suffix meaning **paralysis**

a. paralysis of one (limb)

_____/_____
                    p   s

b. paralysis of two (limbs)

_____/_____
                    p   s

c. paralysis of four (limbs)

_____/_____
                    p   s

d. half paralysis

_____/_____
                    p   s

e. nerve paralysis

_____/_____/_____
                    r   cv   s

f. paralysis of two like parts of a pair (lower limbs)

_____/_____
                    p   s

---

12. pont/o–combining form meaning **pons**

The pons is another part of the brainstem; connects cerebellum to rest of brain (see again Figure 14.2)

a. pertaining to pons

_____/_____
                    r   s

b. pertaining to pons and cerebellum

_____/_____/_____/_____
     r   cv   r   s

c. pertaining to pons and medulla oblongata

_____/_____/_____/_____
     r   cv   r   s

13. thalam/o–combining form meaning **thalamus**

Thalamus is part of brain located just below bulk of cerebrum; relays incoming sensory information to correct area of cerebrum (see again Figure 14.2)

a. pertaining to thalamus   _____ / _____
                                                          r   *s*

b. cutting into thalamus   _____ / _____
                                                          r   *s*

Neurology Vocabulary

The neurology terms presented in this section include eponyms, modern English words, and those that contain Latin or Greek word parts but are not constructed solely from these word parts. When you recognize word parts within a term, they will give you a hint about the word's meaning. In these instances, look for the word parts to follow the term.

Term	Explanation
Alzheimer disease	Chronic brain condition involving progressive disorientation, speech and gait disturbances, and loss of memory
amyotrophic lateral sclerosis (ALS) **a-** = without **my/o** = muscle **-trophic** = development **scler/o** = hardening **-osis** = abnormal condition	Disease with muscular weakness and atrophy due to degeneration of motor neurons of spinal cord; commonly called *Lou Gehrig disease*
anticonvulsant **anti-** = against	Medication to reduce excitability of neurons and to prevent uncontrolled neuron activity associated with seizures
brain tumor	Intracranial mass, either benign or malignant; benign tumor of brain can still be fatal because it will grow and cause pressure on normal brain tissue

Glioma

A   **B**

14.8 (A) Illustration of a large brain tumor and (B) PET scan image revealing brain tumor in the frontal lobe of the brain
Source: (B) Courtesy of Dr. Giovanni DiChiro and Dr. Ramesh Raman of the Neuroimaging Branch, National Institute of Neurological Disorders and Stroke, National Institutes of Health.

Term	Explanation
cerebral contusion **cerebr/o** = cerebrum **-al** = pertaining to	Bruising of brain from impact; symptoms last longer than 24 hours and include unconsciousness, dizziness, vomiting, unequal pupil size, and shock **TERMINOLOGY TIDBIT** The term *contusion* comes from the Latin word *contundere* meaning "to bruise or crush."
cerebral palsy (CP) **cerebr/o** = cerebrum **-al** = pertaining to	Nonprogressive brain damage resulting from defect in fetal development or trauma or oxygen deprivation during or shortly after birth **TERMINOLOGY TIDBIT** The term *palsy* comes from the Old French word *paralisie* meaning "paralysis."
cerebrospinal fluid analysis **cerebr/o** = cerebrum **spin/o** = spine **-al** = pertaining to	Laboratory examination of clear, watery, colorless fluid from within brain and spinal cord; detects infections or bleeding of brain
cerebrovascular accident (CVA) **cerebr/o** = cerebrum **vascul/o** = blood vessels **-ar** = pertaining to	Development of brain infarct due to loss in blood supply to brain; can be caused by ruptured blood vessel (hemorrhage), floating clot (embolus), stationary clot (thrombosis), or compression; extent of damage depends on size and location of infarct and can include dysphasia and hemiplegia; commonly called *stroke* Cerebral hemorrhage: cerebral artery ruptures and bleeds into brain tissue Cerebral embolism: embolus from another area lodges in cerebral artery and blocks blood flow Cerebral thrombosis: blood clot forms in cerebral artery and blocks blood flow Compression: pressure from tumor squeezes adjacent blood vessel and blocks blood flow **14.9** The four common causes of cerebrovascular accidents: hemorrhage, embolism, thrombosis, and compression
coma	Profound unconsciousness or stupor resulting from illness or injury **TERMINOLOGY TIDBIT** The term *coma* comes from the Greek word *koma* meaning "deep sleep or trance."

Term	Explanation
computed tomography (CT scan) **tom/o** = to cut **-graphy** = process of recording	Diagnostic imaging technique that produces a cross-sectional view of body; X-rays taken from multiple angles are compiled by a computer to construct a composite cross-sectional view of the body **14.10** CT scan of brain showing multiple brain tumors Source: Semnic/Shutterstock
concussion	Injury to brain when brain is shaken inside skull because of impact; symptoms last 24 hours or less and can include dizziness, vomiting, unequal pupil size, and shock **TERMINOLOGY TIDBIT** The term *concussion* comes from the Latin word *concutere* meaning "to shake violently."
dementia	Progressive impairment of intellectual function that interferes with performing activities of daily living
epilepsy	Recurrent disorder of brain; seizures and loss of consciousness occur as result of uncontrolled neuron electrical activity **TERMINOLOGY TIDBIT** The term *epilepsy* comes from the Greek word *epilepsia* meaning "seizure or attack."
hydrocephalus **hydr/o** = water **cephal/o** = head	Buildup of cerebrospinal fluid within brain; if congenital, causes head to enlarge; treated by creating shunt from brain to abdomen to drain excess fluid **A** Bulging fontanel / Enlarged ventricles / Blocked aqueduct **B** Catheter tip in ventricle / Valve / Shunt **14.11** (A) A child with the enlarged ventricles of hydrocephalus; (B) the same child with a shunt to send the excess cerebrospinal fluid to the abdominal cavity

Term	Explanation
lumbar puncture (LP) **lumb/o** = low back **-ar** = pertaining to	Puncture with needle into lumbar vertebral area (usually space between fourth and fifth lumbar vertebrae) to withdraw fluid for examination or for injection of medication; also called *spinal puncture* or *spinal tap*

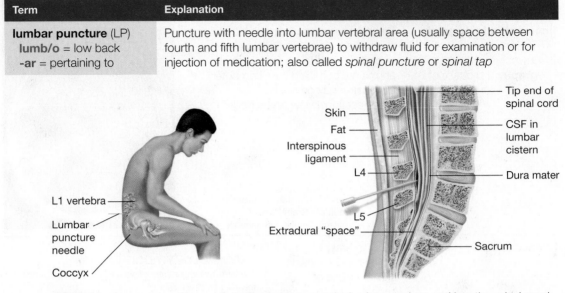

14.12 A lumbar puncture: the needle is inserted between the lumbar vertebrae and into the spinal canal

Term	Explanation
migraine	Specific type of headache characterized by severe head pain, sensitivity to light, dizziness, and nausea
multiple sclerosis (MS) **scler/o** = hardening **-osis** = abnormal condition	Inflammatory autoimmune disease of central nervous system; immune system damages myelin around neurons and results in extreme weakness and numbness
myasthenia gravis **my/o** = muscle **-asthenia** = weakness	Autoimmune disease with severe muscular weakness and fatigue due to difficulty of electrical impulse passing across synapse from one nerve to the next
paralysis	Temporary or permanent loss of muscle function and movement
Parkinson disease	Chronic disorder of the nervous system with fine tremors, muscular weakness, rigidity, and shuffling gait
positron emission tomography (PET)	Diagnostic imaging technique that uses positive radionuclides to reconstruct brain sections; measurement of oxygen and glucose uptake, cerebral blood flow, and blood volume can be taken; amount of glucose brain uses indicates its metabolic activity (see again Figure 14.6B)
seizure	Sudden, uncontrollable onset of symptoms, such as in epileptic seizure; *absence seizure* (petit mal seizure) appears as loss of awareness and absence of activity; *tonic-clonic seizure* (grand mal seizure) is characterized by muscle convulsions
shingles	Eruption of painful blisters on the body along nerve path; thought to be caused by varicella zoster virus infection of nerve root; also called *herpes zoster*

TERMINOLOGY TIDBIT

The term *shingles* comes from the Latin word *cingulum* meaning "girdle." This word describes how the blisters form in a line that encircles the body.

Term	Explanation
spina bifida	Congenital defect in walls of spinal canal in which two sides of vertebra do not meet or close; can result in *meningocele* or *myelomeningocele*

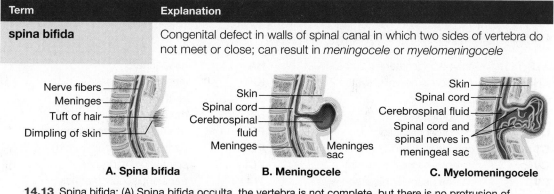

A. Spina bifida **B. Meningocele** **C. Myelomeningocele**

14.13 Spina bifida: (A) Spina bifida occulta, the vertebra is not complete, but there is no protrusion of nervous system structures; (B) meningocele, the meninges protrude through the opening in the vertebra; (C) myelomeningocele, the meninges and spinal cord protrude through the opening in the vertebra

Term	Explanation
spinal cord injury (SCI) **spin/o** = spine **-al** = pertaining to	Damage to spinal cord as result of trauma; spinal cord can be bruised or completely severed
subdural hematoma **sub-** = beneath, under **-al** = pertaining to **hemat/o** = blood **-oma** = mass, tumor	Mass of blood forming underneath dura mater when meninges are torn by trauma; can exert fatal pressure on brain if hematoma is not drained by surgery

— Torn cerebral vein
— Subdural hematoma
— Compressed brain tissue
— Dura mater
— Arachnoid layer

14.14 A subdural hematoma: a meningeal vein has ruptured and blood has accumulated in the subdural space, producing pressure on the brain

Term	Explanation
syncope	Fainting

> **TERMINOLOGY TIDBIT**
> The term *syncope* comes from the Greek word *sunkope* meaning "to cut short or swoon."

Term	Explanation
transient ischemic attack (TIA) **-ic** = pertaining to	Temporary reduction of blood supply to brain; causes temporary symptoms such as syncope, numbness, and hemiplegia; can eventually lead to cerebrovascular accident

Neurology Abbreviations

The following list presents common neurology abbreviations.

ALS	amyotrophic lateral sclerosis	**HA**	headache
ANS	autonomic nervous system	**ICP**	intracranial pressure
CNS	central nervous system	**LP**	lumbar puncture
CP	cerebral palsy	**MS**	multiple sclerosis
CSF	cerebrospinal fluid	**PET**	positron emission tomography
CT scan	computed tomography scan	**PNS**	peripheral nervous system
CVA	cerebrovascular accident	**SCI**	spinal cord injury
CVD	cerebrovascular disease	**TIA**	transient ischemic attack
EEG	electroencephalogram, electroencephalography		

CASE STUDY

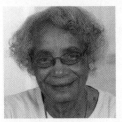

Source: Brian Eichhorn/ Shutterstock

History of Present Illness
A 73-year-old African American female is brought to the ER via ambulance. She was found lying on the floor of her kitchen by her daughter. Patient is awake but unable to speak or move her left extremities. Daughter reports she has witnessed her mother have two short spells of numbness and clumsiness with her left hand over the past three months. She urged her mother to see her family physician but does not believe she has followed through. Medication for hypertension and NSAIDs for arthritis were brought to ER by the daughter, who states she believes her mother is hoarding her medication and not taking it as often as prescribed.

Past Medical History
Hypertension; arthritis in right hip requiring occasional use of quad cane for walking long distances; had hysterectomy at age 46 for endometriosis.

Family and Social History
Patient is widowed and lives alone. She is a retired school bus driver. Daughter reports she is active in her church and tends a large vegetable garden each year. Multiple family members are hypertensive, but history is negative for neurological diseases.

Physical Examination
Patient is awake and calm. She is unable to answer any questions and does not follow any commands for moving left extremities and does not spontaneously move left extremities. Follows all commands with right extremities, and muscle strength appears normal for her age. Her blood pressure was 168/108.

Diagnostic Imaging
MRI of head shows area of cerebral hemorrhage on right side of brain. X-rays of head, spine, and hips were negative for fractures.

Diagnosis
Right CVA with left hemiplegia

Plan of Treatment
1. Admit to ICU and monitor for additional bleeding and worsening of symptoms
2. Aggressive medical treatment to reduce blood pressure

3. Begin rehabilitation with PT, OT, and speech therapy
4. Referral to medical social worker to begin discussions with patient, family, and rehabilitation therapists to determine alternate living arrangements

Critical Thinking Questions

Answer the following questions regarding this case study. Do not just copy words out of the case study but translate all medical terms. To answer some of these questions, you may need to look up information from another chapter of this text, in a medical dictionary, or online. Answers are found at the back of the book.

1. In ER the patient was unable to speak or move the left extremities. What are the medical terms for these symptoms?

   _____

   _____

2. The patient's daughter reported that her mother has had short spells of numbness and clumsiness with the left hand. Review the conditions described in the Neurology Vocabulary and suggest a possible name for these episodes.

   _____

   _____

3. Which of the following is NOT one of the patient's previous medical diagnoses and operations?
   a. Endometrial tissue found throughout pelvic cavity
   b. High blood pressure
   c. Stomach protruding through hole in diaphragm
   d. Joint pain

4. What are NSAIDs, and why was this patient taking them? (*Hint*: Check the orthopedics chapter.)

   _____

   _____

5. Define the following abbreviations used in this medical record: ER, MRI, ICU, PT, OT.

   _____

   _____

6. Why do you think taking skeletal X-rays was a necessary part of this patient's evaluation?

   _____

   _____

7. Explain why the bleeding was found on the right side of the brain, but the paralysis was of the left extremities.

   _____

   _____

PRACTICE

Sound It Out

The following are some of the key terms from this chapter written as their phonetic spelling. Sound out each term and write it in the blank. Pronunciations for all terms are included in the audio glossary at www.mymedicalterminologylab.com.

1. men-in-JYE-tis _____

2. noo-ROH-mah _____

3. ah-FAY-zee-ah _____

4. SER-eh-broh-mah-LAY-she-ah _____

5. en SEFF-ah-low-skle-ROH-sis _____

6. kon-KUSH-un _____

7. en-seff-ah-LYE-tis _____

8. dee-MEN-she-ah _____

9. an-es-THEE-zee-ah _____

10. dis-FAY-zee-ah _____

11. MY-eh-LOP-ah-thee _____

12. noo-REK-toh-mee _____

13. EP-ih-lep-see _____

14. hem-ee-PLEE-jee-ah _____

15. high-droh-SEFF-ah-lus _____

16. meh-NING-goh-seel _____

17. MY-grain _____

18. my-eh-LOG-rah-fee _____

19. NOOR-oh-plas-tee _____

20. pah-RAL-ih-sis _____

21. en-seff-ah-LOW-mah _____

22. pol-ee-noo-RYE-tis _____

23. my-eh-LYE-tis _____

24. SER-eh-broh-VASS-kyoo-lar _____

25. SIN-koh-pee _____

Transcription Practice

Each of the following sentences is written in common English. Underline any words or phrases that can be replaced by a medical term. Then rewrite the entire sentence using medical terms. Answers can be found at the back of the book.

1. Jon took medication to reduce neuron excitability to control his epileptic sudden, uncontrolled onset of symptoms.

   _____

   _____

2. As a result of the development of a brain infarct due to loss in blood supply, Mr. van Pelt was in a profound state of unconsciousness.

   _____

   _____

3. The auto accident victim developed paralysis of all four limbs following a severing of the spinal cord as a result of trauma.

_____

_____

4. During the temporary reduction of blood supply to the brain, Mr. Edelstein had the inability to speak.

_____

_____

5. Ilina's paralysis of one limb was caused by an inflammatory autoimmune disease of the central nervous system.

_____

_____

6. Antonio went to the physician who studies nerves because he was having severe headaches with sensitivity to light, dizziness, and nausea.

_____

_____

7. An image made using positive radionuclides was completed to see whether the tumor was in the largest part of the brain or the second largest part of the brain.

_____

_____

8. A puncture with a needle into the lumbar vertebral area was performed to analyze cerebrospinal fluid for signs of brain inflammation.

_____

_____

9. Mr. Larsen's severe leg pain was caused by inflammation of many nerves.

_____

_____

10. The elderly gentleman with chronic brain condition involving progressive speech and gait disturbances and loss of memory eventually developed impaired intellectual function that interfered with activities of daily living.

_____

_____

Labeling Exercise

Write the name of each structure on the numbered line. Also use this space to write the combining form where appropriate.

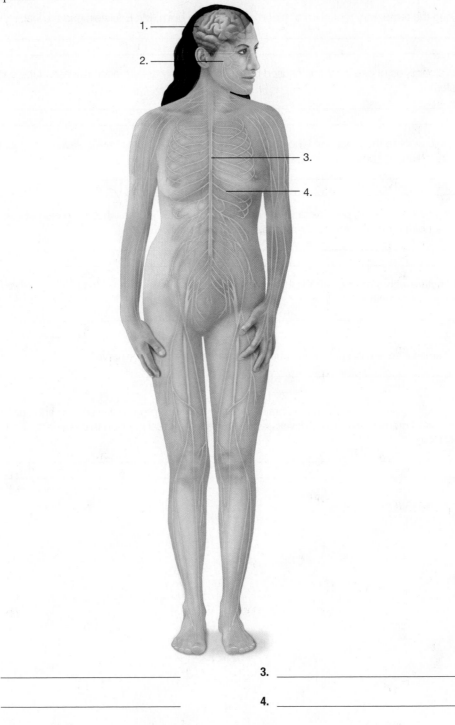

1. _____

2. _____

3. _____

4. _____

Build Medical Terms

Use each of the following word parts to build the indicated medical terms.

The combining form *neur/o* means nerve.

1. nerve pain _____

2. nerve tumor _____

3. study of nerves _____

4. surgical repair of nerves _____

5. nerve disease _____

The combining form *thalam/o* means thalamus.

6. pertaining to thalamus _____

7. cutting into thalamus _____

The suffix *-plegia* means paralysis.

8. paralysis of two (limbs) _____

9. half paralysis _____

The combining form *mening/o* means meninges.

10. pertaining to meninges _____

11. meninges inflammation _____

The combining form *myel/o* means spinal cord.

12. record of spinal cord _____

13. abnormal softening of spinal cord _____

14. spinal cord hardening _____

15. spinal cord inflammation _____

MyMedicalTerminologyLab™

MyMedicalTerminologyLab is a premium online homework management system that includes a host of features to help you study. Registered users will find:

- A multitude of activities and assignments built within the MyLab platform
- Powerful tools that track and analyze your results—allowing you to create a personalized learning experience
- Videos and audio pronunciations to help enrich your progress
- Streaming lesson presentations and self-paced learning modules
- A space where you and your instructors can view and manage your assignments

Fill in the Blank

Fill in the blank to complete each of the following sentences.

1. Amyotrophic lateral sclerosis causes degeneration of the _____ of the spinal cord.

2. Because his dizziness and vomiting lasted less than 24 hours, Ali had a _____ rather than a cerebral _____,

3. The medical term for fainting is _____.

4. The four sections of the brain are the _____, _____, _____, and _____.

5. The protective sac around the brain and spinal cord is called the _____.

6. _____ is brain damage caused by trauma or oxygen deprivation during or shortly after birth.

7. A tonic-clonic seizure used to be called a _____ seizure.

8. _____ is due to electrical impulses having difficulty crossing synapses from one nerve to the next.

9. _____ disease is recognized by fine tremors, muscular weakness, rigidity, and a shuffling gait.

10. _____ is caused by a *herpes zoster* virus of a nerve root.

Abbreviation Matching

Match each abbreviation with its definition.

_____ **1.** LP	**A.**	electroencephalogram
_____ **2.** MS	**B.**	transient ischemic attack
_____ **3.** PNS	**C.**	multiple sclerosis
_____ **4.** EEG	**D.**	cerebral palsy
_____ **5.** SCI	**E.**	amyotrophic lateral sclerosis
_____ **6.** TIA	**F.**	spinal cord injury
_____ **7.** CSF	**G.**	intracranial pressure
_____ **8.** CP	**H.**	lumbar puncture
_____ **9.** ICP	**I.**	cerebrospinal fluid
_____ **10.** ALS	**J.**	peripheral nervous system

Medical Term Analysis

Examine each of the following terms. Begin by dividing it into its word parts and writing them in the indicated blanks (*P = prefix*; *WR = word root*; *CF = combining form*; *S = suffix*). Follow with the definition of each word part and then finally the meaning of the full term.

1. **cerebellar**

   WR _____

   means _____

   S _____

   means _____

   Term meaning: _____

   _____

2. **meningocele**

   CF _____

   means _____

   S _____

   means _____

   Term meaning: _____

   _____

3. **cerebrospinal**

   CF _____

   means _____

   WR _____

   means _____

   S _____

   means _____

   Term meaning: _____

   _____

4. **anesthesia**

   P _____

   means _____

   S _____

   means _____

   Term meaning: _____

   _____

5. **meningomyelitis**

   CF _____

   means _____

   WR _____

   means _____

   S _____

   means _____

   Term meaning: _____

   _____

6. **encephaloma**

   WR _____

   means _____

   S _____

   means _____

   Term meaning: _____

   _____

7. dysphasia

P _____

means _____

S _____

means _____

Term meaning: _____

_____

8. neurology

CF _____

means _____

S _____

means _____

Term meaning: _____

_____

9. pontomedullary

CF _____

means _____

WR _____

means _____

S _____

means _____

Term meaning: _____

_____

10. cerebrotomy

WR _____

means _____

S _____

means _____

Term meaning: _____

_____

Spelling

Some of the following terms are misspelled. Identify the incorrect terms and spell them correctly in the blank provided.

1. neurorhaphy _____

2. encephalalgia _____

3. cerebromalacia _____

4. meningoitis _____

5. quadraplegia _____

6. pontine _____

7. electroencepalography _____

8. hydrocephalus _____

9. myesthenia gravis _____

10. syncope _____

Photomatch Challenge

Each combining form below stands for an area of the central nervous system. Write the name of the area in the blank following the combining form. Then translate the medical term on the second line.

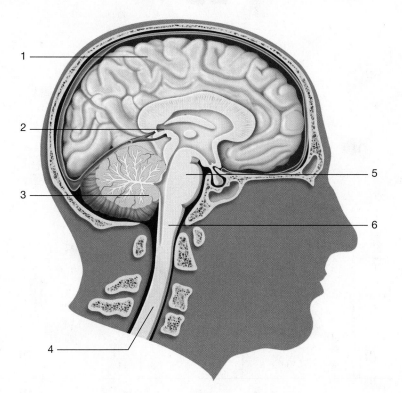

Word Bank:

1. cerebr/o _____

cerebromalacia _____

2. thalam/o _____

thalamotomy _____

3. cerebell/o _____

cerebellitis _____

4. myel/o _____

myelogram _____

5. pont/o _____

pontine _____

6. medull/o _____

medullary _____

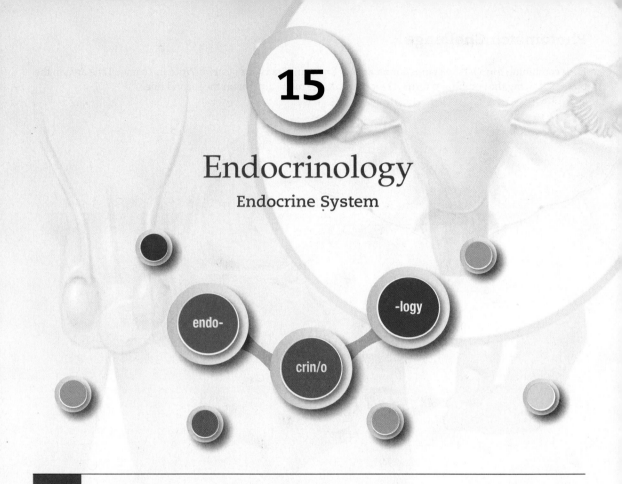

15

Endocrinology

Endocrine System

endo-

crin/o

-logy

Learning Objectives

Upon completion of this chapter, you will be able to:

15-1 Describe the medical specialty of endocrinology.

15-2 Understand the function of the endocrine system.

15-3 Define endocrinology-related combining forms, prefixes, and suffixes.

15-4 Identify the organs treated in endocrinology.

15-5 Build endocrinology medical terms from word parts.

15-6 Explain endocrinology medical terms.

15-7 Use endocrinology abbreviations.

A Brief Introduction to Endocrinology

Endocrinology is a subspecialty of internal medicine. **Endocrinologists** diagnose and treat diseases and conditions that develop as a result of a hormone imbalance. If a gland releases too much hormone, **hypersecretion**, or too little hormone, **hyposecretion**, the target organ functions improperly because it did not receive the correct message.

The **endocrine system** plays a vital role in maintaining **homeostasis**, a stable internal body environment. This system consists of a group of **glands** that secrete chemical messengers called **hormones** directly into the bloodstream. Hormones travel through the blood to **target organs** to adjust their activity to regulate factors such as growth, reproduction, metabolic rate, bone growth, and sugar levels. The endocrine system is made up of the following: two **adrenal glands**, two **ovaries** in the female, four **parathyroid glands**, the **pancreas**, the **pineal gland**, the **pituitary gland**, two **testes** in the male, the **thymus gland**, and the **thyroid gland**.

> **TERMINOLOGY TIDBIT**
> The term *endocrine* literally means "to secrete within." This describes how these glands release their chemicals into the inside of the body by secreting directly into the bloodstream. On the other hand, exocrine glands, such as sweat glands, release their secretions to the outside of the body.

Endocrinology Combining Forms

The following list presents combining forms closely associated with the endocrine system and used for building and defining endocrinology terms.

aden/o	gland	pancreat/o	pancreas
adren/o	adrenal gland	parathyroid/o	parathyroid gland
adrenal/o	adrenal gland	pineal/o	pineal gland
crin/o	to secrete	pituitar/o	pituitary gland
glyc/o	sugar	testicul/o	testes
glycos/o	sugar	thym/o	thymus gland
oophor/o	ovary	thyr/o	thyroid gland
orchi/o	testes	thyroid/o	thyroid gland
ovari/o	ovary		

The following list presents combining forms that are not specific to the endocrine system but are also used for building and defining endocrinology terms.

acr/o	extremities	ophthalm/o	eye
carcin/o	cancer	toxic/o	poison
cyt/o	cell		

Suffix Review

These suffixes introduced in Chapter 2 are being reviewed in this chapter because they are especially important for building endocrinology terms.

-al	pertaining to	-logy	study of
-an	pertaining to	-malacia	abormal softening
-ar	pertaining to	-megaly	enlarged
-centesis	puncture to withdraw fluid	-oid	resembling
-cyte	cell	-oma	tumor, mass
-dipsia	thirst	-osis	abnormal condition
-ectomy	surgical removal	-otomy	cutting into
-edema	swelling	-pathy	disease
-emia	blood condition	-pexy	surgical fixation
-ic	pertaining to	-plasty	surgical repair
-ism	state of	-rrhexis	rupture
-itis	inflammation	-uria	urine condition
-logist	one who studies		

Prefix Review

These prefixes introduced in Chapter 3 are being reviewed here because they are especially important for building endocrinology terms.

endo-	within, inner		**hypo-**	below, insufficient
ex-	outward		**poly-**	many
hyper-	excessive			

Organs Commonly Treated in Endocrinology

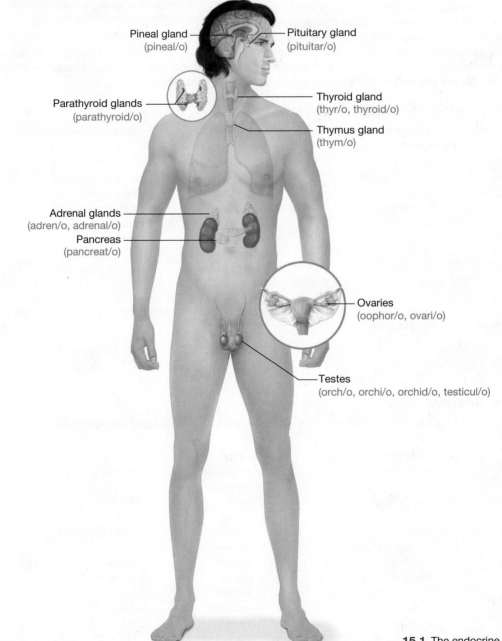

Pineal gland (pineal/o)

Pituitary gland (pituitar/o)

Parathyroid glands (parathyroid/o)

Thyroid gland (thyr/o, thyroid/o)

Thymus gland (thym/o)

Adrenal glands (adren/o, adrenal/o)

Pancreas (pancreat/o)

Ovaries (oophor/o, ovari/o)

Testes (orch/o, orchi/o, orchid/o, testicul/o)

15.1 The endocrine system

Building Endocrinology Terms

This section presents word parts most often used to build endocrinology terms. Following the explanation of the term, you have the opportunity to begin building your own vocabulary. Read the meaning for each term and then fill in the blanks to build a single medical term. Use the slashes to divide prefixes, word roots, combining vowels, and suffixes. To help you out you will find a key to the word parts underneath the blanks: **r** for word roots, **p** for prefix, **cv** for combining vowel, and **s** for suffix. Remember that not every term will contain all these word parts; it's up to you to decide which to use. As you gain experience, this process becomes easier. Answers can be found at the back of the book.

1. **aden/o**–combining form meaning **gland**

   A gland is a group of cells that work together to produce and secrete substances such as hormones; endocrine glands secrete their substances (hormones) directly into the bloodstream; exocrine glands, such as sweat glands, secrete into a duct

   a. cancerous tumor in gland
   _____/_____/_____/_____
                r   *cv*   *r*   *s*

   b. gland cell
   _____/_____/_____
                r   *cv*   *s*

   c. resembling gland
   _____/_____
                r   *s*

   d. abnormal softening of gland
   _____/_____/_____
                r   *cv*   *s*

---

2. **adren/o**–combining form meaning **adrenal gland**

   Each of two adrenal glands sits on top of a kidney; divided into outer **adrenal cortex** and inner **adrenal medulla**; adrenal cortex secretes **aldosterone** to regulate sodium levels in the body, **cortisol** to regulate carbohydrate metabolism, and sex hormones such as **estrogen** and **testosterone**; adrenal medulla secretes **epinephrine** (also called *adrenaline*) to help body respond to emergency situations (see again Figure 15.1)

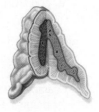

   15.2 The adrenal gland

   > **TERMINOLOGY TIDBIT**
   > The term *cortex* is frequently used in anatomy to indicate the outer portion of an organ such as the adrenal gland or the kidney. The word *cortex* is Latin and means "bark" as in the bark of a tree. The word *medulla* means "marrow." Because marrow is found in the inner cavity of bones, the term came to stand for the middle of an organ.

   a. pertaining to the adrenal gland
   _____/_____
                r   *s*

   b. enlarged adrenal gland
   _____/_____/_____
                r   *cv*   *s*

---

3. **adrenal/o**–combining form meaning **adrenal gland**

   a. surgical removal of adrenal gland
   _____/_____
                r   *s*

   b. adrenal gland inflammation
   _____/_____
                r   *s*

   c. adrenal gland disease
   _____/_____/_____
                r   *cv*   *s*

---

4. **crin/o**–combining form meaning **to secrete**

Refers to glands releasing substances such as hormones

a. study of (the glands that) secrete within

_____/_____/_____/_____
     p   *r*   *cv*   *s*

b. one who studies (the glands that) secrete within

_____/_____/_____/_____
     p   *r*   *cv*   *s*

c. tumor that secretes within

_____/_____/_____
     p   *r*   *s*

d. disease that secretes within

_____/_____/_____/_____
     p   *r*   *cv*   *s*

---

5. **glyc/o**–combining form meaning **sugar**

Even though this combining form means sugar, it usually refers to **glucose**, the primary sugar the body uses for energy production

a. excessive sugar blood condition

_____/_____/_____
     p   *r*   *s*

b. insufficient sugar blood condition

_____/_____/_____
     p   *r*   *s*

---

6. **glycos/o**–combining form meaning **sugar**

a. condition of sugar in urine

_____/_____
               r   *s*

---

7. **oophor/o**–combining form meaning **ovary**

An ovary is one of a pair of almond-shaped organs in female pelvic cavity; releases ova for reproduction; secretes female sex hormones such as **estrogen** (produces female secondary sexual characteristics and regulates menstrual cycle) and **progesterone** (maintains uterine environment for pregnancy) (see again Figure 15.1)

a. ovary inflammation

_____/_____
               r   *s*

b. surgical repair of ovary

_____/_____/_____
               r   *cv*   *s*

c. cutting into ovary

_____/_____
               r   *s*

d. surgical removal of ovary

_____/_____
               r   *s*

---

8. **orchi/o**–combining form meaning **testes**

The testes (also called the **testicles**) are a pair of oval-shaped glands located in scrotum of males; singular forms are *testis* and *testicle*; release sperm for reproduction and male sex hormone **testosterone** (produces male secondary sexual characteristics and regulates sperm production) (see again Figure 15.1)

a. surgical removal of testes

_____/_____
               r   *s*

b. surgical fixation of testes

_____/_____/_____
               r   *cv*   *s*

c. cutting into testes

_____/_____
               r   *s*

---

9. **ovari/o**–combining form meaning **ovary**

   a. pertaining to ovary

   _____/_____
   r   s

   b. puncture of ovary to remove fluid

   _____/_____/_____
   r   cv   s

   c. ruptured ovary

   _____/_____/_____
   r   cv   s

- -

10. **pancreat/o**–combining form meaning **pancreas**

    Pancreas is located in abdominal cavity along lower curvature of stomach; is only gland that is both an endocrine and exocrine gland; endocrine cells, called **pancreatic islets** (or _islets of Langerhans_), secrete **insulin** and **glucagon** to regulate blood sugar levels; insulin lowers blood sugar levels by allowing sugar to enter individual cells; glucagon raises blood sugar by stimulating liver to release stored sugar back into the bloodstream; exocrine portion secretes digestive enzymes into the pancreatic duct, which carries them to the duodenum (see again Figure 15.1)

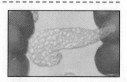

15.3 The pancreas

    a. pertaining to pancreas

    _____/_____
    r   s

    b. surgical removal of pancreas

    _____/_____
    r   s

    c. pancreas inflammation

    _____/_____
    r   s

    d. cutting into pancreas

    _____/_____
    r   s

- -

11. **parathyroid/o**–combining form meaning **parathyroid gland**

    Parathyroid glands are four small glands located on posterior surface of thyroid gland; secrete **parathyroid hormone** to raise blood levels of calcium (see again Figure 15.1)

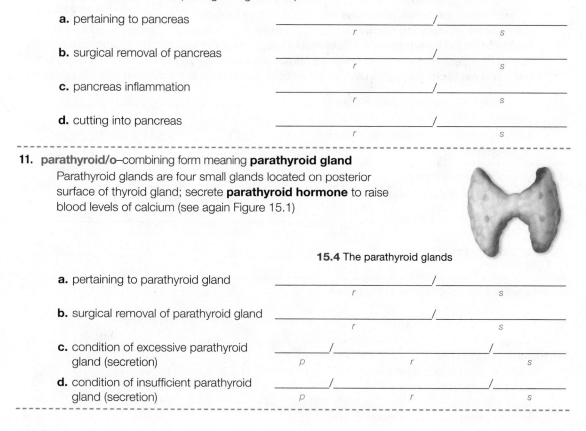

15.4 The parathyroid glands

    a. pertaining to parathyroid gland

    _____/_____
    r   s

    b. surgical removal of parathyroid gland

    _____/_____
    r   s

    c. condition of excessive parathyroid gland (secretion)

    _____/_____/_____
    p   r   s

    d. condition of insufficient parathyroid gland (secretion)

    _____/_____/_____
    p   r   s

- -

12. pineal/o–combining form meaning **pineal gland**

The pineal gland is a small pine cone-shaped gland in thalamus region of brain; secretes **melatonin**, which plays a role in regulating body's circadian rhythm (24-hour clock) (see again Figure 15.1)

15.5 The pineal gland

    a. surgical removal of pineal gland   _____/_____
                                                             r   *s*

---

13. pituitar/o–combining form meaning **pituitary gland**

Pituitary gland is a small marble-shaped gland that hangs down from underside of brain; often referred to as *master gland* because some of its hormones regulate other endocrine glands; divided into **anterior lobe** and **posterior lobe**; anterior lobe secretes **growth hormone** (stimulates body to grow larger), **thyroid-stimulating hormone** (regulates activity of thyroid gland), **adrenocorticotropic hormone** (regulates activity of adrenal cortex), **prolactin** (stimulates milk production by breast), **melanocyte-stimulating hormone** (stimulates melanocytes to produce more melanin), and **follicle-stimulating hormone** and **luteinizing hormone** (work together to regulate activity of ovaries or testes); posterior lobe secretes **antidiuretic hormone** (regulates volume of water in body) and **oxytocin** (stimulates uterine contractions during labor and birth) (see again Figure 15.1)

15.6 The pituitary gland

    a. condition of insufficient pituitary gland (secretion)   _____/_____/_____
                                         p   *r*   *s*

    b. condition of excessive pituitary gland (secretion)   _____/_____/_____
                                         p   *r*   *s*

---

14. poly-–prefix meaning **many**

Often used to indicate "too much" of a substance

    a. many (too much) thirst   _____/_____
                                                 p   *s*

    b. many (too much) urine condition   _____/_____
                                                 p   *s*

---

15. testicul/o–combining form meaning **testes**

    a. pertaining to testes   _____/_____
                                       r   *s*

---

16. thym/o–combining form meaning **thymus gland**

Thymus gland is located in mediastinum of chest behind sternum and above heart; secretes **thymosin**, which is important for immune system's development; begins to shrink in size around puberty and eventually becomes replaced by fatty tissue (see again Figure 15.1)

15.7 The thymus gland

    a. pertaining to thymus gland   _____/_____
                                             r   *s*

    b. surgical removal of thymus gland   _____/_____
                                             r   *s*

c. thymus gland inflammation

_____/_____
r s

d. thymus gland tumor

_____/_____
r s

- -

17. thyr/o–combining form meaning **thyroid gland**

Thyroid gland is located in neck; has two lobes on either side of trachea; secretes **thyroxine** and **triiodothyronine**, which regulate body's metabolic rate; also secretes **calcitonin**, which lowers blood calcium levels (see again Figure 15.1)

15.8 The thyroid gland

a. enlarged thyroid gland

_____/_____/_____
r cv s

b. cutting into thyroid gland

_____/_____
r s

- -

18. thyroid/o–combining form meaning **thyroid gland**

a. pertaining to thyroid gland

_____/_____
r s

b. thyroid gland inflammation

_____/_____
r s

c. surgical removal of thyroid gland

_____/_____
r s

d. condition of excessive thyroid gland (secretion)

_____/_____/_____
p r s

e. condition of insufficient thyroid gland (secretion)

_____/_____/_____
p r s

Endocrinology Vocabulary

The endocrinology terms presented in this section include eponyms, modern English words, and those that contain Latin or Greek word parts but are not constructed solely from these word parts. When you recognize word parts within a term, they will give you a hint about the word's meaning. In these instances, look for the word parts to follow the term.

Term	Explanation
acromegaly **acr/o** = extremities **-megaly** = enlarged	Chronic condition developing in adults with excessive growth hormone; results in elongation and enlargement of bones of head and extremities **15.9** Series of pictures of a woman with acromegaly; as she ages, the bones of her hands and face grow larger, but she will not grow taller

Term	Explanation
adrenal feminization **adren/o** = adrenal gland **-al** = pertaining to	Development of female secondary sexual characteristics (such as breasts) in male as result of increased estrogen secretion by adrenal cortex
adrenal virilism **adren/o** = adrenal gland **-al** = pertaining to **-ism** = state of	Development of male secondary sexual characteristics (such as deeper voice and facial hair) in female as result of increased androgen secretion by adrenal cortex
blood serum test	Blood test to measure level of substances such as hormones in bloodstream; used to study function of endocrine glands
congenital hypothyroidism **hypo-** = insufficient **thyroid/o** = thyroid gland **-ism** = state of	Condition present at birth that results in lack of thyroid hormones; results in poor physical and mental development; formerly called *cretinism*
corticosteroids	In addition to its normal function, these hormones secreted by adrenal cortex also have strong anti-inflammatory action; can be used to treat severe chronic inflammatory diseases such as rheumatoid arthritis
Cushing syndrome	Condition resulting from hypersecretion of adrenal cortex; can be product of adrenal gland tumor; symptoms include weakness, edema, excess hair growth, skin discoloration, and osteoporosis
diabetes insipidus (DI)	Condition caused by insufficient antidiuretic hormone secreted by posterior lobe of pituitary gland; symptoms include polyuria and polydipsia
diabetes mellitus (DM)	Chronic disorder of sugar metabolism; symptoms include hyperglycemia and glycosuria; two different forms of diabetes mellitus: *insulin-dependent diabetes mellitus* (IDDM) or *type 1,* and *noninsulin-dependent diabetes mellitus* (NIDDM) or *type 2.*
dwarfism **-ism** = state of	Being excessively short in height; can result from lack of growth hormone
exophthalmos **ex-** = outward **ophthalm/o** = eye	Condition in which eyeballs protrude, such as in Graves disease; commonly caused by hypersecretion of thyroid hormones

TERMINOLOGY TIDBIT

The term *cretinism* comes from the French word *crestin,* which means "Christian." The intent of using this term was to remind people that persons with poor mental development were still people.

TERMINOLOGY TIDBIT

The term *diabetes* comes from the Greek word meaning "siphon" and was chosen to describe conditions in which large amounts of urine were excreted. The term *mellitus* comes from the Latin term meaning "sweet." Urine from persons with diabetes mellitus is sweet due to the large amount of glucose being released.

15.10 Exophthalmos, a common symptom of hyperthyroidism

Term	Explanation
fasting blood sugar (FBS)	Blood test to measure amount of sugar in bloodstream after a 12-hour fast
gigantism **-ism** = state of	Excessive growth of body due to hypersecretion of growth hormone in a child or teenager
glucose tolerance test (GTT)	Test for initial diagnosis of diabetes mellitus; patient is given dose of glucose; then blood samples are taken at regular intervals to determine patient's ability to use glucose properly
goiter	Enlargement of the thyroid gland **TERMINOLOGY TIDBIT** The term *goiter* comes from the Latin word *guttur* meaning "throat." This word was used to describe the greatly enlarged throat region seen in persons with a goiter. **15.11** A male with a very large goiter Source: Eugene Gordon/Pearson Education
Graves disease	Condition resulting from hypersecretion of thyroid hormones; symptoms include exophthalmos and goiter
Hashimoto disease	Chronic autoimmune form of thyroiditis, results in hyposecretion of thyroid hormones
hormone replacement therapy	Artificial replacement of hormones in patients with hyposecretion disorders; available in pill, injection, or adhesive skin patch forms
insulin-dependent diabetes mellitus (IDDM)	Also called *type 1 diabetes mellitus*; tends to develop early in life; pancreas stops producing insulin; can be autoimmune disease; patient must take insulin injections **15.12** (A) Female checking her blood sugar level with a glucometer before using an insulin pen (an insulin injection system); (B) A person wearing an insulin pump, which delivers small amounts of insulin throughout the day Source: (A) Ron May/Pearson Education (B) Michal Heron/Pearson Education
myxedema **-edema** = swelling	Condition resulting from hyposecretion of thyroid hormones in adult; symptoms include anemia, slow speech, swollen facial features, puffy and dry skin, drowsiness, and mental sluggishness

Term	Explanation
noninsulin-dependent diabetes mellitus (NIDDM)	Also called *type 2 diabetes mellitus*; typically develops later in life; pancreas produces normal to high levels of insulin but cells fail to respond; patients can take medication to improve insulin function
pheochromocytoma **cyt/o** = cell **-oma** = tumor	Usually benign tumor of adrenal medulla; secretes excessive amount of epinephrine; symptoms include anxiety, heart palpitations, dyspnea, hypertension, profuse sweating, headache, and nausea
radioactive iodine uptake (RAIU)	Test of thyroid function that measures how much radioactively tagged iodine is removed from the bloodstream by thyroid gland
radioimmunoassay (RIA)	Test used to measure levels of hormones in plasma of blood
tetany	Nerve irritability and painful muscle cramps resulting from hypocalcemia; hypoparathyroidism is one cause
thyroid function test (TFT)	Blood test to measure levels of thyroxine, triiodothyronine, and thyroid-stimulating hormone in the bloodstream to evaluate thyroid function
thyroid scan	Test in which radioactive iodine is administered and localizes in the thyroid gland; gland is visualized with scanning device; able to detect thyroid gland tumors

TERMINOLOGY TIDBIT

The term *tetany* comes from the Greek word *tetanos* meaning "muscular spasm."

— Goiter

15.13 Radioactive iodine concentrates in the neck of a patient with a goiter; the actual scan is superimposed on a line drawing of the neck region

Term	Explanation
thyrotoxicosis **thyr/o** = thyroid gland **toxic/o** = poison **-osis** = abnormal condition	Condition resulting from extreme hypersecretion of thyroid hormones; symptoms include rapid heart action, tremors, enlarged thyroid gland, exophthalmos, and weight loss

Endocrinology Abbreviations

The following list presents common endocrinology abbreviations.

ACTH	adrenocorticotropic hormone	**Na⁺**	sodium
ADH	antidiuretic hormone	**NIDDM**	noninsulin-dependent diabetes mellitus
DI	diabetes insipidus		
DM	diabetes mellitus	**NPH**	neutral protamine Hagedorn (insulin)
FBS	fasting blood sugar	**PRL**	prolactin
FSH	follicle-stimulating hormone	**PTH**	parathyroid hormone
GH	growth hormone	**RAIU**	radioactive iodine uptake
GTT	glucose tolerance test	**RIA**	radioimmunoassay
IDDM	insulin-dependent diabetes mellitus	**T₃**	triiodothyronine
K⁺	potassium	**T₄**	thyroxine
LH	luteinizing hormone	**TFT**	thyroid function test
MSH	melanocyte-stimulating hormone	**TSH**	thyroid-stimulating hormone

The abbreviations with subscripts are T_3 (triiodothyronine) and T_4 (thyroxine); superscripts are Na^+ (sodium) and K^+ (potassium).

CASE STUDY

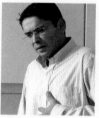

Source: Ronald Sumners/Shutterstock

History of Present Illness

A 32-year-old male presented to ER thinking he was having a heart attack. States he monitors his blood pressure at home because he has hypertension and it has been higher than normal today. Also reports elevated heart rate, heart palpitations, diaphoresis, hand tremors, and extreme anxiety. States his father died of heart attack in his 50s, and he is quite concerned he is having a heart attack.

Past Medical History

Tonsillectomy at age 7. Fractured right femur at age 12 in bicycle accident. Appendectomy at age 19. Currently taking blood pressure medication for mild hypertension.

Social and Family History

Patient has a sedentary job at an accounting firm. Works out three times a week for weight control. He does not smoke and reports drinking about three beers per week. He is married with no children. Father died at age 52 from myocardial infarction. Mother is alive and well.

Physical Examination

Male patient who appears stated age. He is alert and answers all questions appropriately. BP is 184/98, pulse is 110 bpm, RR is 22 breaths/min. Height is 5'11" and weight is 220 lb. He is sweating profusely. He denies any dyspnea; however, patient appears very anxious and unable to sit or lie still on examination table.

Diagnostic Procedures

EKG, cardiac enzymes, and CXR were normal.
Blood tests show increased epinephrine.
Abdominal MRI reveals tumor in right adrenal medulla.

Diagnosis

Probable pheochromocytoma, right adrenal medulla

Plan of Treatment
1. Additional medication to control hypertension and slow down heart rate was started
2. Scheduled appointment with endocrinologist for follow-up care consisting of biopsy to verify diagnosis and determine whether tumor is malignant or benign, continued medical control of symptoms, and surgical removal of tumor

Critical Thinking Questions
Answer the following questions regarding this case study. Do not just copy words out of the case study but translate all medical terms. To answer some of these questions, you may need to look up information from another chapter of this text, in a medical dictionary, or online. Answers are found at the back of the book.

1. List and briefly describe each of the patient's presenting symptoms in the ER.

2. Which of the following is NOT part of this patient's medical history?
   a. Broken arm bone
   b. Removal of tonsils
   c. Removal of appendix
   d. High blood pressure

3. Read the information found at the following National Institutes of Health website, www.nlm.nih.gov/medlineplus/ency/article/002341.htm, and look up the normal range for blood pressure, respiratory rate, and heart rate.

4. Define the following abbreviations: ER, EKG, CXR, BP, and bpm.

5. The patient's denial of dyspnea was noted; define the term.

6. What is the difference between malignant and benign?

7. What are the two purposes for performing a biopsy?

8. What is the term to describe the surgical removal of the adrenal gland?

Sound It Out

The following are some of the key terms from this chapter written as their phonetic spelling. Sound out each term and write it in the blank. Pronunciations for all terms are included in the audio glossary at www.mymedicalterminologylab.com.

1. thigh-roh-MEG-ah-lee _____
2. AD-eh-no-mah-LAY-she-ah _____
3. ad-ree-noh-MEG-ah-lee _____
4. PAN-kree-ah-TYE-tis _____
5. pair-ah-thigh-royd-EK-toh-mee _____
6. ak-roh-MEG-ah-lee _____
7. eks-off-THAL-mohs _____
8. ad-ree-nal-EK-toh-mee _____
9. glye-kohs-YOO-ree-ah _____
10. GOY-ter _____
11. or-kee-EK-toh-mee _____
12. HIGH-per-pih-TOO-ih-tuh-rizm _____
13. JYE-gan-tizm _____

14. high-poh-THIGH-royd-izm _____
15. pol-ee-YOO-ree-ah _____
16. OR-kee-oh-PECK-see _____
17. PAN-kree-ah-TEK-toh-mee _____
18. HIGH-per-gli-SEE-mee-ah _____
19. PIN-ee-ah-LEK-toh-mee _____
20. pol-ee-DIP-see-ah _____
21. TET-ah-nee _____
22. thigh-MY-tis _____
23. thigh-royd-EK-toh-mee _____
24. thigh-roh-toks-ih-KOH-sis _____
25. oh-off-oh-REK-toh-mee _____

Transcription Practice

Each of the following sentences is written in common English. Underline any words or phrases that can be replaced by a medical term. Then rewrite the entire sentence using medical terms. Answers can be found at the back of the book.

1. Gladys' blood test taken after she was given a dose of glucose confirmed the diagnosis of chronic disorder of sugar metabolism.

   _____

   _____

2. When Dr. Nguyen noted protruding eyeballs, she suspected a condition resulting from hypersecretion of thyroid hormones.

   _____

   _____

3. A surgical removal of the adrenal gland was necessary to treat the benign tumor of the adrenal medulla secreting excessive amounts of epinephrine.

_____

_____

4. Insufficient parathyroid gland (secretion) condition is one cause of nerve irritability resulting from hypocalcemia.

_____

_____

5. Two diagnostic tests were ordered: a scanned image of the thyroid gland after administering radioactive iodine and a blood test to measure levels of thyroxine, triiodothyronine, and thyroid-stimulating hormone.

_____

_____

6. Hypersecretion of growth hormone produces excessive body growth in a child or teenager, and lack of growth hormone can produce excessive shortness in height.

_____

_____

7. A person with a condition caused by insufficient antidiuretic hormone often has excessive thirst and frequent urination.

_____

_____

8. When Mrs. Ruiz developed facial hair and a deeper voice, a condition in which male secondary sexual characteristics appear in a female was suspected.

_____

_____

9. Adrenal cortex hormones with strong anti-inflammatory action were prescribed for the patient with rheumatoid arthritis.

_____

_____

10. Mr. McDonald's enlarged adrenal gland was caused by a cancerous glandular tumor.

_____

_____

Build Medical Terms

Use each of the following word parts to build the indicated medical terms.

The combining form *thyroid/o* means thyroid gland.

1. pertaining to thyroid gland _____

2. thyroid gland inflammation _____

3. surgical removal of thyroid gland _____

4. excessive thyroid gland condition _____

5. insufficient thyroid gland condition _____

The combining form *glyc/o* means sugar.

6. excessive sugar blood condition _____

7. insufficient sugar blood condition _____

The prefix *poly-* means many (too much).

8. many (too much) thirst _____

9. many (too much) urine condition _____

The combining form *aden/o* means gland.

10. cancerous tumor in gland _____

11. resembling a gland _____

12. abnormal softening of gland _____

The combining form *pancreat/o* means pancreas.

13. pertaining to pancreas _____

14. pancreas inflammation _____

15. cutting into the pancreas _____

MyMedicalTerminologyLab™

MyMedicalTerminologyLab is a premium online homework management system that includes a host of features to help you study. Registered users will find:

- A multitude of activities and assignments built within the MyLab platform
- Powerful tools that track and analyze your results—allowing you to create a personalized learning experience
- Videos and audio pronunciations to help enrich your progress
- Streaming lesson presentations and self-paced learning modules
- A space where you and your instructors can view and manage your assignments

Labeling Exercise

Write the name of each structure on the numbered line. Also use this space to write the combining form where appropriate.

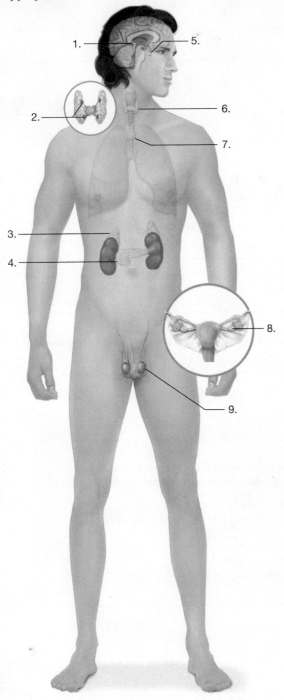
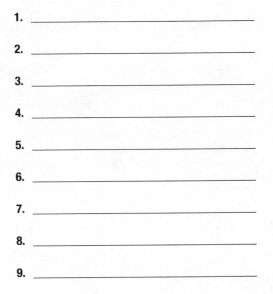

1. _____

2. _____

3. _____

4. _____

5. _____

6. _____

7. _____

8. _____

9. _____

Spelling

Some of the following terms are misspelled. Identify the incorrect terms and spell them correctly in the blank provided.

1. hyperthyroidism _____

2. ovariocentesus _____

3. myxadema _____

4. pheochromocytoma _____

5. radioimmunoassay _____

6. teteny _____

7. exopthalmos _____

8. dwarfism _____

9. corticosteroids _____

10. virilizm _____

Fill in the Blank

Fill in the blank to complete each of the following sentences.

1. The endocrine system plays a vital role in maintaining a stable internal body environment, referred to as _____.

2. Endocrine glands secrete chemical messengers called _____, which travel through the bloodstream to reach their _____.

3. Having too much of a hormone is called _____; having too little is called _____.

4. The adrenal glands sit on top of each _____ and are divided into the outer adrenal _____ and the inner adrenal _____.

5. _____ is secreted by the ovary and regulates the _____ cycle.

6. The two hormones secreted by the pancreas are _____ and _____.

7. Parathyroid hormone works to raise blood levels of _____.

8. The pineal gland secretes _____ that works to regulate the body's _____ rhythm.

9. The _____ gland is often referred to as the *master gland*.

10. The _____ gland is important for normal development of the immune system.

Abbreviation Matching

Match each abbreviation with its definition.

_____ **1.** PRL   **A.** noninsulin-dependent diabetes mellitus

_____ **2.** RAI   **B.** radioimmunoassay

_____ **3.** Na$^+$ **C.** radioactive iodine

_____ **4.** TFT   **D.** thyroxine

_____ **5.** RIA   **E.** prolactin

_____ **6.** LH   **F.** antidiuretic hormone

_____ **7.** T$_4$ **G.** fasting blood sugar

_____ **8.** NIDDM   **H.** sodium

_____ **9.** FBS   **I.** luteinizing hormone

_____ **10.** ADH   **J.** thyroid function test

Medical Term Analysis

Examine each of the following terms. Begin by dividing it into its word parts and writing them in the indicated blanks (*P = prefix*; *WR = word root*; *CF = combining form*; *S = suffix*). Follow with the definition of each word part and then finally the meaning of the full term.

1. orchiopexy

CF _____

means _____

S _____

means _____

Term meaning: _____

_____

2. thyromegaly

CF _____

means _____

S _____

means _____

Term meaning: _____

_____

3. adenocarcinoma

CF _____

means _____

WR _____

means _____

S _____

means _____

Term meaning: _____

_____

4. **hypoparathyroidism**

P _____

means _____

WR _____

means _____

S _____

means _____

Term meaning: _____

_____

5. **thyrotoxicosis**

CF _____

means _____

WR _____

means _____

S _____

means _____

Term meaning: _____

_____

6. **pinealectomy**

WR _____

means _____

S _____

means _____

Term meaning: _____

_____

7. **ovariorrhexis**

CF _____

means _____

S _____

means _____

Term meaning: _____

_____

8. **thymitis**

WR _____

means _____

S _____

means _____

Term meaning: _____

_____

9. **hyperglycemia**

P _____

means _____

WR _____

means _____

S _____

means _____

Term meaning: _____

_____

10. **oophoroplasty**

CF _____

means _____

S _____

means _____

Term meaning: _____

_____

Photomatch Challenge

This illustration shows the pituitary gland and its target organs. For each target, give its combining form. On the second line build the medical term.

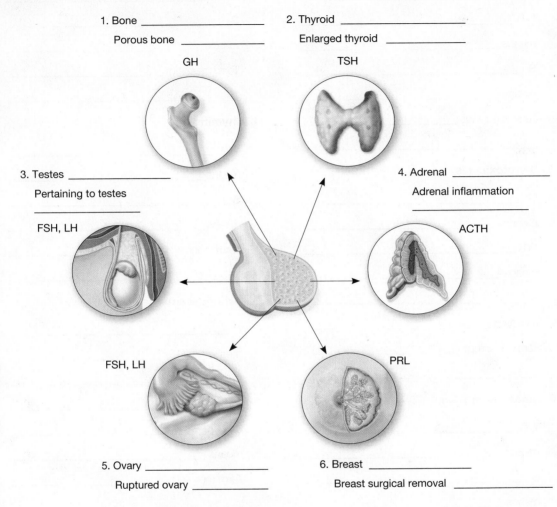

1. Bone _____
   Porous bone _____
   GH

2. Thyroid _____:
   Enlarged thyroid _____
   TSH

3. Testes _____
   Pertaining to testes
   _____
   FSH, LH

4. Adrenal _____
   Adrenal inflammation
   _____
   ACTH

FSH, LH

PRL

5. Ovary _____
   Ruptured ovary _____

6. Breast _____
   Breast surgical removal _____

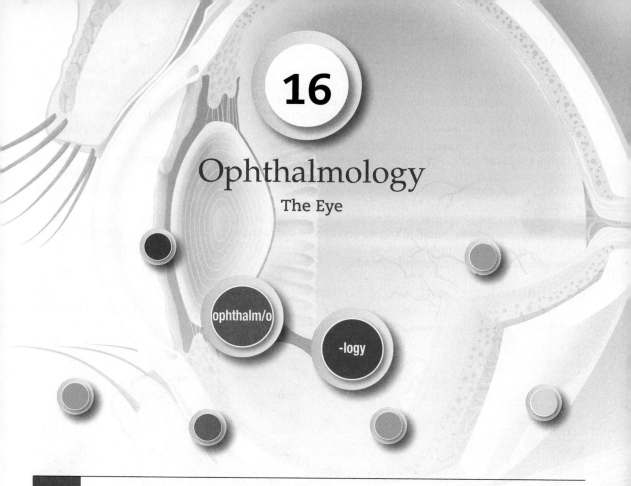

16

Ophthalmology

The Eye

ophthalm/o

-logy

⌄ Learning Objectives

Upon completion of this chapter, you will be able to:

16-1 Describe the medical specialties of ophthalmology and optometry.

16-2 Understand the function of the eye.

16-3 Define ophthalmology-related combining forms, prefixes, and suffixes.

16-4 Identify the structures treated in ophthalmology.

16-5 Build ophthalmology medical terms from word parts.

16-6 Explain ophthalmology medical terms.

16-7 Use ophthalmology abbreviations.

A Brief Introduction to Ophthalmology

The two medical specialties providing eye care are ophthalmology and optometry. There is some degree of confusion regarding the difference in these two professions. **Ophthalmology** (Ophth) is the diagnosis and treatment of diseases and conditions of the eye and vision. **Ophthalmologists** are medical doctors (MD or DO) who have completed at least four years of specialized training after completing medical school. They are involved in all aspects of eye care including vision examinations, corrective lens prescription, diagnosis and treatment of eye diseases and conditions, and eye surgery.

Optometry specializes in assessing vision and prescribing corrective lens, treating glaucoma, corneal damage, and visual skill problems, providing pre- and post-surgical care, as well as screening for other eye diseases. An **optometrist** obtains a doctor of optometry (OD) degree after completing four years at a school of optometry.

The **eyeball** is one of the special sense organs and is responsible for **vision**. Light rays entering the eyeball travel through the **cornea**, **pupil**, **iris**, **lens**, and land on the **retina** to produce an image. The image is then carried to the brain by the **optic nerve**. Accessory structures provide protection for the eye and include the **conjunctivas**, **eyelids**, and **lacrimal glands**.

Ophthalmology Combining Forms

The following list presents combining forms closely associated with the eye and used for building and defining ophthalmology terms.

aque/o	water	**lacrim/o**	tears
blephar/o	eyelid	**ocul/o**	eye
choroid/o	choroid layer	**ophthalm/o**	eye
conjunctiv/o	conjunctiva	**opt/o**	eye, vision
core/o	pupil	**phac/o**	lens
corne/o	cornea	**pupill/o**	pupil
cycl/o	ciliary body	**retin/o**	retina
dacry/o	tears	**scler/o**	sclera
ir/o	iris	**ton/o**	tension, pressure
irid/o	iris	**vitre/o**	glassy
kerat/o	cornea		

The following list presents combining forms that are not specific to the eye but are also used for building and defining ophthalmology terms.

aden/o	gland	**dipl/o**	double
ambly/o	dull, dim	**myc/o**	fungus
angi/o	vessel	**nas/o**	nose
chrom/o	color	**phot/o**	light
cry/o	cold	**xer/o**	dry
cyst/o	sac, urinary bladder		

Suffix Review

These suffixes introduced in Chapter 2 are being reviewed in this chapter because they are especially important for building ophthalmology terms.

-al	pertaining to	**-ectomy**	surgical removal
-ar	pertaining to	**-graphy**	process of recording
-ary	pertaining to	**-ia**	state, condition

-ic	pertaining to	-otomy	cutting into
-ician	specialist	-ous	pertaining to
-itis	inflammation	-pathy	disease
-lith	stone	-pexy	surgical fixation
-logist	one who studies	-phobia	fear
-logy	study of	-plasty	surgical repair
-lysis	to destroy	-plegia	paralysis
-malacia	abnormal softening	-ptosis	drooping
-meter	instrument for measuring	-rrhea	discharge, flow
-metry	process of measuring	-sclerosis	hardening
-opia	vision	-scope	instrument for viewing
-osis	abnormal condition	-scopy	process of visually examining

Prefix Review

These prefixes introduced in Chapter 3 are being reviewed here because they are especially important for building ophthalmology terms.

a-	without	hyper-	excessive
an-	without	intra-	within
hemi-	half	micro-	small

Structures of the Eye and Orbit

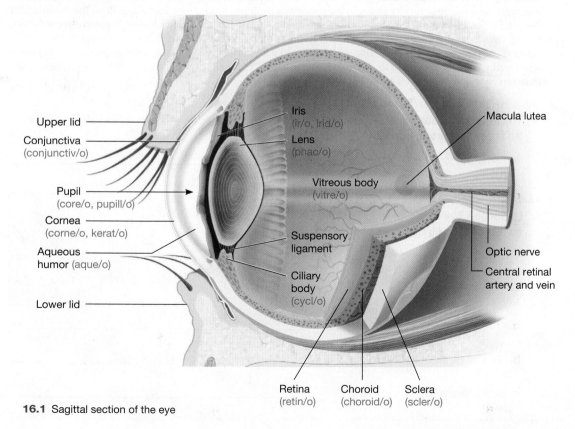

16.1 Sagittal section of the eye

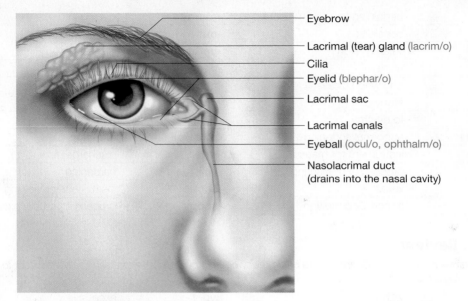

16.2 Anterior view of the eye orbit

Eyebrow

Lacrimal (tear) gland (lacrim/o)

Cilia

Eyelid (blephar/o)

Lacrimal sac

Lacrimal canals

Eyeball (ocul/o, ophthalm/o)

Nasolacrimal duct
(drains into the nasal cavity)

Building Ophthalmology Terms

This section presents word parts most often used to build ophthalmology terms. Following the explanation of the term, you have the opportunity to begin the process of building your own vocabulary. Read the meaning for each term and then fill in the blanks to build a single medical term. Use the slashes to divide prefixes, word roots, combining vowels, and suffixes. To help you out you will find a key to the word parts underneath the blanks: **r** for word roots, **p** for prefix, **cv** for combining vowel, and **s** for suffix. Remember that not every term will contain all these word parts; it's up to you to decide which to use. As you gain experience, this process becomes easier. Answers can be found at the back of the book.

1. **aque/o**–combining form meaning **water**

   The **anterior chamber** is the open area of the eye anterior to the lens and is filled with a watery fluid called **aqueous humor**

   a. pertaining to water

   _____/_____
                      r   s

- -

2. **blephar/o**–combining form meaning **eyelid**

   Upper and lower eyelids are folds of skin that close to protect anterior surface of eyeball; eyelashes are called **cilia** (see again Figure 16.1)

   16.3 The eyelid

   a. drooping eyelid

   _____/_____/_____
                      r   cv   s

   b. surgical repair of the eyelid

   _____/_____/_____
                      r   cv   s

   c. eyelid paralysis

   _____/_____/_____
                      r   cv   s

- -

3. **choroid/o**–combining form meaning **choroid layer**

Choroid layer is middle layer of wall of eyeball; contains many blood vessels (see again Figure 16.1)

   a. pertaining to choroid layer
   _____/_____
   r   s

   b. choroid layer inflammation
   _____/_____
   r   s

4. **conjunctiv/o**–combining form meaning **conjunctiva**

Conjunctiva is a mucous membrane that protects anterior surface of eyeball and turns underneath to line eyelids (see again Figure 16.1)

   a. conjunctiva inflammation
   _____/_____
   r   s

   b. pertaining to conjunctiva
   _____/_____
   r   s

5. **core/o**–combining form meaning **pupil**

Pupil is opening in center of iris; becomes larger or smaller to control amount of light entering inside of eyeball (see again Figure 16.1)

   a. instrument for measuring pupil
   _____/_____/_____
   r   cv   s

   b. process of measuring pupil
   _____/_____/_____
   r   cv   s

6. **corne/o**–combining form meaning **cornea**

Cornea is anterior portion of sclera; transparent to allow light through and curved to bend light rays so that they focus on retina (see again Figure 16.1)

16.4 The cornea

   a. pertaining to cornea
   _____/_____
   r   s

7. **cycl/o**–combining form meaning **ciliary body**

Ciliary body is a ring of muscle around outer edge of lens; attached to lens by **suspensory ligaments**; pulls on edges of lens to change its shape to focus image onto retina (see again Figure 16.1)

   a. ciliary body paralysis
   _____/_____/_____
   r   cv   s

   b. cutting into ciliary body
   _____/_____
   r   s

8. **dacry/o**–combining form meaning **tears**

Tears are watery fluid secreted by lacrimal glands that moisten and cleanse anterior surface of eyeball; **lacrimal glands** are located superior and lateral to eyeball and under orbital bone; tears collect in corner of eye and flow through **lacrimal canals** to **lacrimal sac** (see again Figure 16.2)

   a. tear stone
   _____/_____/_____
   r   cv   s

b. tear flow

_____ / _____ / _____
r   cv   s

c. tear gland inflammation

_____ / _____ / _____ / _____
r   cv   r   s

d. tear sac inflammation

_____ / _____ / _____ / _____
r   cv   r   s

----

9. **ir/o**–combining form meaning **iris**

   Iris is colored portion of eye; made of muscle and contracts or relaxes to change size of pupil (see again Figure 16.1)

16.5 The iris

   a. iris inflammation

_____ / _____
r   s

----

10. **irid/o**–combining form meaning **iris**

   a. iris paralysis

_____ / _____ / _____
r   cv   s

   b. cutting into iris

_____ / _____
r   s

----

11. **kerat/o**–combining form meaning **cornea**

   a. instrument for measuring cornea

_____ / _____ / _____
r   cv   s

   b. process of measuring cornea

_____ / _____ / _____
r   cv   s

   c. surgical removal of cornea

_____ / _____
r   s

   d. cornea inflammation

_____ / _____
r   s

   e. cutting into cornea

_____ / _____
r   s

   f. surgical repair of cornea

_____ / _____ / _____
r   cv   s

----

12. **lacrim/o**–combining form meaning **tears**

   a. pertaining to tears

_____ / _____
r   s

   b. pertaining to nose and tears

_____ / _____ / _____ / _____
r   cv   r   s

----

13. **ocul/o**–combining form meaning **eye**

The eye is a complex sensory organ that allows people to see; hollow (but not empty) sphere; wall of eye composed of three layers: **sclera**, **choroid**, and **retina** (see again Figure 16.1)

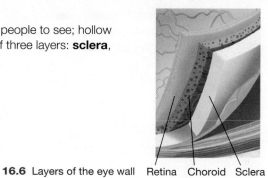

16.6 Layers of the eye wall   Retina   Choroid   Sclera

a. pertaining to inside the eye

_____/_____/_____
                 p   r   s

b. abnormal condition of eye fungus

_____/_____/_____/_____
              r   cv   r   s

c. pertaining to eye

_____/_____
                        r   s

14. **ophthalm/o**–combining form meaning **eye**

a. pertaining to eye

_____/_____
                        r   s

b. study of eye

_____/_____/_____
                    r   cv   s

c. one who studies eye

_____/_____/_____
                    r   cv   s

d. instrument for viewing the eye

_____/_____/_____
                    r   cv   s

e. process of visually examining eye

_____/_____/_____
                    r   cv   s

f. eye paralysis

_____/_____/_____
                    r   cv   s

g. dry eye state/condition

_____/_____/_____
            r   r   s

15. **-opia**–suffix meaning **vision**

a. without half of vision

_____/_____/_____
                    p   p   s

b. double vision

_____/_____
                        r   s

16. **opt/o**–combining form meaning **vision**

a. pertaining to vision

_____/_____
                        r   s

b. instrument for measuring vision

_____/_____/_____
                    r   cv   s

c. process of measuring vision

_____/_____/_____
                    r   cv   s

17. **phac/o**–combining form meaning **lens**

The lens is a transparent structure lying behind iris and pupil; bends light rays passing through it so that they are focused on retina (see again Figure 16.1)

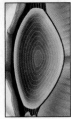

16.7 The lens

a. abnormal softening of lens

_____/_____/_____
r   cv   s

b. to destroy lens

_____/_____/_____
r   cv   s

c. hardening of lens

_____/_____/_____
r   cv   s

18. **pupill/o**–combining form meaning **pupil**

a. pertaining to pupil

_____/_____
r   s

b. instrument for measuring pupil

_____/_____/_____
r   cv   s

19. **retin/o**–combining form meaning **retina**

Retina is inner layer of eyeball; contains light receptors called **rods** and **cones**; rods function in dim light and see in gray tones, cones see color in bright light; area on posterior wall of eyeball, directly opposite lens, called **macula lutea**; small pit in center of macula called **fovea centralis** contains only cones and is point of clearest vision (see again Figure 16.1)

a. pertaining to retina

_____/_____
r   s

b. retina disease

_____/_____/_____
r   cv   s

c. retina inflammation

_____/_____
r   s

d. surgical fixation of retina using cold

_____/_____/_____/_____/_____
r   cv   r   cv   s

20. **scler/o**–combining form meaning **sclera**

Sclera is outermost layer of eye, commonly called *white of eye*; very fibrous and tough (see again Figure 16.1)

a. pertaining to sclera

_____/_____
r   s

b. cutting into sclera

_____/_____
r   s

c. abnormal softening of sclera

_____/_____/_____
r   cv   s

d. sclera inflammation

_____/_____
r   s

21. ton/o–combining form meaning **tension**, **pressure**

    a. instrument for measuring pressure   _____ / _____ / _____

                                             r   *cv*   *s*

    b. process of measuring pressure   _____ / _____ / _____

                                             r   *cv*   *s*

- -

22. vitre/o–combining form meaning **glassy**

    Refers to gel-like shiny substance, **vitreous humor**, that fills **posterior chamber**, the large open cavity between lens and retina

    a. pertaining to glassy   _____ / _____

                                           r   *s*

Ophthalmology Vocabulary

The ophthalmology terms presented in this section include eponyms, modern English words, and those that contain Latin or Greek word parts but are not constructed solely from these word parts. When you recognize word parts within a term, they will give you a hint about the word's meaning. In these instances, look for the word parts to follow the term.

Term	Explanation
accommodation (Acc)	Ability of eye to adjust to variations in distance
achromatopsia **a-** = without **chrom/o** = color	Profound inability to see in color from birth; also called *color blindness*
amblyopia **ambyl/o** = dim **-opia** = vision	Loss of vision not due to any disease; not correctable with glasses; persons with amblyopia wear a patch over one eye to force affected eye to work; commonly called *lazy eye*

16.8 Young girls wearing eye patches under their glasses; the patch covers the strong eye to force the "lazy eye" to work
Source: Courtesy of the National Eye Institute, www.nei.nih.gov

Term	Explanation
astigmatism (As, Ast)	Uneven bending of light rays caused by irregular curvature of cornea; image is fuzzy; corrected with cylindrical lenses

> **TERMINOLOGY TIDBIT**
> The term *astigmatism* comes from the Greek word *stigma* meaning "point" combined with the prefix **a-** meaning "without." "Without a point" describes the fuzzy vision characteristic of astigmatism.

Term	Explanation
cataract	Lens becomes cloudy or opaque; results in whole vision field becoming blurry; treatment is usually surgical removal of cataract and replacement of lens with artificial lens **16.9** Photograph of person with a cataract in the right eye Source: Arztsamui/Shutterstock
color vision tests	Use of multicolored charts to determine ability of patient to recognize color **16.10** Color vision test: a person with red-green color blindness will not be able to see the green 27 embedded in the red colored circles

corneal abrasion
  corne/o = cornea
  -al = pertaining to
	Scraping away of outer layer of cornea

cryoextraction **cry/o** = cold	Procedure to remove lens with cataract using an extremely cold probe

diabetic retinopathy
  retin/o = retina
  -pathy = disease
	Development of small hemorrhages and edema in retina as result of diabetes mellitus; dark spots appear in visual field; laser surgery may be necessary for treatment

fluorescein	Bright green fluorescent dye dropped onto surface of eyeball to highlight corneal abrasions

fluorescein angiography
  angi/o = vessel
  -graphy = process of recording
	Procedure using intravenous bright green fluorescent dye, fluorescein, to examine movement of blood through blood vessels of eye

glaucoma	Condition resulting from increase in intraocular pressure, which, if untreated, can result in atrophy of optic nerve and blindness; patient notices that vision becomes blurry around edges; treated with medication and surgery

TERMINOLOGY TIDBIT

The term *glaucoma* comes from the Greek word *glaukos* meaning "gray-green." The inside of the eyeball appears gray-green when viewed through the pupil.

Term	Explanation
hyperopia **hyper-** = excessive **-opia** = vision	Visual condition in which person can see things in distance but has trouble reading material at close range; also known as *farsightedness*; corrected by convex lens 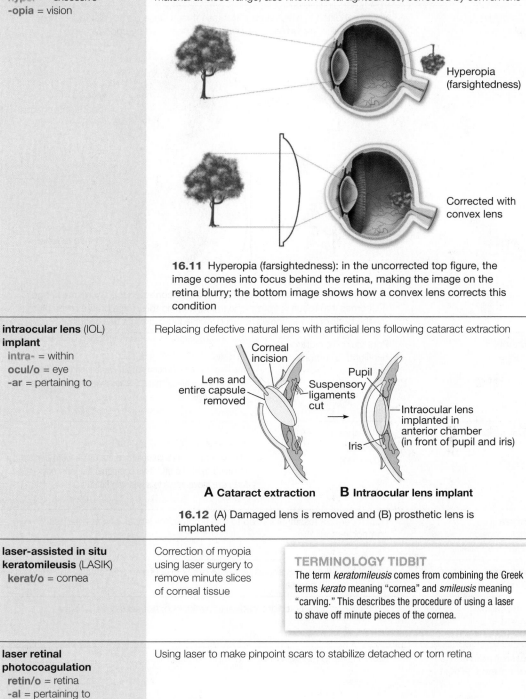 **16.11** Hyperopia (farsightedness): in the uncorrected top figure, the image comes into focus behind the retina, making the image on the retina blurry; the bottom image shows how a convex lens corrects this condition
intraocular lens (IOL) **implant** **intra-** = within **ocul/o** = eye **-ar** = pertaining to	Replacing defective natural lens with artificial lens following cataract extraction **16.12** (A) Damaged lens is removed and (B) prosthetic lens is implanted
laser-assisted in situ keratomileusis (LASIK) **kerat/o** = cornea	Correction of myopia using laser surgery to remove minute slices of corneal tissue **TERMINOLOGY TIDBIT** The term *keratomileusis* comes from combining the Greek terms *kerato* meaning "cornea" and *smileusis* meaning "carving." This describes the procedure of using a laser to shave off minute pieces of the cornea.
laser retinal photocoagulation **retin/o** = retina **-al** = pertaining to **phot/o** = light	Using laser to make pinpoint scars to stabilize detached or torn retina

Term	Explanation
macular degeneration	Deterioration of macula lutea of retina; patient notices loss of vision in center of visual field
myopia (MY) **-opia** = vision	Visual condition in which person can see things close up but distance vision is blurred; also known as *nearsightedness*; corrected by concave lens

Myopia
(nearsightedness)

Corrected with
concave lens

16.13 Myopia (nearsightedness): in the uncorrected top figure, the image comes into focus in front of the retina, making the image on the retina blurry; the bottom image shows how a concave lens corrects this condition

Term	Explanation
nyctalopia **-opia** = vision	Poor vision at night or in dim light; commonly called *night blindness* **TERMINOLOGY TIDBIT** The term *nyctalopia* comes from combining three Greek words: *nux* meaning "night," *alaos* meaning "blind," and *ops* meaning "eye."
nystagmus	Jerky-appearing involuntary eye movement **TERMINOLOGY TIDBIT** The term *nystagmus* comes from the Greek word *nustagmos* meaning "nodding off." This compares the jerky back-and-forth eye movements to a nodding head.
optician **opt/o** = vision **-ician** = specialist	Health care professional trained to make corrective lenses and fit eyeglasses and contact lenses
phacoemulsification **phac/o** = lens	Use of high-frequency sound waves to break up cataract, which is then removed by suction with needle
photophobia **phot/o** = light **-phobia** = fear	Excessive sensitivity to light leading to avoidance; not actual fear of light
photorefractive keratectomy (PRK) **phot/o** = light **kerat/o** = cornea **-ectomy** = surgical removal	Use of laser to reshape cornea to improve visual acuity

Term	Explanation
radial keratotomy (RK) **kerat/o** = cornea **-otomy** = cutting into	Surgery with spokelike incisions in cornea to flatten it, done to correct nearsightedness
refractive error	Defect in ability of eye to bend light rays to focus image properly on fovea centralis (refraction); occurs in myopia and hyperopia
retinal detachment **retin/o** = retina **-al** = pertaining to	Occurs when retina becomes separated from choroid layer; this separation seriously damages blood vessels and nerves, resulting in blindness **16.14** Illustration of normal retina (A) and detached retina (B); note "wavy" lines are caused by retina pulling away from the wall of the eyeball, losing its blood supply and dying **A** Normal retina **B** Detached retina
slit lamp microscope **micro-** = small **-scope** = instrument for viewing	Instrument used in ophthalmology for examining posterior surface of cornea **16.15** Examination of the interior of the eye using an ophthalmoscope Source: Pearson Education
Snellen chart	Chart used for testing visual acuity; contains letters of varying sizes and is shown from distance of 20 feet; average person who can read at this distance is said to have 20/20 vision
strabismus	Weakness of external eye muscle; results in eyes looking in different directions at same time; can be corrected with glasses, eye exercises, and/or surgery; commonly called *cross-eyed* if eye is turned toward the nose **16.16** Illustration of child with strabismus in the right eye, which turns in **TERMINOLOGY TIDBIT** The term *strabismus* comes from the Greek word *strabizein* meaning "to squint."
strabotomy **-otomy** = cutting into	Incision into eye muscles to correct strabismus

Term	Explanation
stye	Small purulent infection of sebaceous gland of eye; treated with hot compresses or surgical incision and drainage; also called *hordeolum*
visual acuity test (VA)	Measurement of sharpness of patient's vision; usually, Snellen chart is used for this test and patient identifies letters from distance of 20 feet; term 20/20 vision means person is able to see at 20 feet what a person with normal vision would expect to see at 20 feet; term such as 20/200 would indicate person's degree of myopia, that is, he or she must be 20 feet away from object to see it when a person with normal vision could see object from 200 feet away

Ophthalmology Abbreviations

The list below presents common ophthalmology abbreviations.

Acc	accommodation		**MY**	myopia
As, Ast	astigmatism		**OD**	doctor of optometry
c.gl.	correction with glasses		**Ophth**	ophthalmology
cyl	cylindrical lens		**PERRLA**	pupils equal, round, reactive to light and accommodation
D	diopter (lens strength)			
DO	doctor of osteopathic medicine		**PRK**	photorefractive keratectomy
ECCE	extracapsular cataract extraction		**REM**	rapid eye movement
ICCE	intracapsular cataract extraction		**RK**	radial keratotomy
IOL	intraocular lens		**s.gl.**	without correction or glasses
IOP	intraocular pressure		**VA**	visual acuity
LASIK	laser-assisted in situ keratomileusis		**VF**	visual field
MD	doctor of medicine			

CASE STUDY

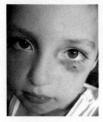

Source: Varina and Jay Patel/Shutterstock

History of Present Illness
An 8-year-old boy was seen by an ophthalmologist in the ER following being struck in the left eye while playing basketball. Symptoms included pain, excessive tearing, decreased visual acuity, and photophobia.

Past Medical History
Fractured right femur in a bike accident at age 5. Hydrocele was surgically repaired shortly after birth with no further problems. Patient is taking no regular medications.

Family and Social History
Patient is a third-grade student. He is active in sports. Patient lives at home with his mother, father, and one older sister. All are healthy.

Physical Examination
Healthy-appearing 8-year-old male in obvious distress from inflamed left eye.

Diagnostic Tests

Snellen chart revealed visual acuity of 20/200 in left eye and 20/20 in right eye. A slit lamp microscope examination showed a conjunctival reddening in the left eye. Corneal examination after applying fluorescein dye revealed a 7-mm corneal abrasion. No ulcer was observed. Examination of the retina was unremarkable.

Diagnosis

Traumatic corneal abrasion in the left eye.

Plan of Treatment

1. Treat abrasion with antibiotic and pain with anesthetic eye drops
2. Use a lubricating ointment if his eye is too dry when he wakes up in the morning
3. Wear an eye patch if he is outside in the sun
4. See an ophthalmologist for a follow-up reexamination in 24 hrs

Critical Thinking Questions

Answer the following questions regarding this case study. Do not just copy words out of the case study but translate all medical terms. In order to answer some of these questions, you may need to look up information from another chapter of this text, in a medical dictionary, or online. Answers are found at the back of the book.

1. List and describe the symptoms that brought this patient to the ER.

   _____

   _____

2. What is the common name for the bone this patient fractured at age 5?

   _____

   _____

3. Explain the results of the visual acuity examination.

   _____

   _____

4. Explain the purpose of using a fluorescein dye.

   _____

   _____

5. Fluorescein dye identified a corneal abrasion but no ulcer. Explain the difference between an abrasion and an ulcer.

   _____

   _____

6. Explain the purpose of each of the two medications used to treat the patient.

   _____

   _____

7. In addition to the medications, what additional recommendations were made?

   _____

   _____

Sound It Out

The following are some of the key terms from this chapter written as their phonetic spelling. Sound out each term and write it in the blank. Pronunciations for all terms are included in the audio glossary at www.mymedicalterminologylab.com.

1. KAIR-ah-toh-plass-tee _____
2. ok-yoo-loh-my-KOH-sis _____
3. kon-junk-tih-VYE-tis _____
4. ir-ih-DOT-oh-mee _____
5. dip-LOH-pee-ah _____
6. glau-KOH-mah _____
7. hem-ee-ah-NOP-ee-ah _____
8. ah-STIG-mah-tizm _____
9. blef-ah-rop-TOH-sis _____
10. high-per-OH-pee-ah _____
11. in-trah-OCK-yoo-lar _____
12. koh-ree-OM-eh-tree _____
13. cry-oh-RET-ih-noh-pek-see _____

14. kair-ah-TYE-tis _____
15. am-blee-OH-pee-ah _____
16. fak-oh-LYE-sis _____
17. my-OH-pee-ah _____
18. KAT-ah-rakt _____
19. nik-tah-LOH-pee-ah _____
20. sigh-kloh-PLEE-jee-ah _____
21. niss-TAG-mus _____
22. fak-oh-skle-ROH-sis _____
23. foh-toh-FOH-bee-ah _____
24. strah-BIZ-mus _____
25. hor-DEE-oh-lum _____

Transcription Practice

Each of the following sentences is written in common English. Underline any words or phrases that can be replaced by a medical term. Then rewrite the entire sentence using medical terms. Answers can be found at the back of the book.

1. Dr. Cohen decided to use a procedure using an extremely cold probe to remove the patient's opaque lens rather than a procedure using high-frequency sound waves.

_____

_____

2. Mr. Blair's nearsightedness was corrected by making spokelike incisions to flatten the cornea.

_____

_____

3. The head injury caused the inner layer of the eyeball to become separated from the choroid layer, which required repair by using a device that emits an intense beam of light to make pinpoint scars.

_____

_____

4. Because the anterior portion of the sclera was abnormally curved, light rays were not evenly bent, resulting in a condition of distorted vision.

_____

_____

5. Examination of the eye with an instrument for viewing inside the eye did not reveal any reason for Mr. Mendez's fear of light.

_____

_____

6. Mrs. Capers made an appointment with the doctor of optometry because of an inflamed outer white layer of the eye and double vision.

_____

_____

7. The baby's mother was concerned about her infant when she noticed inflamed conjunctiva and excessive tear flow.

_____

_____

8. Mr. Carpenter decided that it was no longer safe for him to drive after he developed poor night vision and deterioration of the macula lutea.

_____

_____

9. A patient's sharpness of vision can be evaluated using a chart with letters of varying sizes.

_____

_____

10. A scraping away of the outer layer of Karen's cornea occurred when sand became trapped under her contact lens that was identified by using bright green fluorescent dye.

_____

_____

Fill in the Blank

Fill in the blank to complete each of the following sentences.

1. _____ is the development of small hemorrhages and edema in the retina as a result of having diabetes mellitus.

2. _____ results from a chronic increase in intraocular pressure.

3. _____ was diagnosed using color vision tests.

4. Another word for stye is _____.

5. Involuntary, jerky eye movements are called _____.

6. _____ is commonly referred to as *nearsightedness*.

7. A strabotomy is the surgical procedure that makes an incision in eye muscles to correct _____.

8. A _____ chart is used to test visual acuity.

9. _____ is commonly called *night blindness*.

10. In _____, light rays are bent unevenly due to an abnormally curved cornea.

Abbreviation Matching

Match each abbreviation with its definition.

_____	1. OD	A.	rapid eye movement
_____	2. MY	B.	intraocular lens
_____	3. REM	C.	diopter
_____	4. s.gl.	D.	cylindrical lens
_____	5. D	E.	doctor of optometry
_____	6. ECCE	F.	visual acuity
_____	7. IOL	G.	without correction or glasses
_____	8. VA	H.	radial keratotomy
_____	9. RK	I.	myopia
_____	10. cyl	J.	extracapsular cataract extraction

Labeling Exercise

Write the name of each structure on the numbered line. Also use this space to write the combining form where appropriate.

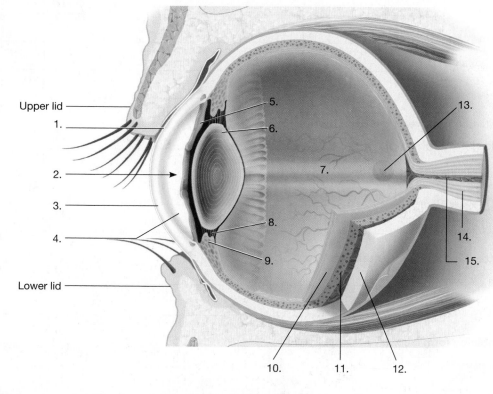

Upper lid —

1. ___

2. ___

3. ___

4. ___

Lower lid —

5.

6.

7.

8.

9.

10.

11.

12.

13.

14.

15.

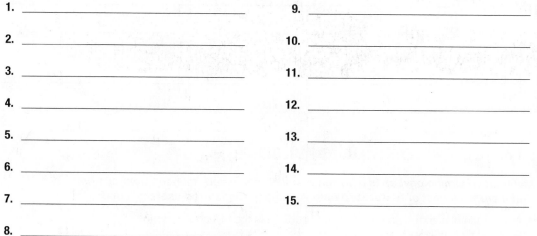

1. _____

2. _____

3. _____

4. _____

5. _____

6. _____

7. _____

8. _____

9. _____

10. _____

11. _____

12. _____

13. _____

14. _____

15. _____

Build Medical Terms

Use each of the following word parts to build the indicated medical terms.

The combining form *ophthalm/o* **means eye.**

1. study of eye _____

2. instrument for viewing eye _____

3. eye paralysis _____

4. pertaining to eye _____

The combining form *kerat/o* **means cornea.**

5. surgical removal of cornea _____

6. cutting into the cornea _____

7. instrument for measuring cornea _____

8. surgical repair of cornea _____

The combining form *retin/o* **means retina.**

9. retina disease _____

10. retina inflammation _____

The combining form *blephar/o* **means eyelid.**

11. surgical repair of eyelid _____

12. eyelid paralysis _____

13. eyelid drooping _____

The suffix *-opia* **means vision.**

14. double vision _____

15. dim vision _____

MyMedicalTerminologyLab™

MyMedicalTerminologyLab is a premium online homework management system that includes a host of features to help you study. Registered users will find:

- A multitude of activities and assignments built within the MyLab platform
- Powerful tools that track and analyze your results—allowing you to create a personalized learning experience
- Videos and audio pronunciations to help enrich your progress
- Streaming lesson presentations and self-paced learning modules
- A space where you and your instructors can view and manage your assignments

Medical Term Analysis

Examine each of the following terms. Begin by dividing it into its word parts and writing them in the indicated blanks (*P = prefix*; *WR = word root*; *CF = combining form*; *S = suffix*). Follow with the definition of each word part and finally the meaning of the full term.

1. blepharoptosis

CF _____

means _____

S _____

means _____

Term meaning: _____

_____

2. dacryoadenitis

CF _____

means _____

WR _____

means _____

S _____

means _____

Term meaning: _____

_____

3. nasolacrimal

CF _____

means _____

WR _____

means _____

S _____

means _____

Term meaning: _____

_____

4. intraocular

P _____

means _____

WR _____

means _____

S _____

means _____

Term meaning: _____

_____

5. cryoretinopexy

CF _____

means _____

CF _____

means _____

S _____

means _____

Term meaning: _____

_____

6. choroiditis

WR _____

means _____

S _____

means _____

Term meaning: _____

_____

7. keratoplasty

CF _____

means _____

S _____

means _____

Term meaning: _____

_____

8. optometry

CF _____

means _____

S _____

means _____

Term meaning: _____

_____

9. ophthalmoscope

CF _____

means _____

S _____

means _____

Term meaning: _____

_____

10. phacosclerosis

CF _____

means _____

S _____

means _____

Term meaning: _____

_____

Spelling

Some of the following terms are misspelled. Identify the incorrect terms and spell them correctly in the blank provided.

1. stie _____

2. nystagmus _____

3. hordoleum _____

4. miopia _____

5. nyctalopia _____

6. cryoextraction _____

7. dacrolith _____

8. oculomycosis _____

9. coreometer _____

10. strabismis _____

Photomatch Challenge

A person with no eye conditions would see the picture in the center. Examine each of the other photos and provide a description of the visual problem. Then, referring to the Ophthalmology Vocabulary section for assistance, match each photo to its condition in the Word Bank.

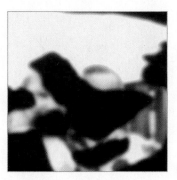

Source: National Eye Institute

1. Describe visual problem

_____

Pathology _____

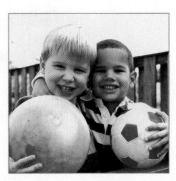

Source: National Eye Institute

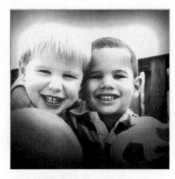

Source: National Eye Institute

2. Describe visual problem

_____

Pathology _____

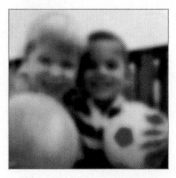

Source: National Eye Institute

3. Describe visual problem

_____

Pathology _____

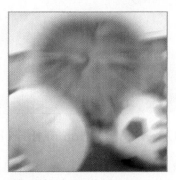

Source: National Eye Institute

4. Describe visual problem

_____

Pathology _____

Word Bank

cataract

diabetic retinopathy

glaucoma

macular degeneration

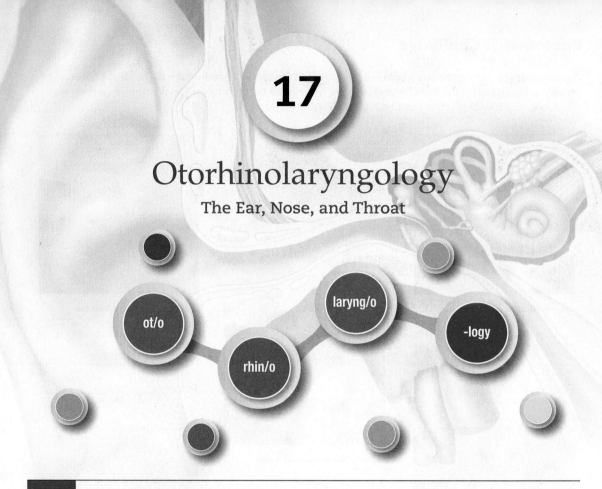

17

Otorhinolaryngology
The Ear, Nose, and Throat

ot/o

rhin/o

laryng/o

-logy

∨ Learning Objectives

Upon completion of this chapter, you will be able to:

17-1   Describe the medical specialty of otorhinolaryngology.

17-2   Understand the function of the ear, nose, and throat.

17-3   Define otorhinolaryngology-related combining forms, prefixes, and suffixes.

17-4   Identify the organs treated in otorhinolaryngology.

17-5   Build otorhinolaryngology medical terms from word parts.

17-6   Explain otorhinolaryngology medical terms.

17-7   Use otorhinolaryngology abbreviations.

A Brief Introduction to Otorhinolaryngology

Otorhinolaryngologists (ENTs, or ear, nose, and throat doctors) are physicians who specialize in diagnosing and treating conditions affecting these organs. A family physician or an internist can also treat these conditions, but the ENT physician is a specialist in treating problems with hearing, balance, swallowing, and voice as well as head and neck tumors and problems affecting the airways.

This medical specialty of **otorhinolaryngology** (ENT) focuses on a specific region of the body, the head and the neck, rather than on a whole body system, such as gastroenterology is to the gastrointestinal system or neurology is to the nervous system. As a group, the organs in the head and neck are responsible for two main functions: to house sensory receptors and to provide passageways for air, food, and drink.

These organs and their functions include the:

- **Ear** – hearing and equilibrium (balance)
- **Nose** – smell and entrance for air into the body
- **Pharynx** – carries air to the larynx and trachea, and food and drink to the esophagus
- **Larynx** – speech
- **Trachea** – brings air to the lungs

Otorhinolaryngology Combining Forms

The following list presents combining forms closely associated with the head and neck region and used for building and defining otorhinolaryngology terms.

adenoid/o	adenoids	**nas/o**	nose
audi/o	hearing	**ot/o**	ear
audit/o	hearing	**pharyng/o**	pharynx (throat)
aur/o	ear	**rhin/o**	nose
cochle/o	cochlea	**sinus/o**	sinus
epiglott/o	epiglottis	**tonsill/o**	tonsils
laryng/o	larynx (voice box)	**trache/o**	trachea (windpipe)
myring/o	tympanic membrane (eardrum)	**tympan/o**	tympanic membrane (eardrum)

The following list presents combining forms that are not specific to the ear, nose, or throat but are also used for building and defining otorhinolaryngology terms.

gastr/o	stomach	**neur/o**	nerve
myc/o	fungus	**py/o**	pus

Suffix Review

These suffixes introduced in Chapter 2 are being reviewed in this chapter because they are especially important suffixes in otorhinolaryngology terms.

-al	pertaining to		**-ory**	pertaining to
-algia	pain		**-osis**	abnormal condition
-ar	pertaining to		**-osmia**	smell
-eal	pertaining to		**-otomy**	cutting into
-ectomy	surgical removal		**-phonia**	voice
-gram	record		**-plasty**	surgical repair
-ic	pertaining to		**-plegia**	paralysis
-itis	inflammation		**-rrhea**	discharge, flow
-logist	one who studies		**-rrhexis**	rupture
-logy	study of		**-sclerosis**	hardening
-megaly	enlarged		**-scope**	instrument for viewing
-meter	instrument for measuring		**-scopy**	process of visually examining
-metry	process of measuring		**-spasm**	involuntary muscle contraction
-oma	tumor, mass		**-stenosis**	narrowing

Prefix Review

These prefixes introduced in Chapter 3 are being reviewed here because they are especially important for building otorhinolaryngology terms.

a-	without		**endo-**	within, inner
an-	without		**pan-**	all
de-	without		**para-**	beside; two like parts of a pair
dys-	abnormal, difficult, painful			

Organs Commonly Treated in Otorhinolaryngology

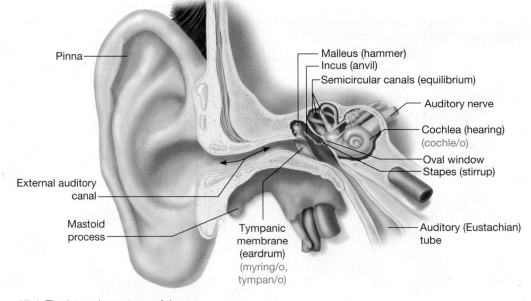

17.1 The internal structures of the ear

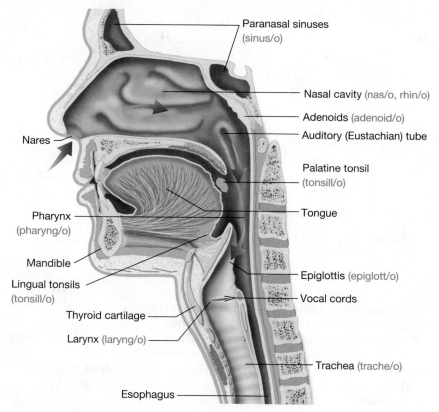

17.2 Sagittal section of head and neck showing the organs of the upper respiratory system: nasal cavity, pharynx, larynx, and trachea

Labels in figure:
- Paranasal sinuses (sinus/o)
- Nasal cavity (nas/o, rhin/o)
- Adenoids (adenoid/o)
- Auditory (Eustachian) tube
- Palatine tonsil (tonsill/o)
- Tongue
- Epiglottis (epiglott/o)
- Vocal cords
- Trachea (trache/o)
- Nares
- Pharynx (pharyng/o)
- Mandible
- Lingual tonsils (tonsill/o)
- Thyroid cartilage
- Larynx (laryng/o)
- Esophagus

Building Otorhinolaryngology Terms

This section presents word parts most often used to build otorhinolaryngology terms. Following the explanation of the term, you have the opportunity to begin building your own vocabulary. Read the meaning for each term and then fill in the blanks to build a single medical term. Use the slashes to divide prefixes, word roots, combining vowels, and suffixes. To help you out you will find a key to the word parts underneath the blanks: **r** for word roots, **p** for prefix, **cv** for combining vowel, and **s** for suffix. Remember that not every term will contain all these word parts; it's up to you to decide which to use. As you gain experience, this process becomes easier. Answers can be found at the back of the book.

1. **adenoid/o**–combining form meaning **adenoids**

    Adenoids are one of three pairs of **tonsils** located in pharynx; also called **pharyngeal tonsils**; tonsils house large number of white blood cells that protect body by removing foreign invaders from air, food, and drink passing through pharynx (see again Figure 17.2)

    a. surgical removal of adenoids   _____/_____
      rs

    b. adenoids inflammation   _____/_____
      rs

2. **audi/o**–combining form meaning **hearing**

    a. study of hearing

                                   _____/_____/_____
                                            r   *CV*   *S*

    b. one who studies hearing

                                     _____/_____/_____
                                            r   *CV*   *S*

    c. process of measuring hearing

                                     _____/_____/_____
                                            r   *CV*   *S*

    d. instrument for measuring hearing

                                     _____/_____/_____
                                            r   *CV*   *S*

    e. record of hearing

                                     _____/_____/_____
                                            r   *CV*   *S*

---

3. **audit/o**–combining form meaning **hearing**

    a. pertaining to hearing

                                     _____/_____
                                            r   *S*

---

4. **aur/o**–combining form meaning **ear**

    The ear is responsible for both **hearing** and **equilibrium** (balance); divided into **external ear, middle ear**, and **inner ear**; **pinna** (**auricle**) captures sound waves and funnels them into **external auditory canal**; sound waves strike **tympanic membrane** (eardrum), causing it to vibrate; three tiny bones (ossicles) in middle ear—the **malleus**, **incus**, and **stapes**—conduct this vibration across middle ear from tympanic membrane to **oval window**; oval window movement initiates vibrations in fluid inside inner ear; vibrating fluid bends hair cells in **cochlea**, which stimulates nerve endings; **auditory nerve** sends message to brain; inner ear also contains organs for equilibrium, **semicircular canals** (see again Figure 17.1)

    a. pertaining to ear

                                       _____/_____
                                            r   *S*

---

5. **cochle/o**–combining form meaning **cochlea**

    Cochlea is part of inner ear containing hair cells responsible for hearing; shaped like a coiled snail shell (see again Figure 17.1)

    17.3 The cochlea

    a. pertaining to cochlea

                                       _____/_____
                                            r   *S*

---

6. **epiglott/o**–combining form meaning **epiglottis**

    Epiglottis is cartilage flap that sits above larynx; rotates to cover larynx with each swallow; prevents food or drink from entering larynx and trachea (see again Figure 17.2)

    17.4 The epiglottis

    a. pertaining to epiglottis

                                       _____/_____
                                            r   *S*

    b. epiglottis inflammation

                                      _____/_____
                                            r   *S*

---

7. **laryng/o**–combining form meaning **larynx**

Larynx, commonly called *voice box*, is located between pharynx and trachea; contains paired **vocal cords** that vibrate as air passes through them to produce sound (see again Figure 17.2)

a. pertaining to larynx

_____/_____
r   s

b. larynx inflammation

_____/_____
r   s

c. process of visually examining larynx

_____/_____/_____
r   cv   s

d. instrument for viewing larynx

_____/_____/_____
r   cv   s

e. surgical removal of larynx

_____/_____
r   s

f. surgical repair of larynx

_____/_____/_____
r   cv   s

g. larynx paralysis

_____/_____/_____
r   cv   s

h. involuntary muscle contraction of larynx

_____/_____/_____
r   cv   s

---

8. **myring/o**–combining form meaning **tympanic membrane**

Located at end of external auditory canal, tympanic membrane converts sound waves striking it into vibrations that move ossicles of middle ear; commonly called *eardrum* (see again Figure 17.1)

a. inflammation of eardrum

_____/_____
r   s

b. surgical removal of eardrum

_____/_____
r   s

c. surgical repair of eardrum

_____/_____/_____
r   cv   s

d. hardening of eardrum

_____/_____/_____
r   cv   s

e. cutting into eardrum

_____/_____
r   s

---

9. **nas/o**–combining form meaning **nose**

Air enters nose through two openings called **nares**, passes through **nasal cavity**, and enters pharynx; divided down middle by cartilage plate called **nasal septum**; lined by **mucous membrane**; air is warmed, moisturized, and cleansed as it passes through; houses sensory receptors for sense of smell (see again Figure 17.2)

17.5 The nose

a. pertaining to nose

_____/_____
r   s

b. pertaining to nose and stomach

_____/_____/_____/_____
r   cv   r   s

c. pertaining to nose and throat

_____/_____/_____/_____
r   cv   r   s

10. -osmia–suffix meaning **smell**

      Sensory receptors for smell are located in roof of nasal cavity

      a. without smell   _____/_____

                                                      p   *s*

---

11. ot/o–combining form meaning **ear**

17.6 An otoscope (A) can be used to examine both the ears (B) and nasal cavity (C)
Source: (A) Patrick Watson/Pearson Education
(B and C) Michal Heron/Pearson Education

      a. pertaining to the ear   _____/_____
                                        r   *s*

      b. ear inflammation   _____/_____
                                        r   *s*

      c. ear pain   _____/_____
                                        r   *s*

      d. study of the ear   _____/_____/_____
                                        r   *cv*   *s*

      e. one who studies the ear   _____/_____/_____
                                        r   *cv*   *s*

      f. process of visually examining the ear   _____/_____/_____
                                        r   *cv*   *s*

      g. instrument for viewing the ear   _____/_____/_____
                                        r   *cv*   *s*

      h. surgical repair of the ear   _____/_____/_____
                                        r   *cv*   *s*

      i. abnormal condition of ear fungus   _____/_____/_____/_____
                                       r   *cv*   *r*   *s*

      j. discharge of pus from the ear   _____/_____/_____/_____/_____
                                     r   *cv*   *r*   *cv*   *s*

---

12. pharyng/o–combining form meaning **pharynx**

      Pharynx is a muscular tube that receives air from nasal cavity and delivers it to larynx; also receives food from oral cavity and transports it to esophagus; location for three sets of tonsils (adenoids, **palatine tonsils**, and **lingual tonsils**); **auditory** (Eustachian) **tube**, which opens with each swallow to equalize air pressure in middle ear, connects middle ear to pharynx; commonly called the *throat* (see again Figure 17.2)

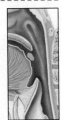

17.7 The pharynx

      a. pertaining to the pharynx   _____/_____
                                        r   *s*

      b. pharynx inflammation   _____/_____
                                        r   *s*

c. surgical repair of pharynx

_____/_____/_____
r　　　　　　cv　　　　s

d. involuntary muscle contraction of pharynx

_____/_____/_____
r　　　　　　cv　　　　s

e. cutting into pharynx

_____/_____
r　　　　　　s

---

13. **-phonia**–suffix meaning **voice**

　a. without voice

_____/_____
p　　　　　　s

　b. abnormal, difficult voice

_____/_____
p　　　　　　s

---

14. **rhin/o**–combining form meaning **nose**

　a. nose inflammation

_____/_____
r　　　　　　s

　b. surgical repair of nose

_____/_____/_____
r　　　　　　cv　　　　s

　c. discharge from nose

_____/_____/_____
r　　　　　　cv　　　　s

　d. abnormal condition of nose fungus

_____/_____/_____/_____
r　　　cv　　　　r　　　　s

---

15. **sinus/o**–combining form meaning **sinuses**

　Paranasal sinuses (para- = beside) are air-filled cavities located within facial bones and con-
　nected to nasal cavity; lined with mucous membrane; act as echo chamber for sound production
　(see again Figure 17.2)

　a. sinus inflammation

_____/_____
r　　　　　　s

　b. inflammation of all sinuses

_____/_____/_____
p　　　　　　r　　　　s

　c. nose and sinus inflammation

_____/_____/_____/_____
r　　　cv　　　　r　　　　s

---

16. **tonsill/o**–combining form meaning **tonsils** (see again Figure 17.2)

　a. pertaining to tonsils

_____/_____
r　　　　　　s

　b. tonsil inflammation

_____/_____
r　　　　　　s

　c. surgical removal of tonsils

_____/_____
r　　　　　　s

17. trache/o–combining form meaning **trachea**

Trachea is a tube that carries air from larynx to lungs; lined with mucous membrane that warms, moisturizes, and cleanses air; commonly called *windpipe* (see again Figure 17.2)

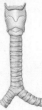

17.8 The trachea

a. pertaining to trachea

_____/_____
r   s

b. enlarged trachea

_____/_____/_____
r   cv   s

c. surgical repair of trachea

_____/_____/_____
r   cv   s

d. cutting into trachea

_____/_____
r   s

e. narrowing of trachea

_____/_____/_____
r   cv   s

f. pertaining to within trachea

_____/_____/_____
p   r   s

17.9 A tracheotomy tube is inserted through an opening in the front of the neck and anchored within the trachea

Epiglottis

Thyroid cartilage — Larynx

Trachea —

Esophagus

Tracheotomy tube —

18. tympan/o–combining form meaning **tympanic membrane** (eardrum) (see again Figure 17.1)

a. pertaining to eardrum

_____/_____
r   s

b. process of measuring eardrum

_____/_____/_____
r   cv   s

c. instrument for measuring eardrum

_____/_____/_____
r   cv   s

d. eardrum record

_____/_____/_____
r   cv   s

e. surgical repair of the eardrum

_____/_____/_____
r   cv   s

f. eardrum rupture

_____/_____/_____
r   cv   s

g. cutting into eardrum

_____/_____
r   s

Otorhinolaryngology Vocabulary

The otorhinolaryngology terms presented in this section include eponyms, modern English words, and those that contain Latin or Greek word parts but are not constructed solely from these word parts. When you recognize word parts within a term, they will give you a hint about the word's meaning. In these instances, look for the word parts to follow the term.

Term	Explanation
acoustic neuroma **neur/o** = nerve **-oma** = tumor	Benign tumor of auditory nerve sheath; symptoms include tinnitus, headache, vertigo, and progressive hearing loss
cochlear implant **cochle/o** = cochlea **-ar** = pertaining to	Hearing device surgically placed under skin behind ear; converts sound signals into magnetic impulses to stimulate auditory nerve **17.10** Photograph of a child with a cochlear implant; this device sends electrical impulses directly to the brain Source: George Dodson/Pearson Education **TERMINOLOGY TIDBIT** The term *cochlea* comes from the Latin word *cochlea* meaning "snail shell." This describes coiled shape of the cochlea.
croup	Acute respiratory condition common in infants and children; symptoms include barking cough
deafness	Inability to hear or having some degree of hearing impairment
decongestant **de-** = without	Medication to reduce nasal and sinus stuffiness and congestion
diphtheria	Bacterial upper respiratory infection; characterized by formation of thick membranous film across throat and high mortality rate; uncommon now due to diphtheria, pertussis, tetanus (DPT) vaccine **TERMINOLOGY TIDBIT** The term *diphtheria* comes from the Greek word *diphthera* meaning "leather hide." This describes the thick membranous film that forms across the throat.
endotracheal (ET) **intubation** **endo-** = within **trache/o** = trachea **-al** = pertaining to	Inserting tube through mouth and into trachea; creates open upper respiratory airway **17.11** Endotracheal intubation: (A) a lighted scope is used to identify the larynx from the esophagus; (B) the tube is placed through the pharynx and larynx into the trachea; (C) the scope is removed, leaving the tube in place

Term	Explanation
epistaxis	Nosebleed
falling test	Group of tests to evaluate balance and equilibrium; for example, balancing on one foot, heel-toe walking, and walking forward with eyes open; test is repeated with patient's eyes closed; swaying and falling with eyes closed can indicate an equilibrium malfunction
hearing aid	Device used by persons with impaired hearing to amplify sound; also called an *amplification device*
Ménière disease	Acute or chronic inner ear condition; can lead to a progressive hearing loss; symptoms include vertigo, hearing loss, and tinnitus
nasal cannula **nas/o** = nose **-al** = pertaining to	Two-pronged plastic device for delivering oxygen directly into nose; one prong is inserted into each naris

TERMINOLOGY TIDBIT

The term *cannula* comes from the Latin word *canna* meaning "reed." Reeds are hollow and can be used like a snorkel to breathe while underwater. This describes the hollow tube shape of a cannula.

17.12 (A) Two-pronged nasal cannula and (B) patient using a nasal cannula
Source: (A) Floyd Jackson/Pearson Education (B) Michal Heron/Pearson Education

Term	Explanation
otitis externa (OE) **ot/o** = ear **-itis** = inflammation	External ear infection; frequently caused by fungus; also called *otomycosis*; common name is *swimmer's ear*
otitis interna **ot/o** = ear **-itis** = inflammation	Inflammation of inner ear; can affect both hearing and equilibrium; also called *inner ear infection*
otitis media (OM) **ot/o** = ear **-itis** = inflammation	Bacterial or viral infection of middle ear; common in children; often preceded by upper respiratory infection during which pathogens move from pharynx to middle ear through auditory tube; commonly referred to as a *middle ear infection*

Fluid collecting in middle ear cavity

Inflamed eardrum

Auditory tube swollen shut

17.13 Otitis media; note inflamed eardrum, swollen auditory tube, and fluid accumulating in middle ear cavity

Term	Explanation
pertussis	Bacterial infection of upper respiratory tract; uncommon now due to diphtheria, pertussis, tetanus (DPT) vaccine; commonly called *whooping cough* due to "whoop" sound made when coughing

> **TERMINOLOGY TIDBIT**
> The term *pertussis* comes from the Latin word *tussis* meaning "cough." Pertussis, or whooping cough, is recognized by its characteristic cough.

Term	Explanation
pressure-equalizing tube (PE tube)	Small tube surgically placed in eardrum; assists in draining trapped fluid and equalizing pressure between middle ear cavity and atmosphere

Eardrum
Pressure-equalizing tube through eardrum
Trapped fluid in middle ear cavity

17.14 Illustration of a PE tube in place through the eardrum

Term	Explanation
Rinne and Weber tuning fork tests	Tests to assess both function of auditory nerve and ability of ear structures to conduct sound waves to inner ear; physician holds tuning fork against or near bones on side of patient's head

17.15 Physician placing a tuning fork behind a patient's ear as part of the Rinne and Weber tuning fork tests
Source: Patrick Watson/Pearson Education

Term	Explanation
tinnitus	Ringing in the ears

> **TERMINOLOGY TIDBIT**
> The term *tinnitus* comes from the Latin word *tinnire* meaning "to ring, tinkle." It is used to describe a ringing sensation in the ear.

Term	Explanation
vertigo	Sensation of spinning or whirling around; incorrectly used to mean dizziness

> **TERMINOLOGY TIDBIT**
> The term *vertigo* comes from the Latin word *verto* meaning "whirling." Typically a person with vertigo perceives the world as spinning around in a circle.

Otorhinolaryngology Abbreviations

The following list presents common otorhinolaryngology abbreviations.

DPT	diphtheria, pertussis, tetanus	**OE**	otitis externa
EENT	eye, ear, nose, throat	**OM**	otitis media
ENT	ear, nose, and throat; otorhinolaryngology	**Oto**	otology
		PE tube	pressure-equalizing tube
ET	endotracheal	**T&A**	tonsillectomy and adenoidectomy
HEENT	head, eye, ear, nose, throat	**URI**	upper respiratory infection

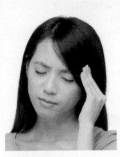

Source: Leungchopan/
Shutterstock

History of Present Illness
A 30-year-old female reports a history of chronic fatigue and headaches for at least 10 years. Headaches are centered above her eyes and occasionally radiate into the teeth of her upper jaw. Recently she became concerned when she noted that she was unable to smell fish she was cooking. She denies fever or cough.

Past Medical History
Patient has no history of hypertension, dental problems, or neurological problems. No known allergies. No prior hospitalizations except for birth of child.

Family and Social History
Patient is a police officer. She is married with one healthy child. She does not drink alcohol but does smoke one to one and a half packs of cigarettes per day. Family history is noncontributory.

Physical Examination
Well-developed and well-nourished female who appears her stated age and is in no obvious distress. Temperature is 99°F, blood pressure is 115/65, pulse is 110 bpm, and breathing rate is 14 breaths per minute. There is tenderness over her brow ridge bilaterally. Examination with otoscope revealed normal-appearing tympanic membranes and no evidence of otitis externa or otitis media. There was no cervical lymphadenopathy.

Diagnostic Tests
Sinus cultures were positive for bacteria and negative for fungus.

Diagnosis
Pansinusitis, potentially chronic based on patient's chronic symptoms

Plan of Treatment
1. Long-term course of oral antibiotic
2. Corticosteroid nose spray
3. Repeat culture in three months
4. Strongly recommend patient seek medical assistance to stop smoking
5. Refer to allergist to investigate whether she has allergies, which may have contributed to development of chronic infections

Critical Thinking Questions
Answer the following questions regarding this case study. Do not just copy words out of the case study but translate all medical terms. To answer some of these questions, you may need to look up information from another chapter of this text, in a medical dictionary, or online. Answers are found at the back of the book.

1. Explain the history of this patient's present illness in your own words.

   _____

   _____

2. What is the medical term for the inability to smell?

   _____

   _____

3. Which of the following conditions was NOT mentioned in her past medical history?

   a. Problems with brain, spinal cord, or nerves

   b. Problems with the thyroid gland

   c. High blood pressure

   d. Problems with the teeth

4. Refer to the immunology chapter and explain what cervical lymphadenopathy means.

_____

_____

5. What does "**pan-**" mean in pansinusitis?

_____

_____

6. Go to National Institutes of Health Medline Plus Medical Encyclopedia at http://www.nlm.nih.gov/ medlineplus/encyclopedia.html. Click on the "V," scroll down the list, and click on "Vital Signs." Compare this patient's vital signs to the normal ranges for the average healthy adult and note whether any of her vital signs are outside the normal ranges.

_____

_____

7. What is a culture? Explain the results of the sinus culture.

_____

_____

8. Describe what you think the purpose of each treatment is.

_____

_____

PRACTICE

Sound It Out

The following are some of the key terms from this chapter written as their phonetic spelling. Sound out each term and write it in the blank. Pronunciations for all terms are included in the audio glossary at www.mymedicalterminologylab.com.

1. oh-TAL-jee-ah _____

2. aw-dee-OM-eh-ter _____

3. dif-THEAR-ee-ah _____

4. fair-IN-goh-spazm _____

5. my-RIN-goh-skle-ROH-sis _____

6. dis-FOH-nee-ah _____

7. ADD-eh-noy-DEK-toh-mee _____

8. OH-toh-plas-tee _____

9. lair-in-JYE-tis _____

10. lair-RING-goh-plee-gee-ah _____

11. lair-RING-go-scope _____

12. mir-IN-goh-plass-tee _____

13. VER-tih-goh _____

14. TIM-pan-oh-gram _____

15. tim-pah-NOM-eh-tree _____

16. oh-TOSS-koh-pee _____

17. pan-sigh-nus-EYE-tis _____

18. per-TUH-sis _____

19. rye-NYE-tis _____

20. rye-noh-REE-ah _____

21. tin-EYE-tus _____

22. ton-sih-LEK-toh-mee _____

23. AW-dee-oh-gram _____

24. tray-kee-oh-steh-NOH-sis _____

25. tim-pan-oh-REK-sis _____

Transcription Practice

Each of the following sentences is written in common English. Underline any words or phrases that can be replaced by a medical term. Then rewrite the entire sentence using medical terms. Answers can be found at the back of the book.

1. The new parents were quite concerned when their baby developed an acute respiratory condition with a barking cough.

_____

_____

2. Meilin's inability to hear was caused by a benign tumor of the auditory nerve sheath.

_____

_____

3. The DPT vaccination protects children against a bacterial upper respiratory infection characterized by formation of a thick membranous film across the throat and whooping cough.

_____

_____

4. The physician ordered supplemental oxygen to be delivered by a two-pronged plastic device directly in the nose.

_____

_____

5. His physician became concerned when Mr. Janssen reported a sensation of spinning along with ringing in the ears.

_____

_____

6. Carmen's physician recommended to her parents that she have tubes surgically placed in the eardrums because of her repeated bacterial infections of the middle ear.

_____

_____

7. The paramedics had to quickly determine whether the patient's condition required a cutting into the trachea or a tube placed through the mouth and into the trachea.

_____

_____

8. Ursula went to see a specialist in the study of the ear, nose, and throat because of her repeated nosebleeds.

_____

_____

9. For his inability to hear, Tariq needed a hearing device surgically placed under the skin behind the ear rather than a device that amplifies sound.

_____

_____

10. After examining the external auditory canal with an instrument for examining the ear, it was obvious Jackson had swimmer's ear caused by a fungal infection.

_____

_____

Fill in the Blank

Fill in the blank to complete each of the following sentences.

1. The ear is responsible for the sense of _____ and _____.

2. The _____ prevents food and drink from entering the larynx.

3. The _____ is commonly called the *voice box*.

4. The pharyngeal tonsils are also called the _____.

5. Sound waves traveling down the external auditory canal strike _____.

6. The _____ nerve sends hearing messages to the brain.

7. Air enters the nasal cavity through two holes called the _____.

8. The common name for epistaxis is _____.

9. A hearing aid is also referred to as a(n) _____.

10. The three small ossicles in the middle ear are the _____, _____, and _____.

Abbreviation Matching

Match each abbreviation with its definition.

_____ 1. URI	A.	otorhinolaryngology
_____ 2. OM	B.	otology
_____ 3. ENT	C.	tonsillectomy and adenoidectomy
_____ 4. HEENT	D.	diphtheria, pertussis, tetanus
_____ 5. Oto	E.	upper respiratory infection
_____ 6. PE tube	F.	otitis externa
_____ 7. OE	G.	head, eye, ear, nose, throat
_____ 8. T&A	H.	endotracheal
_____ 9. ET	I.	otitis media
_____ 10. DPT	J.	pressure-equalizing tube

Labeling Exercise

Write the name of each structure on the numbered line. Also use this space to write the combining form where appropriate.

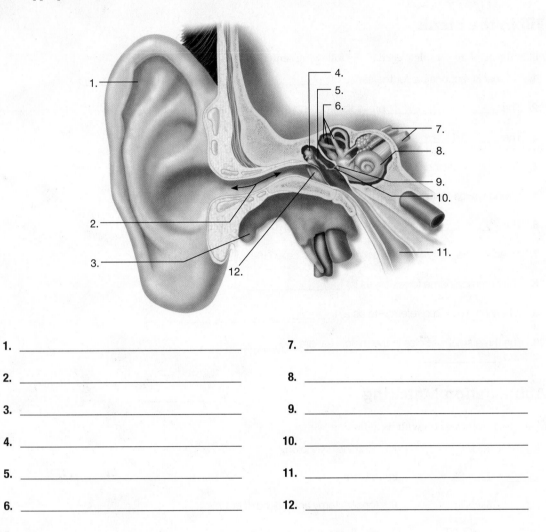

1. _____	7. _____
2. _____	8. _____
3. _____	9. _____
4. _____	10. _____
5. _____	11. _____
6. _____	12. _____

Build Medical Terms

Use each of the following word parts to build the indicated medical terms.

The combining form *ot/o* means ear.

1. study of ear _____

2. abnormal condition of ear fungus _____

3. surgical repair of ear _____

4. ear inflammation _____

5. process of visually examining ear _____

The combining form *pharyng/o* means pharynx.

6. involuntary muscle contraction of pharynx _____

7. pertaining to the pharynx _____

The suffix *-phonia* means voice.

8. without voice _____

9. abnormal, difficult voice _____

The combining form *trache/o* means trachea.

10. narrowing of the trachea _____

11. cutting into the trachea _____

12. enlarged trachea _____

The combining form *tympan/o* means tympanic membrane (eardrum).

13. surgical repair of the eardrum _____

14. instrument for measuring the eardrum _____

15. rupture of the eardrum _____

MyMedicalTerminologyLab™

MyMedicalTerminologyLab is a premium online homework management system that includes a host of features to help you study. Registered users will find:

- A multitude of activities and assignments built within the MyLab platform
- Powerful tools that track and analyze your results—allowing you to create a personalized learning experience
- Videos and audio pronunciations to help enrich your progress
- Streaming lesson presentations and self-paced learning modules
- A space where you and your instructors can view and manage your assignments

Medical Term Analysis

Examine each of the following terms. Begin by dividing it into its word parts and writing them in the indicated blanks (*P = prefix*; *WR = word root*; *CF = combining form*; *S = suffix*). Follow with the definition of each word part and then finally the meaning of the full term.

1. **tympanotomy**

   WR _____

   means _____

   S _____

   means _____

   Term meaning: _____

2. **cochlear**

   WR _____

   means _____

   S _____

   means _____

   Term meaning: _____

3. **nasogastric**

   CF _____

   means _____

   WR _____

   means _____

   S _____

   means _____

   Term meaning: _____

4. **endotracheal**

   P _____

   means _____

   WR _____

   means _____

   S _____

   means _____

   Term meaning: _____

5. **rhinomycosis**

   CF _____

   means _____

   WR _____

   means _____

   S _____

   means _____

   Term meaning: _____

6. **tonsillectomy**

   WR _____

   means _____

   S _____

   means _____

   Term meaning: _____

7. anosmia

P _____

means _____

S _____

means _____

Term meaning:_____

_____

8. laryngoplegia

CF _____

means _____

S _____

means _____

Term meaning: _____

_____

9. pansinusitis

P _____

means _____

WR _____

means _____

S _____

means _____

Term meaning: _____

_____

10. myringosclerosis

CF _____

means _____

S _____

means _____

Term meaning: _____

_____

Spelling

Some of the following terms are misspelled. Identify the incorrect terms and spell them correctly in the blank provided.

1. audiology _____

2. epitaxis _____

3. diptheria _____

4. otopyorhea _____

5. tracheostenosis _____

6. tympanotomy _____

7. vertigo _____

8. canula _____

9. tinnitus _____

10. pertusiss _____

Photomatch Challenge

Match each upper respiratory condition with its name in the Word Bank.

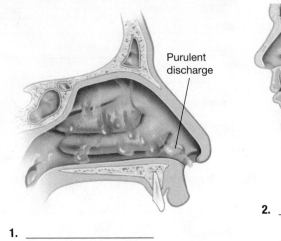

Purulent discharge

1. _____

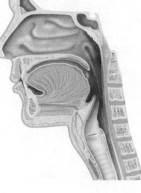

2. _____

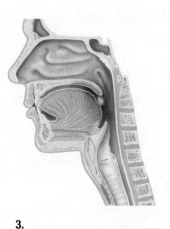

3. _____

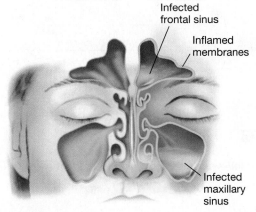

Infected frontal sinus

Inflamed membranes

Infected maxillary sinus

4. _____

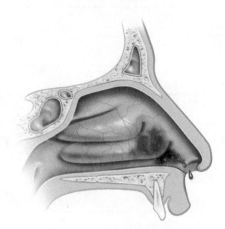

5. _____

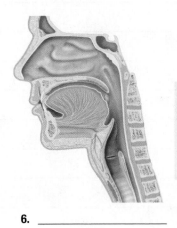

6. _____

Word Bank:

epistaxis	rhinitis
laryngitis	sinusitis
pharyngitis	tonsillitis

Word Parts

Prefixes

a-	without	hetero-	different	peri-	around
an-	without	homo-	same	poly-	many
ante-	before, in front of	hyper-	excessive	post-	after
anti-	against	hypo-	below, insufficient	pre-	before
auto-	self	infra-	below	primi-	first
bi-	two	inter-	between	quadri-	four
brady-	slow	intra-	within	retro-	behind
de-	without	micro-	small	sub-	beneath, under
di-	two	mono-	one	supra-	above
dys-	painful, difficult, abnormal	multi-	many	tachy-	fast
		neo-	new	trans-	across
endo-	within, inner	nulli-	none	tri-	three
epi-	above	pachy-	thick	ultra-	excess
eu-	normal, good	pan-	all	uni-	one
ex-	outward	para-	beside; two like parts of a pair		
extra-	outside of				
hemi-	half	per-	through		

Combining Forms

abdomin/o	abdomen	arthr/o	joint	carp/o	carpus (wrist)
acr/o	extremities	atel/o	incomplete	caud/o	tail
aden/o	gland	ather/o	fatty substance, plaque	cephal/o	head
adenoid/o	adenoids			cerebell/o	cerebellum
adip/o	fat	atri/o	atrium	cerebr/o	cerebrum
adren/o	adrenal gland	audi/o	hearing	cervic/o	neck, cervix
adrenal/o	adrenal gland	audit/o	hearing	chem/o	chemical
albumin/o	albumin	aur/o	ear	chol/e	bile
alveol/o	alveolus (air sac)	azot/o	nitrogen waste	cholangi/o	bile duct
ambly/o	dull, dim	bacteri/o	bacteria	cholecyst/o	gallbladder
amni/o	amnion	balan/o	glans penis	choledoch/o	common bile duct
an/o	anus	bas/o	base	chondr/o	cartilage
angi/o	vessel	bi/o	life	chori/o	chorion
anter/o	front (side of body)	blephar/o	eyelid	choroid/o	choroid layer
		brachi/o	arm	chrom/o	color
aort/o	aorta	bronch/o	bronchus	clavicul/o	clavicle (collar bone)
append/o	appendix	bronchi/o	bronchus		
appendic/o	appendix	bronchiol/o	bronchiole	coagul/o	clotting
aque/o	water	burs/o	bursa	coccyg/o	coccyx (tailbone)
arteri/o	artery	carcin/o	cancer	cochle/o	cochlea
arteriol/o	arteriole	cardi/o	heart	col/o	colon

colon/o	colon	glute/o	buttocks	melan/o	melanin, black
colp/o	vagina	glyc/o	sugar	men/o	menses, menstruation
coni/o	dust	glycos/o	sugar, glucose		
conjunctiv/o	conjunctiva	gynec/o	woman, female	mening/o	meninges
core/o	pupil	hem/o	blood	metacarp/o	metacarpus (hand bones)
corne/o	cornea	hemat/o	blood		
coron/o	heart	hepat/o	liver	metatars/o	metatarsus (foot bones)
corpor/o	body	hidr/o	sweat		
cortic/o	cortex	humer/o	humerus (upper arm bone)	metr/o	uterus
cost/o	rib			muscul/o	muscle
crani/o	skull	hydr/o	water	my/o	muscle
crin/o	to secrete	hyster/o	uterus	myc/o	fungus
cry/o	cold	ichthy/o	scaly	myel/o	bone marrow, spinal cord
crypt/o	hidden	ile/o	ileum		
cubit/o	elbow	ili/o	ilium (part of pelvis)	myring/o	tympanic membrane (eardrum)
cutane/o	skin				
cyan/o	blue	immun/o	protection, immunity		
cycl/o	ciliary body			nas/o	nose
cyst/o	urinary bladder, sac	infer/o	below, lower	nat/o	birth
		inguin/o	groin	necr/o	death
cyt/o	cell	ir/o	iris	nephr/o	kidney
dacry/o	tears	irid/o	iris	neur/o	nerve
derm/o	skin	isch/o	to hold back	neutr/o	neutral
dermat/o	skin	ischi/o	ischium (part of pelvis)	noct/i	night
dipl/o	double			o/o	egg
dist/o	farthest (away from beginning of structure)	jejun/o	jejunum	ocul/o	eye
		kerat/o	keratin, hard, hornlike, cornea	olig/o	scanty
				onych/o	nail
diverticul/o	diverticulum	kyph/o	hump	oophor/o	ovary
dors/o	back (side of body)	lacrim/o	tears	ophthalm/o	eye
		lapar/o	abdomen	opt/o	eye, vision
duoden/o	duodenum	laryng/o	larynx (voice box)	or/o	mouth
electr/o	electricity			orbit/o	eye socket
embol/o	plug	later/o	side	orch/o	testes
embry/o	embryo	leuk/o	white	orchi/o	testes
encephal/o	brain	lip/o	fat	orchid/o	testes
enter/o	intestine	lith/o	stone	orth/o	straight
eosin/o	rosy red	lob/o	lobe	oste/o	bone
epididym/o	epididymis	lord/o	bent backward	ot/o	ear
epiglott/o	epiglottis	lumb/o	low back	ovari/o	ovary
episi/o	vulva	lymph/o	lymph	ox/i	oxygen
erythr/o	red	lymphaden/o	lymph node	pancreat/o	pancreas
esophag/o	esophagus	lymphangi/o	lymph vessel	parathyroid/o	parathyroid gland
femor/o	femur (thigh bone)	mamm/o	breast		
		mandibul/o	mandible (lower jaw)	patell/o	patella (kneecap)
fet/o	fetus			path/o	disease
fibr/o	fibrous	mast/o	breast	pelv/o	pelvis
fibul/o	fibula (thinner lower leg bone)	maxill/o	maxilla (upper jaw)	phac/o	lens
		medi/o	middle	phag/o	eating
gastr/o	stomach	mediastin/o	mediastinum	phalang/o	phalanges (fingers and toes)
genit/o	genitals	medull/o	medulla oblongata		
glomerul/o	glomerulus			pharyng/o	pharynx (throat)

phleb/o	vein	scoli/o	crooked, bent	tonsill/o	tonsils
phot/o	light	seb/o	sebum, oil	toxic/o	poison
pineal/o	pineal gland	semin/i	semen	trache/o	trachea (windpipe)
pituitar/o	pituitary gland	septic/o	infection		
pleur/o	pleura	sigmoid/o	sigmoid colon	trich/o	hair
pneum/o	lung, air	sinus/o	sinus	tympan/o	tympanic membrane (eardrum)
pneumon/o	lung	son/o	sound		
polyp/o	polyp	sperm/o	sperm		
pont/o	pons	spermat/o	sperm	uln/o	ulna (part of forearm)
poster/o	back (side of body)	sphygm/o	pulse		
		spin/o	spine	ungu/o	nail
proct/o	rectum and anus	spir/o	breathing	ur/o	urine
prostat/o	prostate gland	splen/o	spleen	ureter/o	ureter
proxim/o	nearest (to beginning of structure)	spondyl/o	vertebra	urethr/o	urethra
		stern/o	sternum (breast bone)	urin/o	urine
pub/o	pubis (part of pelvis)			uter/o	uterus
		steth/o	chest	vagin/o	vagina
pulmon/o	lung	super/o	above, upper	valv/o	valve
pupill/o	pupil	system/o	system	valvul/o	valve
py/o	pus	tars/o	tarsus (ankle)	varic/o	dilated vein
pyel/o	renal pelvis	ten/o	tendon	vas/o	blood vessel, vas deferens
radi/o	radius (part of forearm)	tendin/o	tendon		
		testicul/o	testes	vascul/o	blood vessel
rect/o	rectum	thalam/o	thalamus	ven/o	vein
ren/o	kidney	thorac/o	chest	ventr/o	belly (side of body)
retin/o	retina	thromb/o	clot		
rhin/o	nose	thym/o	thymus gland	ventricul/o	ventricle
sacr/o	sacrum	thyr/o	thyroid gland	venul/o	venule
salping/o	uterine (fallopian) tube	thyroid/o	thyroid gland	vertebr/o	vertebra (backbone)
		tibi/o	tibia (shin, larger lower leg bone)		
scapul/o	scapula (shoulder blade)			vesic/o	bladder, sac
		tom/o	to cut	vesicul/o	seminal vesicle
scler/o	hardening, sclera	ton/o	tension, pressure	vitre/o	glassy
				xanth/o	yellow
				xer/o	dry

Suffixes

-ac	pertaining to	-cyte	cell	-er	one who
-al	pertaining to	-cytosis	abnormal cell condition (too many)	-esthesia	feeling, sensation
-algia	pain			-genesis	produces, generates
-an	pertaining to	-derma	skin condition		
-ar	pertaining to	-desis	surgical fusing	-genic	producing
-ary	pertaining to	-dipsia	thirst	-gen	that which produces
-asthenia	weakness	-dynia	pain		
-atic	pertaining to	-eal	pertaining to	-globin	protein
-cele	protrusion	-ectasis	dilated	-globulin	protein
-centesis	puncture to withdraw fluid	-ectomy	surgical removal	-gram	record
		-edema	swelling	-graph	instrument for recording
-clasia	surgical breaking	-emesis	vomiting		
-cle	small	-emia	blood condition	-graphy	process of recording
-cyesis	pregnancy				

-gravida	pregnancy	-ole	small	-porosis	porous
-ia	state, condition	-oma	tumor, mass	-ptosis	drooping
-iasis	abnormal condition	-opia	vision	-ptysis	spitting up, coughing up
-iatric	medical specialty	-opsy	view of	-rrhage	excessive, abnormal flow
-iatrist	physician	-ory	pertaining to		
-iatry	treatment, medicine	-ose	pertaining to	-rrhagia	abnormal flow condition
		-osis	abnormal condition		
-ician	specialist	-osmia	sense of smell	-rrhaphy	suture
-ic	pertaining to	-ostomy	surgically create an opening	-rrhea	discharge, flow
-ine	pertaining to			-rrhexis	rupture
-ior	pertaining to	-otomy	cutting into	-sclerosis	hardening
-ism	state of	-ous	pertaining to	-scope	instrument for viewing
-ist	specialist	-oxia	oxygen		
-itis	inflammation	-para	to bear (offspring)	-scopy	process of visually examining
-kinesia	movement	-partum	childbirth		
-lith	stone	-pathy	disease	-spasm	involuntary muscle contraction
-logist	one who studies	-penia	too few		
-logy	study of	-pepsia	digestion	-stasis	stopping
-lysis	to destroy	-pexy	surgical fixation	-stenosis	narrowing
-lytic	destruction	-phagia	eating, swallowing	-therapy	treatment
-malacia	abnormal softening	-phasia	speech	-thorax	chest
		-phil	attracted to	-tic	pertaining to
-manometer	instrument to measure pressure	-phobia	fear	-tome	instrument to cut
		-phonia	voice		
-megaly	enlarged	-plasia	formation of cells	-toxic	poison
-meter	instrument for measuring	-plasm	formation	-tripsy	surgical crushing
		-plasty	surgical repair	-trophic	development
-metry	process of measuring	-plegia	paralysis	-trophy	development
		-pnea	breathing	-ule	small
-nic	pertaining to	-poiesis	formation	-uria	urine condition
-oid	resembling				

Abbreviations and Symbols

Abbreviations and symbols are commonly used when writing medical documents because they are convenient and save time; however, they can certainly be confusing. For example, *DC* may mean discontinue or discharge. Use of an incorrect abbreviation can result in problems for a patient as well as insurance records and processing. If there is ever a concern that an abbreviation may be misinterpreted, it is always best to spell out the word instead.

It is never acceptable to use one's own abbreviations or symbols. All health care facilities have a list of approved abbreviations and symbols, and it is extremely important to become familiar with and follow this list closely. Just as importantly, there is also a list of abbreviations and symbols that should never be used. Abbreviations and symbols that have been shown to be misleading are placed on this list.

This appendix presents the most common abbreviations and symbols used in medical documents. They have been grouped together into categories for ease of learning. However, abbreviations are so essential to learning medical terminology that throughout this book, many of these have already been presented within the chapters immediately following terms. Additionally, a list of common abbreviations for each medical specialty is given in each chapter.

Abbreviations for Health Care Providers, Services, or Units

AuD	Doctor of Audiology
BSN	Bachelor of Science in Nursing
CCS	Certified Coding Specialist
CCU	Coronary Care Unit
CLS	Clinical Laboratory Scientist
CLT	Clinical Laboratory Technician
CMA	Certified Medical Assistant
CNA	Certified Nurse Aide
COTA	Certified Occupational Therapy Assistant
CRT	Certified Respiratory Therapist
CV	Cardiovascular
DC	Doctor of Chiropractic
DDM	Doctor of Dental Medicine
DDS	Doctor of Dental Surgery
Derm	Dermatology
DI	Diagnostic imaging
DO	Doctor of Osteopathic Medicine
DPT	Doctor of Physical Therapy
DTR	Dietetic Technician, Registered

ED	Emergency Department
EMT-B	Emergency Medical Technician–Basic
EMT-I	Emergency Medical Technician–Intermediate
EMT-P	Emergency Medical Technician–Paramedic
ENT	Ear, Nose, and Throat
ER	Emergency Room
GI	Gastrointestinal
GU	Genitourinary
GYN	Gynecology
ICU	Intensive Care Unit
LPN	Licensed Practical Nurse
LVN	Licensed Vocational Nurse
MD	Medical Doctor
MLT	Medical Laboratory Technician
MSN	Master of Science in Nursing
MSW	Medical Social Worker
MT	Medical Technologist
NICU	Neonatal Intensive Care Unit
NP	Nurse Practitioner
OB	Obstetrics
OD	Doctor of Optometry
OPD	Outpatient Department

Ophth	Ophthalmology
OR	Operating room
Orth, Ortho	Orthopedics
OT	Occupational Therapy; Occupational Therapist
OTA	Occupational Therapy Assistant
Path	Pathology
Peds	Pediatrics
Pharm D	Doctor of Pharmacy
PT	Physical Therapy; Physical Therapist
PTA	Physical Therapy Assistant
RD	Registered Dietitian
RDH	Registered Dental Hygienist
Rehab	Rehabilitation Unit
RHIA	Registered Health Information Administrator
RN	Registered Nurse
RPh	Registered Pharmacist
RRT	Registered Respiratory Therapist, Registered Radiologic Technologist
RR	Recovery Room
X-ray	Radiology

Abbreviations Indicating Time or Frequency

ā	before
ac	before meals
ad lib	as desired
am, AM	morning
ante	before
bid	twice a day
d	day
noc, noct	night
p̄	after
pc	after meals
pm, PM	evening
prn	as needed
q	every
qh	every hour
qid	four times a day
STAT, stat	at once/immediately
tid	three times a day
yr	year

Abbreviations for Units of Measurement

cg	centigram
cm	centimeter
dr	dram
ft	foot, feet
g	gram
gm	gram
gr	grain
gt	drop
gtt	drops
h	hour
hr	hour
in	inch
kg	kilogram
L	liter
lb	pound
m	meter
mcg	microgram
mEq	milliequivalent
mg	milligram
min	minutes
mL	milliliter
mm	millimeter
oz	ounce
pt	pint
qt	quart

sec	seconds
T, tbsp	tablespoon
t, tsp	teaspoon
yd	yard

Patient Chart Abbreviations

ADLs	activities of daily living
AK	above knee
AMA	against medical advice
amb	ambulate, walk
BK	below knee
BR	bathroom; bed rest
BRP	bathroom privileges
CA	cancer; chronological age
CBR	complete bed rest
CC	chief complaint
c/o	complains of
DOA	dead on arrival
DOB	date of birth
DNR	do not resuscitate
Dx	diagnosis
Ex	examination
FH	family history
f/u	follow up
h/o	history of
H&P	history and physical
HEENT	head, eye, ear, nose, throat
Hx	history
I&O	intake and output
LA	left arm
LE	lower extremity
LL	left leg
MH	marital history; mental health
MS	mental status
NKA	no known allergies
PE	physical exam; pulmonary embolism
PERRLA	pupils equal, round, reactive to light and accommodation
PI	present illness
PMH	past medical history
pt	patient
RA	right arm
RL	right leg
r/o, R/O	rule out
ROM	range of motion
SH	social history
s/p	status post (previous disease condition)

Sx	symptoms, signs
Tx	treatment
UE	upper extremity
WDWN	well developed, well nourished

Vital Signs Abbreviations

BP	blood pressure
BPM, bpm	beats per minute
ht	height
NTP	normal temperature and pressure
P	pulse
R	respirations
RR	respiratory rate
T	temperature
TPR	temperature, pulse, and respirations
VS, V/S	vital signs
wt	weight

Pharmacy Abbreviations

APAP	acetaminophen (Tylenol™)
ASA	aspirin
cap(s)	capsule(s)
Chemo	chemotherapy
disp	dispense
dtd	give of such a dose
ī	one
ID	intradermal
īī	two
īīī	three
IM	intramuscular
inj	injection
IV	intravenous
no sub	no substitute
non rep	do not repeat
npo, NPO	nothing by mouth
NS	normal saline
OD, od	overdose
oint	ointment
OTC	over-the-counter
PCA	patient-controlled administration
PDR	*Physician's Desk Reference*
po, PO	by mouth
Rx	prescription, treatment
Sig	label as follows/directions

sl	under the tongue
sol	solution
s̄s̄	one-half
Subc	subcutaneous
Subq	subcutaneous
suppos, supp	suppository
tab(s)	tablet
top	apply topically

Miscellaneous Abbreviations

aq	aqueous (water)
ant	anterior
AP	anteroposterior
cont	continue
DC, dc, d/c	discontinue
DISC, disc	discontinue
et	and
ETOH	ethanol
HIPAA	Health Insurance Portability and Accountability Act
L,Ⓛ	left
lat	lateral
mets	metastases
neg	negative
PA	posteroanterior
per	by
p/o	postoperative
pos	positive
post	posterior

post-op	after operation
prep	prepare for
PTA	prior to admission
R,Ⓡ	right
ROS	review of systems
TO	telephone order
VO	verbal order
w/c	wheelchair
WNL	within normal limits
w/u	work up
y/o	years old

Chemical Abbreviations

Ba	barium
C	carbon
$C_6H_{12}O_6$	glucose
Ca	calcium
CO_2	carbon dioxide
Cl	chlorine
Fe	iron
H	hydrogen
HCl	hydrochloric acid
HCO_3^-	bicarbonate
Hg	mercury
H_2O	water
I	iodine
K	potassium
Mg	magnesium
N	nitrogen
Na	sodium
NaCl	sodium chloride (salt)

O_2	oxygen
Pb	lead

Symbols

c̄	with
s̄	without
=	equal
≠	not equal
+	positive
−	negative
±	plus or minus
↑	increase
↓	decrease
#	pounds, number
♀	female
♂	male
→	from–to (in the direction of)
1°	primary
2°	secondary
3°	tertiary
%	percent
°C	degrees Celcius
°F	degrees Fahrenheit
≈	approximately
Δ	change
α	alpha
β	beta
×	times
"	inch
'	feet

Abbreviations to Be Avoided

Abbreviations make writing notes faster, but they also create the possibility of being misunderstood. For this reason, the Joint Commission on Accreditation of Healthcare Organizations (JCAHO) and the Institute for Safe Medication Practices (ISMP) publishes lists of error-prone abbreviations that are not to be used. The following table presents these abbreviations and what should be used instead. The Joint Commission (TJC) has determined that the first seven abbreviations (marked with an *) must appear on an accredited institution's "Do Not Use" list of abbreviations.

Abbreviation	Intended Meaning	Potential Problem	Recommendation
IU*	International unit	Mistaken for "IV" or "10"	Write "international unit"
MS, MSO_4, and $MgSO_4$*	Morphine sulfate, magnesium sulfate	Mistaken for each other	Write "morphine sulfate" or "magnesium sulfate"
Not using a zero before a decimal point (0.X)*	.X mg	Decimal point is missed	Always write a zero before a decimal point (0.X mg)
q.d. or QD*	Every day	Mistaken for "qid"	Write "daily"

Abbreviation	Intended Meaning	Potential Problem	Recommendation
q.o.d. or QOD*	Every other day	Mistaken for "qd" or for "qid"	Write "every other day"
U or u*	Unit	Mistaken for "0," "4," or "cc"	Write "unit"
Using a zero after a decimal point*	X.0 mg	Decimal point is missed	Never write a zero by itself after a decimal point (X mg is correct)
@	at	Mistaken for "2"	Write "at"
&	and	Mistaken for "2"	Write "and"
< and >	lesser than and greater than	Mistakenly read as the opposite symbol	Write "lesser than" and "greater than"
+	and	Mistaken for "4"	Write "and"
°	hour	Mistaken for "0"	Write "hr," "h," or "hour"
i/d	one daily	Mistaken for "tid"	Write "one daily"
μg	microgram	Mistaken for "mg"	Write "mcg"
ʒ	dram	Mistaken for "3"	Write "dram"
AS, AD, AU and OS, OD, OU	Left ear, right ear, both ears and left eye, right eye, both eyes	Mistaken for each other (for example, "AS" and "OS")	Write "left ear," "right ear," "both ears," "left eye," "right eye," and "both eyes"
BT	bedtime	Mistaken for "bid"	Write "bedtime"
cc	Cubic centimeter	Mistaken for "U" (units)	Since a cubic centimeter is equal to a milliliter, write "mL"
D/C	discharge	Mistaken to mean "discontinue"	Write "discharge"
Dose and unit of measure run together (such as 10mg or 100mL)	10 mg or 100 mL	Mistaken for "100 mg" or "1000 mL"	Use adequate space between dose and unit of measure
Drug name and dose run together (such as Inderal40 mg)	Inderal 40 mg	Mistaken for "Inderal 140 mg"	Use adequate space between drug name and dose
hs or HS	Half-strength or at bedtime	Meanings can be mistaken for each other	Write "half-strength" or "at bedtime"
IJ	injection	Mistaken for "IV"	Write "injection"
IN	Intranasal	Mistaken for "IM" or "IV"	Write "intranasal" or "NAS"
Large numbers without proper comma (such as 100000)	100,000	Mistaken for "1,000,000"	Always use commas in large numbers

Abbreviation	Intended Meaning	Potential Problem	Recommendation
o.d. or OD	once daily	Mistaken for "right eye (OD)" or "overdose"	write "daily"
OJ	orange juice	Mistaken for "right eye (OD)"	write "orange juice"
Per os	by mouth	"os" can be mistaken to mean "left eye"	write "PO," "orally," or "by mouth"
Period following abbreviation such as mg. or mL.	mg or mL	Period mistaken for "1"	Write "mg" or "mL"
qhs	every bedtime	Mistaken for "qhr"	Write "bedtime"
qn	every night	Mistaken for "qh"	Write "nightly"
q1d	every day	Mistaken for "qid"	Write "daily"
q6PM	every day at 6:00 p.m.	Mistaken to mean "every 6 hours"	Write "daily at 6 p.m."
SC, SQ, sub q	Subcutaneous	SC mistaken for "SL," SQ mistaken for "5 every," the separate q mistaken for "every"	Write "Subq," "Subc," or "subcutaneous"
ss	sliding scale or one-half	Mistaken for each other and for "55"	Write "sliding scale," "one-half," or "1/2"
SSRI and SSI	sliding scale regular insulin and sliding scale insulin	Mistaken for "selective-serotonin reuptake inhibitor" and "strong solution of iodine"	Write "sliding scale (insulin)"
tiw or TIW	Three times a week	Mistaken for "three times a day" or "twice weekly"	Write "3 times weekly"
UD	as directed (*ut dictum*)	Mistaken for unit dose	Write "as directed"
x3d	for three days	Mistaken to mean "for 3 doses"	Write "for three days"

Selected English/Spanish Glossary

English	Spanish
abdomen (belly)	vientre
acute	agudo
AIDS (Acquired Immune Deficiency Syndrome)	SIDA (Sindrome de Immune Deficiencia Adquirida)
allergy	alergia
anemia	anemia; sangre delgada
angina	angina
ankle	tobillo
anxiety	ansiedad
appendix	apéndice
arm	brazo
artery	arteria
arthritis	artritis
asphyxia	asfixia; sofocación
asthma	asma; ansia
back	espalda; lomo
bad	malo
benign	benigno; de poca gravedad
better	major
black	negro
bladder	vejiga
blood	sangre
blood pressure	presión sanguínea; presión arterial
blood test	prueba de sangre
blue	azul
body	cuerpo
bone	hueso
brain	cerebro
breast	pecho; seno
breathe	respirar; inhalar
bronchitis	bronquitis; catarro de pecho
bruise	contusión; morado
burning	ardiente
cancer	cáncer
capillary	capilar
cardiology	cardiología
cartilage	cartílago
cataract	catarata
cheek	mejilla; cachete
chest	pecho; tórax
chickenpox	varicela; viruela loca
cholesterol	colesterol
chronic	crónico
clavicle	clavícula
closed	cerrado
clot	coágulo; trombo
cold	frío; catarro
common cold	resfriado común
concussion	concusión; conmoción
convulsion	convulsión; ataque
cough	tos
croup	crup
CT scan	tomografía axial computarizada
dark	oscuro
dead	muerto
deaf	sordo(a)
deep breath	rispirar profundo
deficient	deficiente
dermatology	dermatología
diabetes	diabetes
diagnosis	diagnóstico
dialysis	diálisis
diarrhea	diarrea; estómago suelto
difficulty in breathing	dificultad de la respiración
diphtheria	difteria
dizziness	mareo; vértigo
double vision	visión doble; ver doble
dry	seco
dysuria	disuria; emisión de la orina
ear	oreja; oído
earache	dolor de oído
edema	edema
elbow	codo
endocrinology	endocrinología
epilepsy	epilepsia
equilibrium	equilibrio
esophagus	esófago
excessive	excesivo; desmesurado
exhale	exhalar
external	externo
eye	ojo
fainting	desmayo
fast	rápido(a)

English	Spanish	English	Spanish
fatigue	fatiga; cansancio	larynx	laringe
fever	fiebre; calentura	left	izquierdo(a)
finger	dedo de la mano	leg	pierna
foot	pie	ligament	ligarnento
forearm	antebrazo	lips	labios
fracture	fractura	liver	hígado
gallbladder	vesócula biliar	lump	bolita; abultamiento;
gallstones	cálculos biliar		nudo; protuberancia
gastroenterology	gastroenterología	lung	pulmón; bofe
genital	genital	lymph node	nódulo; ganglio linfático
gland	glándula	lymphatic	linfático
glaucoma	glaucoma	malignant	maligno; pernicioso
good	bueno	mandible	mandíbula
gray	gris	maxilla	maxilar
green	verde	measles	sarampión
gums	encías	middle	medio
gynecology	ginecología	mouth	boca
hand	mano	mumps	paperas; parotiditis
hard	duro	murmur	soplo; murmullo del corazón
head	cabeza	muscle	músculo
headache	dolor de cabeza	muscle spasm	espasmo muscular
healthy	sana	narrow	estrecho
hearing	audición; oído	nausea	náusea; mareo
heart	corazón	navel	ombligo
hematology	hematología	neck	cuello; pescuezo
hemorrhage	hemorragia; desangramiento	nephrology	nefrología
hepatitis	hepatitis	nerve	nervio
hip	cadera	neurology	neurologia
hormone	hormona	nose	nariz
hot	caliente; calor	nosebleed	hemorragia nasal
hypertension	hipertensión; presión arterial alta	obstetrics	obstericia
immunology	immunología	oncology	oncología
incision	corte; incisión	open	abierto
infection	infección	ophthalmology	oftalmología
inflammation	inflamación	orange-yellow	cirrho
influenza	gripe; influenza	orthopedics	ortopedia
inhale	inhalar	otorhinolaryngology	otorrinolaringología
injection	inyección; piquete	ovary	ovario
inner	interior	oxygen	oxígeno
insulin	insulina	pain	dolor
internal	interno	palpitation	palpitación
intestine	intestino; tripa	pancreas	páncreas
intravenous	intravenoso	paralysis	parálisis
itching	comezón; picazón	parathyroid	paratiroideo
jaundice	ictericia	pathology	patología
joint	articulación; coyuntura	pelvis	pelvis
kidney	riñón	penis	pene
kidney stone	cálculo renales	phlegm	flemón; inflamación
knee	rodilla; gozne		difusa
large	grande	pituitary	pituitaria

English	Spanish
pneumonia	neumonía; inflamación de los pulmones
pregnancy	embarazo
prostate gland	próstata
pulmonology	neumólogía
pulse	pulso
purple	morado
rash	salpullido; sarpullido; erupción cutánea
rectum	recto; guía de atrás
red	rojo
redness	enrojecimiento; piel colorada
respiration	respiración
rib	costilla
right	derecha
sacrum	sacro; rabadilla
scapula	escápula; hueso de la espaldilla
shoulder	hombro
sick	enfermo(a); mal(a)
side	costado
skeleton	esqueleto
skin	piel; cuero; pellejo; cutis
skull	cráneo; calavera
slow	lento(a); pausado(a)
small	pequeño(a)
soft	blando(a)
sore throat	dolor de garganta
spasm	espasmo
spine	espinazo
spleen	bazo
sprain	torcedura; falseamiento; falseado
sternum	esternón
stiff	tieso(a); rígido(a)
stomach	estómago
stroke	apoplejía; embolia; derrame cerebral
strong	fuerte
surgery	cirugía
swallow	ingerir; pasar; tragar
sweating	sudar
swelling	hinchar
symptom	síntoma

English	Spanish
teeth	dientes
temperature	temperatura
tendon	cuello
test	puerba
testes	testículos; huevos; bolas
tetanus	tétano
thigh	muslo
thorax	tórax
throat	garganta
thyroid	tiroides
toe	dedo del pié
tongue	lengua
tonsil	tonsila; amigdala
tonsillitis	tonsilitis; amigdalitis
trachea	tráquea
treatment	tratamiento
tremor	temblor
tuberculosis	tuberculosis
ulcer	úlcera
ultrasound	ecografía; ultrasonido
unconscious	inconsciente
urethra	uretra; canal
urinalysis	análisis de orina
urination	urinacion
urine	orina; pipí
urology	urología
uterus	útero
vaccination	vacunación
vagina	vagina
vein	vena
vertebral column	columna vertebral
vision	visión
vomit	vómito
weakness	debilidad
white	blanco
whooping cough	tos ferina
worse	peor
wound	herida
wrist	muñeca
x-ray	radiografia; rayos equis
yellow	amarillo

Answer Keys

Chapter 1

Practice Exercises

Recognizing Types of Medical Terms

1. Latin/Greek   2. modern English   3. eponym   4. Latin/Greek   5. Latin/Greek   6. eponym
7. modern English   8. eponym   9. modern English   10. Latin/Greek

Forming Plurals

1. bursae   2. diverticula   3. adenoma   4. ganglia   5. indices   6. diagnosis   7. alveolus

Practice Defining Medical Terms

1. word root, combining vowel, suffix, abnormal softening of the brain   2. prefix, word root, suffix, pertaining to under the skin   3. word root, combining vowel, suffix, surgical fixation of the uterus
4. prefix, word root, suffix, inflammation of all the sinuses   5. word root, combining vowel, suffix, to suture a vessel   6. prefix, word root, suffix, pertaining to between the ventricles

Practice Building Medical Terms

1. laryngoplasty   2. arthroscope   3. subscapular   4. ophthalmology   5. neuroma
6. intramuscular

Chapter 2

Practice Exercises

Recognizing Categories of Suffixes

1. disease/abnormal condition, paralysis   2. diagnostic, process of measuring   3. general, cell
4. surgical, cutting into   5. disease/abnormal condition, stone   6. diagnostic, instrument for viewing   7. general, chest   8. diagnostic, process of recording   9. disease/abnormal condition, vomiting   10. surgical, surgical breaking   11. disease/abnormal condition, to destroy
12. surgical, surgical removal

Matching

1. E   2. L   3. F   4. H   5. C   6. D   7. I   8. A   9. K   10. G   11. B   12. J

Choosing the Correct Adjective Forms

1. cardiac   2. ovarian   3. duodenal   4. ventricular   5. pulmonary   6. esophageal   7. gastric
8. uterine   9. venous   10. hepatic

Build Medical Terms

1. gastrectomy   2. gastroscope   3. gastroscopy   4. gastralgia or gastrodynia   5. cystolith
6. cystoscope   7. cystoscopy   8. cystostomy   9. cystic   10. angioplasty   11. angioma
12. angiography   13. angiogram   14. angiostenosis   15. arteriosclerosis   16. arteriospasm
17. arteriorrhexis   18. arteriole   19. arthritis   20. arthroscope   21. arthroscopy
22. arthroplasty   23. arthrocentesis   24. dermatology   25. dermatologist   26. dermatitis
27. dermatosis   28. hepatitis   29. hepatoma   30. hepatomegaly   31. hepatocyte

32. hepatic   33. rhinorrhea   34. rhinoplasty   35. rhinorrhagia   36. bronchitis
37. bronchoscope   38. bronchoscopy   39. tracheostomy   40. tracheotomy
41. tracheocele   42. tracheomalacia   43. tracheal   44. colostomy   45. colectomy
46. colopexy   47. nephrology   48. nephrologist   49. nephromalacia   50. nephrosis
51. nephropathy   52. nephropexy   53. thoracotomy   54. thoracocentesis   55. thoracodynia
or thoracalgia   56. neurology   57. neurologist   58. neuroplasty   59. neurotripsy   60. neuralgia
or neurodynia   61. myorrhaphy   62. myopathy   63. myalgia or myodynia   64. myotome
65. myograph   66. myogram   67. myography

Chapter 3

Practice Exercises

Recognizing Categories of Prefixes

1. disease/abnormality, painful/difficult/abnormal   2. direction/body position, below or number,
insufficient   3. number, none   4. disease/abnormality, slow   5. disease/abnormality, without
6. time, new   7. direction/body position, between   8. time, after   9. number, small   10. direction/
body position, around   11. direction/body position, above   12. disease/abnormality, against

Matching

1. G   2. D   3. L   4. A   5. J   6. K   7. E   8. B   9. F   10. H   11. I   12. C

Build Medical Terms

1. tachycardia   2. bradycardia   3. endocarditis   4. pericarditis   5. pancarditis
6. intracellular   7. extracellular   8. multicellular   9. unicellular   10. intradermal
11. subdermal   12. epidermal   13. homograft   14. heterograft   15. autograft
16. bilateral   17. unilateral   18. preoperative   19. postoperative   20. intraoperative
21. primipara   22. nullipara   23. multipara   24. aphagia   25. dysphagia   26. polyphagia
27. apepsia   28. dyspepsia   29. bradypepsia   30. atrophy   31. dystrophy   32. hemiplegia
33. quadriplegia   34. monoplegia   35. apnea   36. eupnea   37. tachypnea   38. bradypnea
39. hyperpnea   40. hypopnea   41. infrascapular   42. suprascapular   43. subscapular
44. anuria   45. polyuria   46. dysuria

Chapter 4

Building Directional Terms

1. anterior   2. caudal   3. cephalic   4. distal   6. dorsal   7. inferior   8. lateral   9. medial
10. posterior   12. proximal   14. superior   16. ventral

Building Body Surface Terms

1. abdominal   2. antecubital   4. brachial   5. cervical   6. cranial   7. femoral   8. genital
9. gluteal   10. inguinal   12. nasal   13. orbital   14. oral   15. otic   17. patellar   18. pelvic
21. scapular   22. sternal   23. thoracic   27. vertebral

Practice Exercises

Directional Terms

1. posterior or dorsal   2. cephalic or superior   3. caudal or inferior   4. superficial
5. proximal   6. ventral or anterior   7. superior or cephalic   8. medial   9. lateral   10. anterior or
ventral   11. distal   12. deep   13. inferior or caudal   14. dorsal or posterior   15. prone

Fill in the Blank

1. spinal   2. pleura   3. dorsal   4. kidney   5. thoracic   6. peritoneum   7. brain   8. heart
9. pelvic   10. meninges   11. abdominal   12. mediastinum

Labeling Exercise—External Surface Anatomy

1. Cranial 2. Cervical 3. Thoracic 4. Brachial 5. Abdominal 6. Pelvic 7. Genital
8. Femoral 9. Trunk 10. Scapular 11. Vertebral 12. Gluteal

Matching—Planes and Sections

1. A 2. F 3. B 4. A, B 5. A 6. E 7. C 8. C 9. D

Matching–Organs and Clinical Divisions of the Abdominopelvic Cavity

1. A 2. D 3. C 4. C 5. E 6. A 7. B 8. D 9. C 10. F 11. C 12. E 13. B

Labeling Exercise—Anatomical Divisions of the Abdominopelvic Cavity

1. Right hypochondriac region   2. Right lumbar region   3. Right iliac/inguinal region   4. Epigastric region   5. Umbilical region   6. Hypogastric region   7. Left hypochondriac region   8. Left lumbar region   9. Left iliac/inguinal region

Chapter 5

Building Dermatology Terms

1. a. adenectomy; b. adenitis; c. adenoma; d. adenopathy; e. adenomegaly   2. a. adipose or adipic; b. adipocyte; c. adipoma   3. a. cutaneous; b. subcutaneous; c. percutaneous
4. a. cyanosis; b. cyanotic   5. a. ichthyoderma; b. scleroderma; c. xanthoderma; d. xeroderma; e. pachyderma; f. erythroderma; g. pyoderma; h. leukoderma   6. a. dermal or dermic; b. epidermal; c. intradermal; d. hypodermic; e. transdermal   7. a. dermatitis; b. dermatology; c. dermatologist; d. dermatosis; e. dermatoplasty; f. dermatomycosis; g. dermatopathy; h. dermatosclerosis   8. a. hidrosis; b. anhidrosis; c. hidradenitis; d. hyperhidrosis
9. a. keratoderma; b. keratosis; c. keratogenic   10. a. lipectomy; b. lipoid; c. lipoma; d. lipocyte   11. a. melanoma; b. melanocyte; c. melanotic   12. a. onychectomy; b. onychitis; c. onychomalacia; d. onychomycosis; e. onychophagia; f. hyperonychia   13. a. pyogenic; b. pyorrhea   14. a. seborrhea   15. a. trichomycosis; b. trichophagia   16. a. ungual; b. subungual

Case Study

1. First appeared as painful, reddened, raised spots with pus in them
2. Antibiotic pills taken by mouth, ointments to reduce inflammation rubbed into skin, swirling water baths to clean ulcers
3. Diabetes mellitus
4. A
5. C&S–C means culture, growing bacteria in a petri dish to identify what kind of bacteria it is; S means sensitivity, determining which antibiotic will best kill the bacteria; in this case, penicillin will not kill it, so vancomycin is recommended
6. Staph is common bacteria found on skin and in nose and throat; can become serious infection if it gets down into layers of skin or invades bloodstream, urinary tract, lungs, and heart; some strains of staph have become resistant to many common antibiotics
7. Gangrene occurs when tissue does not have sufficient circulation to keep tissue healthy; as a result, tissue dies
8. Antibiotics to fight infection given into vein, treatments in whirlpool bath to clean up ulcers, go to surgery to remove dead and infected tissue

Practice Exercises

Sound It Out

1. abrasion 2. adipoma 3. cyst 4. anhidrosis 5. biopsy 6. cellulitis 7. ulcer
8. abscess 9. dermatome 10. fissure 11. cyanosis 12. gangrene 13. hypodermic

14. vesicle   15. lipoma   16. nodule   17. macule   18. necrosis   19. papule
20. psoriasis   21. dermatology   22. seborrhea   23. subcutaneous   24. tinea
25. ungual

Transcription Practice

1. The dermatologist took a biopsy to determine that the patient has a nevus rather than malignant melanoma.
2. A culture and sensitivity was performed to determine how best to treat the infected ulcer.
3. The patient had a very large boil (or furuncle) surrounded by a large area of cellulitis.
4. Ms. Marks was lucky, when she tripped off the curb she received only abrasions and contusions.
5. Mr. Brown's chronic exposure to toxins at work had left him with xeroderma, ichthyoderma, and pachyderma.
6. After years of onychophagia, the patient developed onychomalacia and onychomycosis that required onychectomy.
7. To repair the areas of third-degree burns, a skin graft was necessary.
8. Mr. Strong was concerned that the lump he could feel under his skin was an adenoma, but it turned out to only be a lipoma/adipoma, and it was removed with a lipectomy/adipectomy.
9. The plastic surgeon helped Mr. Marsh decide whether to use chemabrasion or dermabrasion for his face lift.
10. New medical students often have difficulty telling the difference between a macule, a papule, and a cyst.

Labeling Exercise

1. Epidermis   2. Dermis   3. Subcutaneous layer   4. Sweat gland **(hidr/o)**   5. Sensory receptors   6. Sebaceous gland **(seb/o)**   7. Arrector pili muscle   8. Hair shaft **(trich/o)**
9. Nerve   10. Vein   11. Artery

Build Medical Terms

1. a. xeroderma; b. erythroderma; c. pyoderma; d. scleroderma; e. pachyderma
2. a. hyperhidrosis; b. anhidrosis   3. a. melanocyte; b. melanoma   4. a. dermatopathy; b. dermatoplasty; c. dermatology   5. a. onychomalacia; b. onychomycosis; c. onychectomy

Spelling

1. impetigo   2. correctly spelled   3. wheal   4. correctly spelled   5. correctly spelled
6. tinea   7. petechiae   8. gangrene   9. correctly spelled   10. necrosis

Fill in the Blank

1. fissure, laceration   2. herpes simplex   3. dermabrasion   4. third-degree   5. macule
6. debridement   7. ecchymosis   8. biopsy   9. papule or nodule, pustule   10. decubitus ulcer

Abbreviation Matching

1. E   2. I   3. H   4. G   5. J   6. B   7. A   8. D   9. F   10. C

Medical Term Analysis

1. **aden/o**, gland, **-megaly**, enlarged, enlarged gland   2. **adip/o**, fat, **-cyte**, cell, fat cell
3. **cyan**, blue, **-osis**, abnormal condition, abnormal condition of blue   4. **hypo-**, below, **derm**, skin, **-ic**, pertaining to, pertaining to below skin   5. **kerat/o**, hard or hornlike, **-genic**, producing, producing hard, hornlike   6. **lip**, fat, **-ectomy**, surgical removal, surgical removal of fat   7. **py/o**, pus, **-rrhea**, discharge or flow, pus discharge   8. **erythr/o**, red, **-derma**, skin condition, red skin condition   9. **trich/o**, hair, **myc**, fungus, **-osis**, abnormal condition, abnormal condition of hair fungus   10. **sub-**, beneath, **cutane**, skin, **-ous**, pertaining to, pertaining to beneath the skin

Photomatch Challenge

1. cyst   2. fissure   3. macule   4. pustule   5. ulcer   6. vesicle

Chapter 6

Building Orthopedic Terms

1. a. iliac; b. subiliac   2. a. carpal; b. costal; c. intercostal; d. femoral; e. humeral; f. ischial; g. metacarpal; h. metatarsal; i. radial; j. sacral; k. sternal; l. substernal; m. tarsal; n. tibial; o. vertebral; p. intervertebral   3. a. clavicular; b. fibular; c. mandibular; d. submandibular; e. patellar; f. scapular; g. subscapular; h. ulnar   4. a. arthrocentesis; b. arthroclasia; c. arthrodesis; d. arthrography; e. arthrogram; f. arthritis; g. arthroscopy; h. arthroscope; i. arthroplasty; j. arthralgia   5. a. maxillary; b. supramaxillary   6. a. bursal; b. bursitis; c. bursectomy   7. a. chondral; b. chondritis; c. chondrectomy; d. chondromalacia; e. chondroma; f. chondroplasty   8. a. cranial; b. intracranial; c. craniotomy; d. cranioplasty   9. a. coccygeal; b. phalangeal   10. a. pubic; b. suprapubic   11. a. bradykinesia; b. dyskinesia; c. hyperkinesia   12. a. muscular; b. intramuscular   13. a. myeloma; b. myelogenic; c. myelopathy   14. a. myalgia; b. myasthenia; c. electromyogram; d. electromyography; e. myopathy; f. myorrhaphy; g. myorrhexis   15. a. ostealgia; b. osteocyte; c. osteogenic; d. osteoarthritis; e. osteochondritis; f. osteochondroma; g. osteoclasia; h. osteomyelitis; i. osteopathy; j. osteotome; k. osteomalacia; l. osteoporosis   16. a. spondylosis; b. spondylitis   17. a. tenalgia; b. tenodynia; c. tenodesis; d. tenorrhaphy   18. a. tendinous; b. tendinitis; c. tendinoplasty; d. tendinosis

Case Study

1. Osteoporosis–means "porous bones"; the thinning and loss of bone density that occurs slowly over time as more minerals such as calcium are removed from bone than are deposited; very common in postmenopausal women
Compression fracture–loss of height of vertebral body; osteoporosis makes bones less strong, and they collapse easily
2. Answers will vary; example of a correct answer is Actonel–slows bone loss and increases bone mass
3. RL–right leg; FX or Fx–fracture; T10–10th thoracic vertebra; NSAIDs–nonsteroidal anti-inflammatory drug; LE–lower extremity; DTRs–deep tendon reflexes; MRI–magnetic resonance imaging; L4-5–between 4th and 5th lumbar vertebrae; HNP–herniated nucleus pulposus
4. B
5. Myocardial infarction–heart attack; renal failure-kidneys stop filtering waste from blood; Alzheimer disease–progressive dementia; spina bifida–vertebrae do not fully form around spinal cord
6. X-ray–radiation is passed through body to produce image by exposing a photographic plate–it showed spondylosis but no arthritis
MRI–image created by strong magnetic field and radiowaves–showed herniated nucleus pulposus at L4-5
7. Pain relief, traction, back strengthening exercises
8. Use of thin catheter tube inserted into intervertebral disk through skin to suck out pieces of herniated or ruptured disk; or laser is used to vaporize disk

Practice Exercises

Sound It Out

1. fibromyalgia   2. chondroplasty   3. electromyogram   4. femoral   5. arthroplasty
6. iliac   7. intervertebral   8. intramuscular   9. lordosis   10. mandibular   11. bursitis
12. metacarpal   13. fibular   14. myeloma   15. arthrocentesis   16. scoliosis

17. patellar   18. prosthesis   19. pubic   20. radiography   21. chondroma
22. osteoporosis   23. tenodynia   24. contracture   25. tibial

Transcription Practice

1. The comminuted fracture required open reduction and internal fixation.
2. Radiography revealed a femoral osteochondroma.
3. The patient's chronic bursitis eventually required a bursectomy.
4. Mary's hand deformities from rheumatoid arthritis were improved by wearing an orthosis.
5. When Otto's osteoarthritis in his knee prevented him from walking he had a total knee arthroplasty.
6. What first appeared to be an oblique fracture turned out to be a spiral fracture.
7. A bone scan was necessary to identify the stress fracture.
8. Jean's vertebral osteoporosis was diagnosed by dual-energy absorptiometry.
9. The child's dyskinesia caused the physician to suspect muscular dystrophy.
10. The ankle strain was severe enough to require a tenodesis.

Labeling Exercise

1. Maxilla–upper jaw **(maxill/o)**   2. Mandible–lower jaw **(mandibul/o)**   3. Sternum–breast bone **(stern/o)**   4. Rib **(cost/o)**   5. Vertebrae **(spondyl/o, vertebr/o)**   6. Sacrum **(sacr/o)**   7. Coccyx–tailbone **(coccyg/o)**   8. Cranium–skull **(crani/o)**   9. Clavicle–collar bone **(clavicul/o)**   10. Scapula–shoulder blade **(scapul/o)**   11. Humerus **(humer/o)**   12. Radius–forearm **(radi/o)**   13. Ulna–forearm **(uln/o)**   14. Carpus–wrist bones **(carp/o)**   15. Metacarpus–hand bones **(metacarp/o)**   16. Phalanges–finger bones **(phalang/o)**   17. Ilium **(ili/o)**   18. Pubis **(pub/o)**   19. Ischium **(ischi/o)**   20. Femur–thigh bone **(femor/o)**   21. Patella–kneecap **(patell/o)**   22. Tibia–shin bone **(tibi/o)**   23. Fibula **(fibul/o)**   24. Tarsus–ankle bones **(tars/o)**   25. Metatarsus–foot bones **(metatars/o)**   26. Phalanges–toe bones **(phalang/o)**

Build Medical Terms

1. arthrocentesis   2. arthritis   3. arthroscope   4. arthroplasty   5. arthrography
6. myasthenia   7. myorrhaphy   8. hyperkinesia   9. bradykinesia   10. osteotome
11. osteoporosis   12. osteogenic   13. chondromalacia   14. chondroma   15. chondroplasty

Fill in the Blank

1. closed or simple   2. osteoporosis   3. kyphosis   4. orthosis   5. Carpal tunnel syndrome
6. prosthesis   7. Greenstick   8. ligaments, tendons   9. internal fixation   10. spasm

Abbreviation Matching

1. D   2. G   3. F   4. J   5. A   6. C   7. I   8. B   9. H   10. E

Medical Term Analysis

1. **arthr/o**, joint, **-desis**, surgical fusion, surgical fusion of joint   2. **burs**, bursa, **-ectomy**, surgical removal, surgical removal of bursa   3. **electr/o**, electricity, **my/o**, muscle, **-gram**, record, record of muscle electricity   4. **intra-**, within, **crani**, skull, **-al**, pertaining to, pertaining to within the skull   5. **oste/o**, bone, **myel**, bone marrow, **-itis**, inflammation, inflammation of bone and bone marrow   6. **ten**, tendon, **-algia**, pain, tendon pain   7. **spondyl**, vertebra, **-osis**, abnormal condition, vertebra abnormal condition   8. **sub-**, below, **stern**, sternum, **-al**, pertaining to, pertaining to below the sternum   9. **inter-**, between, **vertebr**, vertebrae, **-al**, pertaining to, pertaining to between vertebrae   10. **supra-**, above, **maxill**, maxilla, **-ary**, pertaining to, pertaining to above the maxilla

Spelling

1. correctly spelled   2. bursectomy   3. correctly spelled   4. correctly spelled   5. correctly spelled   6. correctly spelled   7. chondrectomy   8. coccygeal   9. dyskinesia   10. spondylosis

Photomatch Challenge

1. transverse fracture   2. oblique fracture   3. spiral fracture   4. comminuted fracture
5. greenstick fracture   6. compression fracture

Chapter 7

Building Cardiology Terms

1. a. angiogram; b. angiography; c. angioma; d. angioplasty; e. angiospasm; f. polyangiitis
2. a. aortic; b. aortoplasty   3. a. arterial; b. arteriogram; c. arteriography; d. arteriorrhaphy;
e. arteriorrhexis; f. arteriostenosis; g. arteriole   4. a. arteriolar   5. a. atherosclerosis;
b. atherectomy   6. a. atrial; b. interatrial; c. atrioventricular   7. a. cardiac; b. cardiodynia;
c. electrocardiogram; d. electrocardiography; e. cardiologist; f. cardiology; g. cardiomegaly;
h. cardiomyopathy; i. cardiorrhexis; j. pericardial; k. endocardial; l. myocardial   8. a. coronary
9. a. embolectomy; b. embolism   10. a. ischemia   11. a. phlebitis; b. phlebotomy; c. phlebogram;
d. phlebography   12. a. arteriosclerosis   13. a. stethoscope   14. a. thrombotic; b. thrombosis;
c. thromboangiitis; d. thrombophlebitis; e. thrombogenic; f. thrombolysis   15. a. valvoplasty;
b. valvotomy; c. valvule   16. a. valvular; b. valvulitis   17. a. varicosis; b. varicose   18. a. vasospasm
19. a. vascular; b. cardiovascular   20. a. venous; b. venogram; c. venography; d. intravenous; e.
venule   21. a. ventricular; b. interventricular   22. a. venular

Case Study

1. SOB—shortness of breath, having difficulty breathing, especially with activity; angina pectoris—
chest pain associated with cardiac ischemia
2. CHF—congestive heart failure, inability of heart to pump blood forcefully enough through body;
swelling in feet
3. Digoxin, or digitalis, is drug given to people with congestive heart failure to make their hearts
beat stronger
4. Heart is beating too fast (153 beats per minute), but there is no abnormality in heartbeat and no
evidence of heart attack
5. Edema is tissue swelling; she has edema in both feet and in her abdomen; she does not have
edema in her hands or face
6. B
7. Final diagnosis is mitral valve prolapse; this means valve between left atrium and left ventricle
is too loose to close tightly, allowing blood to flow backward into atrium; this diagnosis is best
supported by echocardiogram, which showed regurgitation (backflow) of blood into atrium
8. Patient is scheduled to undergo valvoplasty, or surgical repair of mitral valve with an artificial valve.

Practice Exercises

Sound It Out

1. vasospasm   2. angioplasty   3. intravenous   4. cardiomyopathy   5. atherosclerosis
6. bradycardia   7. cardiovascular   8. defibrillation   9. electrocardiography   10. embolism
11. endarterectomy   12. fibrillation   13. hypertension   14. infarct   15. myocardial
16. phlebitis   17. endocarditis   18. sphygmomanometer   19. tachycardia
20. thrombolysis   21. aneurysm   22. cardiomegaly   23. polyangiitis   24. thrombosis
25. stethoscope

Transcription Practice

1. Dr. Jones suspected his patient had had a myocardial infarction, so he ordered an
electrocardiogram and cardiac enzymes.
2. The paramedics applied defibrillation because fibrillation was detected.
3. The patient developed bradycardia and required surgery to implant a pacemaker.
4. Susan wore a Holter monitor for 24 hours to further evaluate her angina pectoris.

5. The patient had a Doppler ultrasonography to assess whether she had heart valve prolapse or heart valve stenosis.
6. During auscultation, the nurse detected a heart murmur caused by mitral valve prolapse.
7. The patient suffered an infarct when an embolus broke off a plaque.
8. A cardiac catheterization was ordered to determine whether the patient requires a percutaneous transluminal coronary angioplasty.
9. The patient experiences angina pectoris because of severe coronary artery disease.
10. This patient's hypertension eventually caused him to develop congestive heart failure.

Spelling

1. tachycardia   2. correctly spelled   3. correctly spelled   4. auscultation   5. atherosclerosis or arteriosclerosis   6. correctly spelled   7. correctly spelled   8. aneurysm   9. angioma 10. correctly spelled

Labeling Exercise

1. Left atrium **(atri/o)**   2. Aortic valve **(valvul/o, valv/o)**   3. Mitral valve **(valvul/o, valv/o)**
4. Left ventricle **(ventricul/o)**   5. Endocardium   6. Myocardium   7. Aorta **(aort/o)**   8. Right atrium **(atri/o)**   9. Pulmonary valve **(valvul/o, valv/o)**   10. Tricuspid valve **(valvul/o, valv/o)**
11. Right ventricle **(ventricul/o)**

Build Medical Terms

1. cardiology   2. cardiomegaly   3. cardiorrhexis   4. cardiogram   5. valvoplasty
6. valvotomy   7. arteriosclerosis   8. atherosclerosis   9. angioma   10. angiospasm
11. arteriorrhaphy   12. arterial   13. arteriography   14. thrombophlebitis   15. thrombolysis

Fill in the Blank

1. aneurysm   2. cardiac arrest   3. stethoscope   4. Holter monitor   5. congenital septal defect
6. venipuncture   7. vegetation   8. clot-busters   9. heart murmur   10. cardiopulmonary resuscitation

Abbreviation Matching

1. D   2. H   3. F   4. B   5. G   6. I   7. A   8. J   9. E   10. C

Medical Term Analysis

1. **aort/o**, aorta, **–plasty**, surgical repair, surgical repair of the aorta   2. **embol**, plug, **–ectomy**, surgical removal, surgical removal of a plug   3. **cardi/o**, heart, **my/o**, muscle, **–pathy**, disease, disease of heart muscle   4. **endo–**, inner, **cardi**, heart, **–al**, pertaining to, pertaining to inner (lining) of heart   5. **thromb/o**, clot, **angi**, vessel, **–itis**, inflammation, inflammation of vessel with clots
6. **ather/o**, fatty substance, **–sclerosis**, hardening, hardening with fatty substance   7. **valvul**, valve, **–otomy**, cutting into, cutting into a valve   8. **inter–**, between, **ventricul**, ventricle, **–ar**, pertaining to, pertaining to between ventricles   9. **cardi/o**, heart, **vascul**, blood vessel, **–ar**, pertaining to, pertaining to blood vessels of the heart   10. **steth/o**, chest, **–scope**, instrument for viewing, instrument for viewing chest

Photomatch Challenge

1. Stress test   2. Venipuncture   3. Electrocardiography   4. Cardiopulmonary resuscitation
5. slow, A   6. fast, B

Chapter 8

Building Hematology Terms

1. a. erythrocyte; b. leukocyte; c. thrombocyte; d. monocyte; e. lymphocyte   2. a. erythrocytosis; b. leukocytosis; c. thrombocytosis   3. a. anemia; b. hyperglycemia; c. hypoglycemia; d. hyperlipemia   4. a. hemocyte; b. hemoglobin; c. hemostasis; d. hemorrhage; e. hemolysis;

f. hemocytolysis; g. hemocytoma; h. hemocytometer; i. hemocytometry   5. a. hematology; b. hematologist; c. hematic; d. hematoma; e. hematopathology; f. hematocytopenia; g. hematopoiesis   6. a. erythropenia; b. leukopenia; c. thrombocytopenia; d. pancytopenia; e. eosinopenia; f. neutropenia   7. a. eosinophil; b. basophil; c. neutrophil   8. a. erythropoiesis; b. leukopoiesis; c. thrombopoiesis   9. a. thrombolysis; b. thrombectomy; c. thrombosis

Case Study

1. Fatigue and dyspnea (shortness of breath) with even light activity; three episodes of sinusitis (sinus inflammation) and pharyngitis (throat inflammation) in past 6 months; easy bruising; two episodes of epistaxis (nosebleed) in last week
2. Complete blood count (CBC); consists of red blood cell count (RBC), white blood cell count (WBC), hemoglobin (Hgb), hematocrit (Hct), white blood cell differential, and platelet count
3. Pancytopenia; fatigue and dyspnea because of low red cell count; recurring infections because of low white cell count; bruising and epistaxis because of low platelet count
4. Appendix removed at age 12; gallbladder removed at age 35; has been pregnant three times with two children born and one child died before it was a viable age
5. She could be exposed to toxic chemicals in her job working with pesticides
6. Respiratory rate is 22 breaths/minute; heart rate is 102 bpm; the patient's results are probably much higher than yours
7. Biopsy removes small sample of tissue for examination under microscope for purpose of making a diagnosis; this patient had her bone marrow biopsied; biopsy revealed low number of blood cells in marrow that are normal in appearance
8. Blood transfusion treats symptoms; long-term antibiotics treat symptoms; medication to stimulate bone marrow treats underlying cause; bone marrow transplant treats underlying cause; washing hands and avoiding sick people treats symptoms

Practice Exercise

Sound It Out

1. hematocrit   2. leukopoiesis   3. coagulate   4. embolus   5. anemia   6. hematopathology   7. hemocytolysis   8. thrombolysis   9. autotransfusion   10. hemolysis   11. erythropenia   12. leukemia   13. erythrocytosis   14. leukocytosis   15. thrombosis   16. pancytopenia   17. hematoma   18. phlebotomy   19. septicemia   20. thalassemia   21. hypoglycemia   22. neutropenia   23. thrombocytosis   24. hemophilia   25. leukopenia

Transcription Practice

1. The formed elements of blood are erythrocytes, leukocytes, and platelets (thrombocytes).
2. The patient had a bone marrow aspiration to determine whether she had leukemia.
3. The blood vessel was blocked by an embolus.
4. Elena received thrombolytic therapy during her heart attack.
5. Because he had diabetes, Ted monitored his blood for hyperglycemia.
6. The patient suffered hemorrhage and hematoma as a result of the auto accident.
7. The hematologist determined that Genevieve had developed pernicious anemia.
8. Following heart surgery, Tran received an autotransfusion.
9. A complete blood count revealed that Marco had pancytopenia.
10. Because septicemia was suspected, a blood culture and sensitivity was ordered.

Abbreviation Matching

1. G   2. J   3. E   4. A   5. I   6. H   7. D   8. B   9. F   10. C

Fill in the Blanks

1. aplastic   2. embolus   3. thrombolytic   4. too many   5. venipuncture   6. culture and sensitivity   7. hematocrit   8. leukemia   9. vitamin B12   10. blood poisoning

Labeling Exercise

1. Plasma 2. Erythrocytes **(erythr/o)** 3. Platelets 4. Neutrophil **(neutr/o)** 5. Lymphocyte **(lymph/o)** 6. Monocyte 7. Basophil **(bas/o)** 8. Eosinophil **(eosin/o)**

Build Medical Terms

1. erythrocyte 2. leukocyte 3. thrombocyte 4. hematology 5. hematopoiesis 6. hematic
7. hematoma 8. hyperglycemia 9. anemia 10. hemostasis 11. hemorrhage
12. hemolysis 13. eosinophil 14. basophil 15. neutrophil

Medical Term Analysis

1. **erythr/o**, red, **-cytosis**, abnormal cell condition, abnormal red cell condition 2. **hemat/o**, blood, **-logist**, one who studies, one who studies blood 3. **hemat/o**, blood, **path/o**, disease, **-logy**, study of, study of blood diseases 4. **hyper-**, excessive, **lip**, fat, **-emia**, blood condition, blood condition of excessive fat 5. **hem/o**, blood, **cyt/o**, cell, **-meter**, instrument to measure, instrument to measure blood cells 6. **leuk/o**, white, **-poiesis**, formation, white [blood cell] formation 7. **lymph/o**, lymph, **-cyte**, cell, lymph cell 8. **hem/o**, blood, **-globin**, protein, blood protein 9. **pan-**, all, **cyt/o**, cells, **-penia**, too few, too few of all cells 10. **thromb**, clot, **-ectomy**, surgical removal, surgical removal of clot

Spelling

1. hypoglycemia 2. correctly spelled 3. correctly spelled 4. septicemia 5. correctly spelled 6. platelet 7. polycythemia vera 8. correctly spelled 9. correctly spelled 10. erythropoiesis

Photomatch Challenge

1. C 2. D 3. E 4. F 5. B 6. A

Chapter 9

Building Immunology Terms

1. a. adenoidectomy; b. adenoiditis 2. a. immunologist; b. immunology; c. immunoglobulin; d. immunogenic; e. immunotherapy 3. a. lymphatic; b. lymphoma; c. lymphedema; d. lymphocyte; e. lymphocytic; f. lymphocytoma; g. lymphogenic; h. lymphoid; i. lymphostasis 4. a. lymphadenectomy; b. lymphadenopathy; c. lymphadenography; d. lymphadenogram; e. lymphadenitis; f. lymphadenosis 5. a. lymphangiitis; b. lymphangiopathy; c. lymphangioma; d. lymphangiography; e. lymphangiogram; f. lymphangiectomy; g. lymphangiectasis; h. lymphangioplasty 6. a. pathogenic; b. pathogen; c. pathology; d. pathologist 7. a. phagocyte; b. phagocytic 8. a. splenic; b. splenitis; c. splenoid; d. splenoma; e. splenectomy; f. splenomegaly; g. splenomalacia; h. splenopexy; i. splenorrhaphy 9. a. thymic; b. thymectomy; c. thymoma 10. a. tonsillar; b. tonsillectomy; c. tonsillitis

Case Study

1. As a heroin addict, he probably shared needles; unsafe sex practices and blood transfusion
2. Yeast
3. Thrush, weight loss, recurring infections (sinusitis and bronchitis), diarrhea, night sweats, extreme fatigue, unexplained fevers, muscular wasting, fever, enlarged cervical and inguinal lymph nodes
4. ELISA; Western blot is considered more precise than ELISA
5. ARC is early in infection and symptoms are milder; AIDS is later stages of infection in which immune system is no longer able to resist infections and person is prone to opportunistic infections
6. Infections that occur when immune system is compromised; PCP and Kaposi sarcoma

7. Zidovudine keeps virus from reproducing; Epivir prevents virus from multiplying; Viracept slows growth of virus
8. If CD4 count is low, immune system is not able to work very well and patient is at higher risk of opportunistic infection; if it remains OK, then HIV medications are working

Practice Exercises

Sound It Out

1. lymphoma   2. allergy   3. pathology   4. immunotherapy   5. inflammation
6. splenomegaly   7. lymphadenectomy   8. antihistamine   9. lymphadenitis
10. lymphadenography   11. lymphangiitis   12. lymphangiogram   13. lymphangioma
14. sarcoidosis   15. lymphostasis   16. mononucleosis   17. pathogenic
18. lymphocytoma   19. splenectomy   20. tonsillectomy   21. splenopexy   22. thymectomy
23. vaccination   24. thymoma   25. adenoiditis

Transcription Practice

1. Marcie's repeated bouts of tonsillitis required her to have a tonsillectomy and adenoidectomy.
2. The lymphangiogram revealed a lymphangioma.
3. The immunologist is a physician who treats autoimmune diseases.
4. Jamar had a history of anaphylactic shock in response to bee stings.
5. Mykos had to take immunosuppressants after his kidney transplant.
6. Joyce's allergy to pollen was treated with antihistamines.
7. The AIDS patient developed pneumocystis pneumonia.
8. Jennifer's allergic reactions consisted of hives and urticaria.
9. Shona's hand pain turned out to be caused by systemic lupus erythematosus.
10. Carlos's lymphadenopathy turned out to be Hodgkin disease.

Build Medical Terms

1. lymphadenectomy   2. lymphadenogram   3. lymphadenopathy   4. immunoglobulin
5. immunologist   6. splenomegaly   7. splenoid   8. splenic   9. tonsillitis   10. tonsillectomy
11. tonsillar   12. lymphangiitis   13. lymphangioplasty   14. lymphangiography
15. lymphangioma

Labeling Exercise

1. Lymphatic vessel **(lymphangi/o)**   2. Lymph nodes **(lymphaden/o)**   3. Tonsils **(tonsill/o, adenoid/o)**   4. Thymus gland **(thym/o)**   5. Spleen **(splen/o)**

Spelling

1. urticaria   2. spelled correctly   3. spelled correctly   4. spelled correctly   5. lymphadenosis
6. immunosuppressants   7. splenomalacia   8. tonsillitis   9. spelled correctly   10. spelled correctly

Fill in the Blank

1. allergist   2. autoimmune   3. lymph vessels, edema   4. wheals   5. Corticosteroids   6. AIDS-related complex   7. immunizations   8. skin   9. Anaphylactic shock or anaphylaxis   10. Western blot test

Abbreviation Matching

1. G   2. C   3. J   4. H   5. D   6. A   7. E   8. I   9. B   10. F

Medical Term Analysis

1. **adenoid**, adenoids, **-itis**, inflammation, adenoid inflammation   2. **lymph/o**, lymph, **-genic**, producing, lymph producing   3. **immun/o**, immunity or protection, **-therapy**, treatment, immunity treatment   4. **lymph/o**, lymph, **cyt**, cell, **-oma**, tumor, lymph cell tumor   5. **phag/o**, eating, **cyt**, cell, **-ic**, pertaining to, pertaining to eating cell   6. **lymphaden/o**, lymph node, **-pathy**, disease,

lymph node disease   7. **path/o**, disease, **-logy**, study of, study of disease   8. **lymphangi**, lymph vessel, **-ectasis**, dilated, dilated lymph vessel   9. **thym**, thymus gland, **-ectomy**, surgical removal, surgical removal of thymus gland   10. **lymph**, lymph, **-edema**, swelling, lymph swelling

Photomatch Challenge

1. B   2. E   3. A   4. F   5. D   6. C

Chapter 10

Building Pulmonology Terms

1. a. alveolar   2. a. bronchogram; b. bronchography; c. bronchitis; d. bronchoscope; e. bronchoscopy; f. bronchospasm; g. bronchogenic   3. a. bronchial; b. bronchiole; c. bronchiectasis   4. a. bronchiolar   5. a. pneumoconiosis   6. a. cyanosis   7. a. lobar; b. lobectomy   8. a. mediastinal; b. mediastinotomy   9. a. orthopnea   10. a. anoxia   11. a. oximeter; b. oximetry   12. a. pleural; b. pleurocentesis; c. pleurodynia; d. pleuralgia; e. pleuritis   13. a. apnea; b. dyspnea; c. eupnea; d. hyperpnea; e. hypopnea; f. bradypnea; g. tachypnea   14. a. pneumogram; b. pneumograph; c. pneumography; d. pneumothorax   15. a. pneumonic; b. pneumonocentesis; c. pneumonectomy; d. pneumonotomy   16. a. pulmonary or pulmonic; b. pulmonology; c. pulmonologist   17. a. hemoptysis   18. a. spirogram; b. spirometer; c. spirometry   19. a. thoracalgia; b. thoracodynia; c. thoracic; d. thoracotomy; e. thoracocentesis; f. thoracostomy   20. a. hemothorax; b. pyothorax; c. pneumothorax   21. a. tracheal; b. tracheoplasty; c. tracheostomy; d. tracheotomy; e. tracheitis; f. endotracheal

Case Study

1. D. pain in the chest region
2. Endometriosis–presence of endometrial tissue outside uterus; she had uterus removed
   cholelithiasis–gallbladder stones; she had gallbladder removed
   lumbar compression fracture due to osteoporosis–collapse of vertebra because her bones were brittle
3. No, it is not important; it does not include lung problems; her brother has high blood pressure, her mother had a stroke (blood vessel disease), and her father had diabetes mellitus (problem with blood sugar levels because pancreas fails to produce enough insulin)
4. Crackles (crackling sound during inhalation), but no rhonchi (whistling sound during inhalation or exhalation)
5. In sputum culture and sensitivity, a sputum specimen is placed in culture medium in an attempt to grow and then identify type of bacteria present and what antibiotic is effective in killing it; this test did not reveal any bacteria in her sputum
   Sputum cytology examines cells in sputum for presence of cancer; this test did identify cancerous cells in patient's sputum
6. Chest radiograph, AP view, is a plain chest X-ray taken from front to back; it showed a suspicious-looking cloudy area in her lung
   Chest CT scan is an X-ray image formed with assistance of a computer to have a cross-sectional view of chest; it shows more detail and revealed that cloudy area was a tumor
7. Thoracic surgeon to open up her chest and remove one lobe of her lung; oncologist (cancer specialist) to determine whether cancer has spread and whether she needs to have chemotherapy treatments

Practice Exercise

Sound It Out

1. tracheotomy   2. apnea   3. asthma   4. bronchitis   5. hemothorax   6. bronchogenic   7. pneumonectomy   8. bronchospasm   9. cyanosis   10. emphysema   11. atelectasis

12. hyperventilation 13. influenza 14. lobectomy 15. oximeter 16. bronchography
17. pleurisy 18. pneumocentesis 19. pneumoconiosis 20. tuberculosis
21. pyothorax 22. spirometry 23. anoxia 24. thoracotomy 25. tracheoplasty

Transcription Practice

1. During auscultation, the physician heard crackles when the patient inhaled.
2. It was unclear from the chest X-ray whether the patient had hemothorax or pyothorax.
3. The results of the arterial blood gases revealed hypoxia.
4. The patient underwent a lobectomy after the discovery of bronchogenic carcinoma.
5. Mr. Scott's hypopnea was so severe because he had cyanosis.
6. Carlyn went to the pulmonologist when she noticed hemoptysis several mornings in a row.
7. The physician ordered a sputum culture and sensitivity because Lars was coughing up purulent sputum.
8. The patient underwent pulmonary function tests using a spirometer and an oximeter.
9. The patient had chronic obstructive pulmonary disease, causing him to have dyspnea and a chronic cough.
10. Pulmonary angiography was ordered to determine whether there was a pulmonary embolism.

Spelling

1. pneumoconiosis 2. correctly spelled 3. correctly spelled 4. ventilator 5. purulent
6. correctly spelled 7. correctly spelled 8. hyperpnea 9. correctly spelled 10. alveolar

Labeling Exercise

1. Trachea **(trache/o)** 2. Lobe **(lob/o)** 3. Right primary bronchus **(bronch/o, bronchi/o)**
4. Right lung **(pneum/o, pneumon/o, pulmon/o)** 5. Mediastinum **(mediastin/o)** 6. Left primary bronchus **(bronch/o, bronchi/o)** 7. Left lung **(pneum/o, pneumon/o, pulmon/o)**
8. Chest **(thorac/o, steth/o)** 9. Diaphragm

Build Medical Terms

1. bronchogram 2. bronchoscopy 3. bronchospasm 4. pneumonocentesis
5. pneumonectomy 6. pneumonic 7. pneumonotomy 8. atelectasis 9. bronchiectasis
10. tracheostomy 11. tracheoplasty 12. tracheitis 13. apnea 14. tachypnea 15. dyspnea

Fill in the Blank

1. asthma 2. bronchoscopy 3. emphysema 4. cystic fibrosis 5. trachea 6. spirometer
7. hyperventilation 8. infant respiratory distress syndrome 9. pneumothorax 10. pulmonary embolism

Abbreviation Matching

1. D 2. H 3. F 4. A 5. J 6. B 7. I 8. E 9. G 10. C

Medical Term Analysis

1. **thorac/o**, chest, **-centesis**, puncture to withdraw fluid, puncture chest to withdraw fluid
2. **cyan**, blue, **-osis**, abnormal condition, abnormal condition of being blue 3. **pneum/o**, air, **-thorax**, chest, air in the chest 4. **endo-**, within, **trache**, trachea, **-al**, pertaining to, pertaining to within the trachea 5. **pneum/o**, lung, **coni**, dust, **-osis**, abnormal condition, abnormal condition of lung dust 6. **ox/i**, oxygen, **-meter**, instrument to measure, instrument to measure oxygen
7. **orth/o**, straight, **-pnea**, breathing, straight breathing 8. **pleur/o**, pleura, **-dynia**, pain, pleura pain 9. **bronchi**, bronchus, **-ectasis**, expansion, bronchus expansion 10. **lob**, lobe, **-ectomy**, surgical removal, surgical removal of lobe

Photomatch Challenge

1. pleural effusion 2. pneumothorax 3. asthma 4. atelectasis 5. pneumonia 6. emphysema

Chapter 11

Building Gastroenterology Terms

1. a. anal 2. a. appendectomy 3. a. appendicitis 4. a. cholelithiasis; b. cholelithotripsy
5. a. cholangiogram; b. cholangiography 6. a. cholecystitis; b. cholecystectomy;
c. cholecystogram; d. cholecystography 7. a. choledocholithiasis; b. choledocholithotripsy
8. a. colostomy; b. colitis; c. colorectal 9. a. colonoscope; b. colonoscopy; c. colonic
10. a. diverticulitis; b. diverticulosis; c. diverticulectomy 11. a. duodenal; b. duodenostomy
12. a. hematemesis; b. hyperemesis 13. a. enteritis; b. enteric 14. a. esophageal;
b. esophagoplasty; c. esophagitis; d. esophagoscope; e. esophagoscopy 15. a. gastric;
b. gastritis; c. gastroenteritis; d. gastrectomy; e. gastrostomy; f. gastroscope; g. gastroscopy;
h. gastrodynia; i. gastralgia; j. gastroenterologist; k. gastroenterology 16. a. hepatitis; b. hepatic;
c. hepatoma 17. a. ileal; b. ileostomy 18. a. jejunal; b. jejunostomy 19. a. laparotomy;
b. laparoscope; c. laparoscopy 20. a. pancreatic; b. pancreatitis 21. a. apepsia; b. dyspepsia;
c. bradypepsia 22. a. aphagia; b. dysphagia; c. polyphagia or hyperphagia 23. a. polyposis;
b. polypectomy 24. a. proctoptosis; b. proctoscope c. proctoscopy; d. proctologist;
e. proctology 25. a. rectocele; b. rectal 26. a. sigmoidoscope; b. sigmoidoscopy

Case Study

1. Increasing upper abdominal pain for past eight months, sharp upper abdominal pain about
   30 minutes after eating
2. Milk and ice cream; spicy foods; over-the-counter antacids (Tums, Rolaids, Zantac)
3. Blood test for *Helicobacter pylori*, a bacteria that can cause stomach ulcers; this test was
   positive, meaning the bacteria are present; esophagogastroduodenoscopy, a visual examination
   of esophagus, stomach, and first section of intestine showed stomach was inflamed, but there
   was no evidence of bleeding or an ulcer
4. In the middle of upper abdomen overlying much of stomach; radiate means pain travels from
   one area of body to another
5. Difficulty swallowing/eating, burning sensation under breast bone, feeling like he is going to
   throw up, actually throwing up, pain in lower abdomen, vomiting blood, dark tarry stool, loose
   watery stool
6. Because his family has had serious GI problems, his mother had cancer of the colon, and his
   brother had liver disease
7. C
8. Patient was put on two medications, one to reduce inflamed stomach and one to kill bacterial
   infection; if he is not better in three months, physician will repeat visual exam of esophagus,
   stomach, and first section of intestine to see what is happening

Practice Exercises

Sound It Out

1. sigmoidoscope 2. rectocele 3. gastritis 4. cholangiogram 5. cirrhosis
6. colitis 7. colonoscopy 8. cholecystectomy 9. dyspepsia 10. esophagoplasty
11. gastroenteritis 12. gastroscope 13. appendicitis 14. hemorrhoids 15. dysentery
16. hyperemesis 17. bradypepsia 18. ileostomy 19. laparoscopy 20. laparotomy
21. dysphagia 22. gastrectomy 23. volvulus 24. sigmoidoscopy 25. appendix

Transcription Practice

1. Mr. Mercado was noted to have jaundice, leading to a diagnosis of hepatitis.
2. Mrs. Mendez underwent an esophagogastroduodenoscopy (EGD) that revealed peptic ulcer
   disease.
3. Mr. Brown's severe diverticulitis resulted in his having a diverticulectomy.

4. The patient presented in the ER with severe nausea and hematemesis.
5. The physician ordered a barium enema (BE, or lower GI series) because of concern that the patient could have polyposis.
6. Because of her cholelithiasis, Ms. Katopolis had a laparotomy and cholecystectomy.
7. Common symptoms of gastroesophageal reflux disease (GERD) include dysphagia and gastrodynia/gastralgia.
8. The patient was found to have an ileus and required a jejunostomy.
9. The BM (or feces) was tested for occult blood and ova and parasites (O&P).
10. To evaluate Mr. Habib's melena, his gastroenterologist performed a proctoscopy, a sigmoidoscopy, and a colonoscopy.

Labeling Exercise

1. Liver **(hepat/o)** 2. Gallbladder **(cholecyst/o)** 3. Colon **(col/o, colon/o)** 4. Appendix **(appendic/o, append/o)** 5. Esophagus **(esophag/o)** 6. Stomach **(gastr/o)** 7. Pancreas **(pancreat/o)** 8. Duodenum **(duoden/o)** 9. Jejunum **(jejun/o)** 10. Ileum **(ile/o)** 11. Sigmoid colon **(sigmoid/o)** 12. Rectum **(rect/o, proct/o)** 13. Anus **(an/o)** 14. Small intestine **(enter/o)**

Build Medical Terms

1. gastritis 2. gastrectomy 3. gastroscope 4. gastralgia or gastrodynia 5. gastrodynia or gastralgia 6. proctoptosis 7. rectocele 8. cholecystitis 9. cholecystectomy 10. duodenostomy 11. colostomy 12. gastrostomy 13. apepsia 14. dyspepsia 15. bradypepsia

Abbreviation Matching

1. H 2. D 3. G 4. I 5. C 6. A 7. B 8. F 9. J 10. E

Fill in the Blank

1. total parenteral nutrition 2. stomach, lower esophagus, duodenum 3. vomit 4. barium swallow 5. liver, gallbladder 6. ascites 7. ileus 8. ulcerative colitis 9. spastic colon 10. gastric bypass

Spelling

1. correctly spelled 2. esophageal 3. pancreatitis 4. correctly spelled 5. gastritis 6. correctly spelled 7. correctly spelled 8. cirrhosis 9. volvulus 10. correctly spelled

Medical Term Analysis

1. **esophag/o**, esophagus, **-plasty**, surgical repair, surgical repair of esophagus 2. **append**, appendix, **-ectomy**, surgical removal, surgical removal of appendix 3. **choledoch/o**, common bile duct, **lith/o**, stone, **-tripsy**, surgical crushing, surgical crushing of stone in common bile duct 4. **hyper-**, excessive, **-emesis**, vomiting, excessive vomiting 5. **gastr/o**, stomach, **enter**, intestine, **-itis**, inflammation, inflammation of stomach and intestine 6. **hepat**, liver, **-oma**, tumor, liver tumor 7. **diverticul**, blind pouch, **-osis**, abnormal condition, abnormal condition of blind pouches 8. **ile**, ileum, **-ostomy**, surgically create an opening, surgically create opening in ileum 9. **lapar/o**, abdomen, **-scope**, instrument for viewing, instrument for viewing abdomen 10. **poly-**, many, **-phagia**, eating, many (excessive) eating

Photomatch Challenge

1. diverticulosis or diverticulitis 2. colostomy 3. laparoscopy 4. polyposis 5. cholelithiasis 6. appendicitis

Chapter 12

Building Urology and Nephrology Terms

1. a. balanitis; b. balanorrhea   2. a. cystalgia; b. cystocele; c. cystectomy; d. cystitis; e. cystoscopy; f. cystogram; g. cystography; h. cystoscope; i. cystic; j. cystolith   3. a. epididymitis; b. epididymal   4. a. lithotripsy; b. ureterolithiasis; c. nephrolithiasis; d. cystolithiasis 5. a. nephrectomy; b. nephritis; c. nephromegaly; d. nephroma; e. nephroptosis; f. nephrotomy; g. nephropathy; h. nephropexy; i. nephrosclerosis; j. glomerulonephritis; k. nephrolith; l. nephrosis   6. a. anorchism; b. orchitis; c. cryptorchism   7. a. orchiopexy; b. orchialgia 8. a. orchidectomy   9. a. cystostomy; b. nephrostomy; c. ureterostomy; d. pyelostomy; e. urethrostomy; f. vasovasostomy   10. a. prostatectomy; b. prostatitis; c. prostatic 11. a. pyelonephritis; b. pyelogram; c. pyelography   12. a. renal; b. renogram; c. renography 13. a. seminal; b. seminuria   14. a. aspermia; b. oligospermia   15. a. spermatogenesis; b. spermatolysis; c. spermatic; d. spermatocyte   16. a. testicular   17. a. urology; b. urologist; c. uremia   18. a. ureteritis; b. ureterostenosis; c. ureteral   19. a. urethroplasty; b. urethralgia; c. urethritis; d. urethroscope; e. urethroscopy; f. urethrostenosis; g. urethrotomy; h. urethral 20. a. glycosuria; b. nocturia; c. oliguria; d. pyuria; e. anuria; f. dysuria; g. hematuria; h. polyuria; i. albuminuria; j. azoturia; k. bacteriuria   21. a. urinary; b. urinometer   22. a. vasectomy; b. vasorrhaphy   23. a. vesiculitis; b. vesiculectomy; c. vesicular

Case Study

1. He has nocturnal hesitancy (difficulty initiating urination during the night) and frequency (urinating more often but without any increase in overall volume of urine); he does not have urinary incontinence (inability to hold back urination) or erectile dysfunction (inability to achieve an erection)
2. D. prostatic cancer
3. Vital signs are routine measures of general health; they include temperature, pulse, respiration rate, and blood pressure
4. Urinalysis (UA), digital rectal exam (DRE), prostate-specific antigen (PSA), computed tomography scan (CT scan), culture and sensitivity (C&S), erectile dysfunction (ED), myocardial infarction (MI), percutaneous transluminal coronary angioplasty (PTCA), hypertension (HTN), biopsy (Bx), red blood cells (RBC)
5. Urinalysis is a physical and chemical examination of urine; it is checked for pH, specific gravity, and presence of substances such as blood and sugar; this patient did have blood present in his urine, but no bacteria were found
6. An oncologist is a physician specializing in diagnosing and treating cancer; oncologist did not recommend that patient have any radiation or chemotherapy treatments because cancer showed no signs of having left prostate gland; however, patient is to continue having a PSA done every three months
7. Two tests were diagnostic images: a bone scan and a CT scan; metastasis is spread of initial cancerous tumor to another site in body
8. Myocardial infarction is a heart attack; part of heart muscle dies because of lack of blood supply; percutaneous transluminal coronary angioplasty is a treatment procedure that uses a balloon to expand a blocked coronary artery and improve blood flow to heart muscle

Practice Exercises

Sound It Out

1. ureterostenosis   2. balanorrhea   3. cryptorchism   4. urinometer   5. aspermia 6. nephroma   7. dysuria   8. epididymitis   9. vesiculitis   10. hematuria   11. hemodialysis 12. gonorrhea   13. pyelonephritis   14. nephrosis   15. lithotripsy   16. nephrosclerosis 17. oligospermia   18. orchidectomy   19. polyuria   20. prostatitis   21. renography 22. vasectomy   23. urinalysis   24. varicocele   25. nephromegaly

Transcription Practice

1. A cystoscopy revealed the presence of a cystolith and the patient underwent a lithotripsy.
2. When noting the balanorrhea and balanitis, the physician knew she needed to determine if the patient had acquired a sexually transmitted disease.
3. A retrograde pyelogram confirmed the diagnosis of pyelonephritis.
4. A semen analysis performed 6 weeks after the vasectomy confirmed aspermia.
5. The patient's polycystic kidney disease had resulted in renal failure, necessitating the use of hemodialysis.
6. The results of the urinalysis showed that there was pyuria, bacteriuria, and glycosuria.
7. After the patient developed anuria a renogram revealed that the patient had developed nephrosclerosis.
8. The elderly gentleman required a circumcision for phimosis.
9. The patient required a ureterostomy following a cystectomy for bladder cancer.
10. Bob developed nephrolithiasis and underwent extracorporeal shockwave lithotripsy.

Abbreviation Matching

1. J   2. G   3. F   4. B   5. A   6. E   7. I   8. H   9. D   10. C

Labeling Exercise

1. Kidney **(ren/o, nephr/o)**   2. Ureter **(ureter/o)**   3. Renal artery   4. Renal vein   5. Urinary bladder **(cyst/o)**   6. Urethra **(urethr/o)**

Build Medical Terms

1. nephrology   2. nephromegaly   3. nephropathy   4. nephroptosis   5. nephropexy
6. spermatolysis   7. spermatic   8. cystogram   9. cystoscopy   10. prostatitis
11. prostatectomy   12. hematuria   13. nocturia   14. dysuria   15. glycosuria

Fill in the Blank

1. varicocele   2. benign prostatic hyperplasia   3. testosterone   4. number, swimming strength, shape   5. voiding cystourethrography   6. circumcision   7. Hesitancy   8. Prostate specific antigen   9. blood urea nitrogen   10. calculus

Spelling

1. epididymitis   2. nephrolithiasis   3. correctly spelled   4. pyelography   5. correctly spelled
6. correctly spelled   7. hydrocele   8. trichomoniasis   9. correctly spelled   10. correctly spelled

Medical Term Analysis

1. **balan**, glans penis, **-itis**, inflammation, inflammation of glans penis   2. **vas**, vas deferens, **-ectomy**, surgical removal, surgical removal of vas deferens   3. **py**, pus, **-uria**, urine condition, urine condition of pus   4. **ureter**, ureter, **-ostomy**, surgically create an opening, surgically create an opening in ureter   5. **nephr/o**, kidney, **lith**, stone, **-iasis**, abnormal condition, abnormal condition of kidney stones   6. **ur/o**, urine, **-logy**, study of, study of urine   7. **testicul**, testes, **-ar**, pertaining to, pertaining to the testes   8. **crypt**, hidden, **orch**, testes, **-ism**, state of, state of hidden testes   9. **prostat**, prostate gland, **-ectomy**, surgical removal, surgical removal of prostate gland   10. **cyst/o**, bladder, **-scope**, instrument for viewing, instrument for viewing bladder

Photomatch Challenge

1. epididymitis   2. varicocele   3. undescended testicle   4. orchitis   5. testicular cancer
6. hydrocele

Chapter 13

Building Obstetrics and Gynecology Terms

1. a. amniotic; b. amniotomy; c. amniorrhea; d. amniocentesis; e. amniorrhexis 2. a. cervical; b. cervicectomy; c. cervicitis; d. endocervicitis; e. cervicoplasty 3. a. chorionic; b. choriocarcinoma 4. a. colposcope; b. colposcopy; c. colpectomy; d. colporrhaphy 5. a. embryonic; b. embryogenic; c. embryology 6. a. episiorrhaphy; b. episioplasty; c. episiotomy 7. a. fetal; b. fetometry; c. fetoscope; d. fetoscopy 8. a. nulligravida; b. primigravida; c. multigravida 9. a. gynecology; b. gynecologist 10. a. hysteropexy; b. hysterorrhexis; c. hysterectomy; d. hysterography; e. hysterogram 11. a. laparotomy; b. laparoscope; c. laparoscopy 12. a. mammary; b. mammogram; c. mammography; d. mammoplasty 13. a. mastalgia; b. mastitis; c. mastectomy 14. a. amenorrhea; b. dysmenorrhea; c. oligomenorrhea; d. menorrhagia 15. a. endometritis; b. metrorrhea; c. metrorrhagia 16. a. natal; b. neonatal; c. neonatology; d. neonatologist 17. a. oocyte; b. oogenesis 18. a. oophoritis; b. oophorectomy; c. oophoropexy 19. a. ovarian; b. ovariosalpingitis 20. a. nullipara; b. primipara; c. multipara 21. a. antepartum; b. postpartum 22. a. salpingectomy; b. salpingitis; c. salpingography; d. salpingogram; e. salpingocyesis 23. a. uterine; b. uteroplasty; c. uteroscope; d. uteroscopy; e. intrauterine 24. a. vaginal; b. vaginitis; c. transvaginal

Case Study

1. Patient is postmenopausal; she had not had any menstrual periods for three years; mild to moderate uterine cramps, lower abdominal pain, and painful intercourse
2. prn = as needed; grav2 = two pregnancies; para2 = two live births; D&C = dilation of cervix and curettage of endometrial lining; EMB = endometrial biopsy, removing a piece of tissue to examine under a microscope
3. Migraine–takes pain medicine as needed; asthma–takes a bronchodilator; hyperlipemia–using no treatment
4. Cervical cancer; she has endometrial cancer, not cervical cancer
5. Blood tests, Hgb = hemoglobin, measures amount of hemoglobin present in blood; HCT = hematocrit, measures volume of red blood cells in blood; anemic because of loss of blood from continuous vaginal bleeding
6. Stage 1: tumor confined to body of uterus; Stage 2: tumor extends to the cervix; Stage 3: tumor has spread to pelvic region; Stage 4: extensive pelvic tumors or tumors have spread to distant organs; if cancer is in pelvic lymph nodes, it would be Stage 3
7. Hysteroscopy is a visual examination of inside of uterus with fiberoptic camera; tumor area was very small, so the D&C missed it
8. Lymphadenectomy means surgical removal of lymph nodes; they will be examined for cancer cells to see whether the cancer has spread

Practice Exercises

Sound It Out

1. amniocentesis 2. cervicoplasty 3. choriocarcinoma 4. colposcopy 5. cystocele 6. dysmenorrhea 7. endometriosis 8. fetometry 9. hysterography 10. intrauterine 11. laparoscopy 12. mammogram 13. mastectomy 14. multipara 15. neonatal 16. nulligravida 17. oophorectomy 18. ovariosalpingitis 19. postpartum 20. primigravida 21. rectocele 22. salpingocyesis 23. transvaginal 24. uteroplasty 25. vaginitis

Transcription Practice

1. Mrs. Scott's dysmenorrhea was treated with a dilation and curettage.
2. Over time Mrs. Martinez had developed a vesicovaginal fistula.
3. The neonatologist assisted with the cesarean section.
4. Jean's infertility was the result of scarring caused by pelvic inflammatory disease.

5. A hysterectomy became necessary because of extensive endometriosis.
6. The new patient at the gynecologist's office was primigravida and nullipara.
7. Maria was happy to find out she had fibrocystic breast disease and not breast cancer.
8. A salpingectomy was necessary following the discovery of an ectopic pregnancy (or salpingocyesis).
9. Following an abnormal Pap smear, Tawanda's cervical cancer was diagnosed by conization.
10. A laparoscopy was conducted to examine the patient for ovarian cancer.

Build Medical Terms

1. hysteropexy   2. hysterectomy   3. hysterorrhexis   4. hysterogram   5. fetal   6. fetometry
7. antepartum   8. postpartum   9. amenorrhea   10. dysmenorrhea   11. oligomenorrhea
12. menorrhagia   13. mastalgia   14. mastitis   15. mastectomy

Spelling

1. hysterectomy   2. spelled correctly   3. spelled correctly   4. spelled correctly
5. premenstrual   6. antepartum   7. menorrhagia   8. spelled correctly   9. amniotomy
10. spelled correctly

Fill in the Blank

1. uterine, fallopian   2. gynecology, obstetrics   3. endometrium, myometrium   4. Chorionic villus sampling   5. fetal heart rate, fetal heart tone   6. hemolytic disease of the newborn   7. fistula
8. tubal ligation   9. cervix   10. stillbirth

Labeling Exercise

1. Milk gland   2. Nipple   3. Areola   4. Milk duct   5. Fat   6. Uterus (**metr/o**, **hyster/o**, **uter/o**)   7. Vagina (**colp/o**, **vagin/o**)   8. Uterine (fallopian) tube (**salping/o**)   9. Ovum (**o/o**)
10. Ovary (**oophor/o**, **ovari/o**)   11. Myometrium   12. Endometrium   13. Cervix (**cervic/o**)

Medical Term Analysis

1. **oophor/o**, ovary, **-pexy**, surgical fixation, surgical fixation of the ovary   2. **colp/o**, vagina, **-scope**, instrument for viewing, instrument for viewing the vagina   3. **chori/o**, chorion, **carcin**, cancer, **-oma**, tumor, chorion cancerous tumor   4. **intra-**, within, **uter**, uterus, **-ine**, pertaining to, pertaining to within the uterus   5. **trans-**, across, **vagin**, vagina, **-al**, pertaining to, pertaining to across the vagina   6. **embry/o**, embryo, **-nic**, pertaining to, pertaining to the embryo
7. **o/o**, egg, **-cyte**, cell, egg cell   8. **cervic/o**, cervix, **-plasty**, surgical repair, surgical repair of cervix   9. **ovari/o**, ovary, **salping**, uterine tube, **-itis**, inflammation, inflammation of ovary and uterine tube   10. **episi**, vulva, **-otomy**, cutting into, cutting into the vulva

Abbreviation Matching

1. F   2. C   3. I   4. A   5. H   6. B   7. J   8. D   9. G   10. E

Photomatch Challenge

1. hysterectomy   2. amniocentesis   3. right salpingo-oophorectomy   4. bilateral hysterosalpingo-oophorectomy   5. laparoscopy   6. bilateral salpingo-oophorectomy

Chapter 14

Building Neurology Terms

1. a. cerebellar; b. cerebellitis   2. a. meningocele; b. meningomyelocele   3. a. cerebral; b. cerebrospinal; c. cerebritis; d. cerebromalacia; e. cerebrosclerosis; f. cerebrovascular; g. cerebrotomy   4. a. encephalic; b. electroencephalogram; c. electroencephalography; d. encephalalgia; e. encephalitis; f. encephalopathy; g. encephaloma; h. encephalomalacia;

i. encephalosclerosis   5. a. anesthesia; b. hyperesthesia   6. a. medullary   7. a. meningeal;
b. meningitis; c. meningomyelitis   8. a. myelogram; b. myelography; c. myelitis; d. myelomalacia;
e. myeloneuritis; f. myelopathy; g. myelosclerosis; h. myelotomy   9. a. neural; b. neuralgia;
c. neurectomy; d. neurology; e. neurologist; f. neuroma; g. neuropathy; h. neuroplasty;
i. polyneuritis; j. neurorrhaphy   10. a. aphasia; b. dysphasia   11. a. monoplegia; b. diplegia;
c. quadriplegia; d. hemiplegia; e. neuroplegia f. paraplegia   12. a. pontine; b. pontocerebellar;
c. pontomedullary   13. a. thalamic; b. thalamotomy

Case Study

1. aphasia, hemiplegia   2. transient ischemic attack   3. c   4. nonsteroidal anti-inflammatory
drugs taken for her arthritis   5. emergency room, magnetic resonance imaging, intensive care unit,
physical therapy, occupational therapy   6. because she was found on the floor and had probably
fallen   7. each side of the brain controls the opposite side of the body

Practice Exercises

Sound It Out

1. meningitis   2. neuroma   3. aphasia   4. cerebromalacia   5. encephalosclerosis
6. concussion   7. encephalitis   8. dementia   9. anesthesia   10. dysphasia
11. myelopathy   12. neurectomy   13. epilepsy   14. hemiplegia   15. hydrocephalus
16. meningocele   17. migraine   18. myelography   19. neuroplasty   20. paralysis
21. encephaloma   22. polyneuritis   23. myelitis   24. cerebrovascular   25. syncope

Transcription Practice

1. Jon took anticonvulsants to control his epileptic seizures.
2. As a result of the cerebrovascular accident, Mr. van Pelt was in a coma.
3. The auto accident victim developed quadriplegia following a spinal cord injury.
4. During the transient ischemic attack, Mr. Edelstein had aphasia.
5. Ilina's monoplegia was caused by multiple sclerosis.
6. Antonio went to the neurologist because he was having migraines.
7. A positron emission tomography was completed to see whether the tumor was in the cerebrum
   or the cerebellum.
8. A lumbar puncture was performed to analyze cerebrospinal fluid for signs of encephalitis.
9. Mr. Larsen's severe leg pain was caused by polyneuritis.
10. The elderly gentleman with Alzheimer disease eventually developed dementia.

Labeling Exercise

1. Brain **(encephal/o)**   2. Cranial nerve **(neur/o)**   3. Spinal cord **(myel/o)**   4. Spinal nerve
(neur/o)

Build Medical Terms

1. neuralgia   2. neuroma   3. neurology   4. neuroplasty   5. neuropathy   6. thalamic
7. thalamotomy   8. diplegia   9. hemiplegia   10. meningeal   11. meningitis   12. myelogram
13. myelomalacia   14. myelosclerosis   15. myelitis

Fill in the Blank

1. motor neurons   2. concussion, contusion   3. syncope   4. cerebrum, cerebellum, thalamus,
brainstem   5. meninges   6. Cerebral palsy   7. grand mal   8. Myasthenia gravis
9. Parkinson   10. Shingles

Abbreviation Matching

1. H   2. C   3. J   4. A   5. F   6. B   7. I   8. D   9. G   10. E

Medical Term Analysis

1. **cerebell**, cerebellum, **-ar**, pertaining to, pertaining to the cerebellum   2. **mening/o**, meninges, **-cele**, protrusion, protrusion of the meninges   3. **cerebr/o**, cerebrum, **spin**, spine, **-al**, pertaining to, pertaining to the cerebrum and spine   4. **an-**, without, **-esthesia**, sensation, without sensation   5. **mening/o**, meninges, **myel**, spinal cord, **-itis**, inflammation, inflammation of meninges and spinal cord   6. **encephal**, brain, **-oma**, tumor, brain tumor   7. **dys-**, difficult, **-phasia**, speech, difficult speech   8. **neur/o**, nerve, **-logy**, study of, study of nerves
9. **pont/o**, pons, **medull**, medulla oblongata, **-ary**, pertaining to, pertaining to the pons and medulla oblongata   10. **cerebr**, cerebrum, **-otomy**, cutting into, cutting into the cerebrum

Spelling

1. neurorrhaphy   2. correctly spelled   3. correctly spelled   4. meningitis   5. quadriplegia
6. correctly spelled   7. electroencephalography   8. correctly spelled   9. myasthenia gravis
10. correctly spelled

Photomatch Challenge

1. cerebrum, abnormal softening of cerebrum   2. thalamus, cutting into thalamus   3. cerebellum, cerebellum inflammation   4. spinal cord, record of spinal cord   5. pons, pertaining to the pons
6. medulla oblongata, pertaining to medulla oblongata

Chapter 15

Building Endocrinology Terms

1. a. adenocarcinoma; b. adenocyte; c. adenoid; d. adenomalacia   2. a. adrenal;
b. adrenomegaly   3. a. adrenalectomy; b. adrenalitis; c. adrenalopathy   4. a. endocrinology;
b. endocrinologist; c. endocrinoma; d. endocrinopathy   5. a. hyperglycemia; b. hypoglycemia
6. a. glycosuria   7. a. oophoritis; b. oophoroplasty; c. oophorotomy; d. oophorectomy
8. a. orchiectomy; b. orchiopexy; c. orchiotomy   9. a. ovarian; b. ovariocentesis;
c. ovariorrhexis   10. a. pancreatic; b. pancreatectomy; c. pancreatitis; d. pancreatotomy
11. a. parathyroidal; b. parathyroidectomy; c. hyperparathyroidism; d. hypoparathyroidism
12. a. pinealectomy   13. a. hypopituitarism; b. hyperpituitarism   14. a. polydipsia; b. polyuria
15. a. testicular   16. a. thymic; b. thymectomy; c. thymitis; d. thymoma   17. a. thyromegaly;
b. thyrotomy   18. a. thyroidal; b. thyroiditis; c. thyroidectomy; d. hyperthyroidism; e. hypothyroidism

Case Study

1. Hypertension, high blood pressure; elevated heart rate, heart beating too fast; heart palpitations, pounding heartbeat; diaphoresis, profuse sweating; hand tremors, uncontrollable shaking of the hands; extreme anxiety, feeling of dread
2. A
3. Blood pressure: 90/60 mmHg to 120/80 mmHg; respiratory rate: 12–18 breaths per minute; heart rate: 60–100 beats per minute
4. Emergency room, electrocardiogram, chest X-ray, blood pressure, beats per minute
5. Difficulty breathing
6. Malignant is cancerous, life-threatening tumor that tends to spread throughout body; *benign* is not cancerous
7. To verify that tumor is a pheochromocytoma and to determine whether tumor is cancerous
8. Adrenalectomy

Practice Exercises

Sound It Out

1. thyromegaly   2. adenomalacia   3. adrenomegaly   4. pancreatitis   5. parathyroidectomy
6. acromegaly   7. exophthalmos   8. adrenalectomy   9. glycosuria   10. goiter

11. orchiectomy 12. hyperpituitarism 13. gigantism 14. hypothyroidism 15. polyuria
16. orchiopexy 17. pancreatectomy 18. hyperglycemia 19. pinealectomy 20. polydipsia
21. tetany 22. thymitis 23. thyroidectomy 24. thyrotoxicosis 25. oophorectomy

Transcription Practice

1. Gladys's glucose tolerance test confirmed the diagnosis of diabetes mellitus.
2. When Dr. Nguyen noted exophthalmos, she suspected Graves disease (or hyperthyroidism).
3. An adrenalectomy was necessary to treat the pheochromocytoma.
4. Hypoparathyroidism is one cause of tetany.
5. Two diagnostic tests were ordered, a thyroid scan and a thyroid function test.
6. Hypersecretion of growth hormone produces gigantism and lack of growth hormone can produce dwarfism.
7. A person with diabetes insipidus often has polydipsia and polyuria.
8. When Mrs. Ruiz developed facial hair and a deeper voice, adrenal virilism was suspected.
9. Corticosteroids were prescribed for the patient with rheumatoid arthritis.
10. Mr. McDonald's adrenomegaly was caused by an adenocarcinoma.

Build Medical Terms

1. thyroidal 2. thyroiditis 3. thyroidectomy 4. hyperthyroidism 5. hypothyroidism
6. hyperglycemia 7. hypoglycemia 8. polydipsia 9. polyuria 10. adenocarcinoma
11. adenoid 12. adenomalacia 13. pancreatic 14. pancreatitis 15. pancreatotomy

Labeling Exercise

1. Pineal gland (**pineal/o**) 2. Parathyroid glands (**parathyroid/o**) 3. Adrenal glands (**adren/o, adrenal/o**) 4. Pancreas (**pancreat/o**) 5. Pituitary gland (**pituitar/o**) 6. Thyroid gland (**thyr/o, thyroid/o**) 7. Thymus gland (**thym/o**) 8. Ovaries (**oophor/o, ovari/o**) 9. Testes (**orch/o, orchi/o, orchid/o, testicul/o**)

Spelling

1. correctly spelled 2. ovariocentesis 3. myxedema 4. correctly spelled 5. correctly spelled 6. tetany 7. exophthalmos 8. correctly spelled 9. correctly spelled 10. virilism

Fill in the Blank

1. homeostasis 2. hormones, target organs 3. hypersecretion, hyposecretion 4. kidney, cortex, medulla 5. Estrogen, menstrual 6. insulin, glucagon 7. calcium 8. melatonin, circadian 9. pituitary 10. thymus

Abbreviation Matching

1. E 2. C 3. H 4. J 5. B 6. I 7. D 8. A 9. G 10. F

Medical Term Analysis

1. **orchi/o**, testes, **-pexy**, surgical fixation, surgical fixation of the testes 2. **thyr/o**, thyroid gland, **-megaly**, enlarged, enlarged thyroid gland 3. **aden/o**, gland, **carcin**, cancer, **-oma**, tumor, cancerous gland tumor 4. **hypo-**, insufficient, **parathyroid**, parathyroid gland, **-ism**, condition, condition of insufficient parathyroid gland 5. **thyr/o**, thyroid gland, **toxic**, poison, **-osis**, abnormal condition, abnormal condition of thyroid poisoning 6. **pineal**, pineal gland, **-ectomy**, surgical removal, surgical removal of pineal gland 7. **ovari/o**, ovary, **-rrhexis**, rupture, ruptured ovary 8. **thym**, thymus gland, **-itis**, inflammation, inflammation of thymus gland 9. **hyper-**, excessive, **glyc**, sugar, **-emia**, blood condition, blood condition of excessive sugar 10. **oophor/o**, ovary, **-plasty**, surgical repair, surgical repair of the ovary

1. **oste/o**, osteoporosis   2. **thyr/o** or **thyroid/o**, thyromegaly   3. **testicul/o**, testicular   4. **adren/o** or **adrenal/o**, adrenalitis   5. **ovari/o**, ovariorrhexis   6. **mamm/o** or **mast/o**, mastectomy

Chapter 16

Building Ophthalmology Terms

1. a. aqueous   2. a. blepharoptosis; b. blepharoplasty; c. blepharoplegia   3. a. choroidal; b. choroiditis   4. a. conjunctivitis; b. conjunctival   5. a. coreometer; b. coreometry   6. a. corneal   7. a. cycloplegia; b. cyclotomy   8. a. dacryolith; b. dacryorrhea; c. dacryoadenitis; d. dacryocystitis   9. a. iritis   10. a. iridoplegia; b. iridotomy   11. a. keratometer; b. keratometry; c. keratectomy; d. keratitis; e. keratotomy; f. keratoplasty   12. a. lacrimal; b. nasolacrimal   13. a. intraocular; b. oculomycosis; c. ocular   14. a. ophthalmic; b. ophthalmology; c. ophthalmologist; d. ophthalmoscope; e. ophthalmoscopy; f. ophthalmoplegia; g. xerophthalmia   15. a. hemianopia; b. diplopia   16. a. optic; b. optometer; c. optometry   17. a. phacomalacia; b. phacolysis; c. phacosclerosis   18. a. pupillary; b. pupillometer   19. a. retinal; b. retinopathy; c. retinitis; d. cryoretinopexy   20. a. scleral; b. sclerotomy; c. scleromalacia; d. scleritis   21. a. tonometer; b. tonometry   22. a. vitreous

Case Study

1. Pain; excessive tearing; decreased visual acuity–fuzzy or cloudy vision; photophobia–increased sensitivity to light
2. Thigh bone
3. Patient had normal 20/20 vision in right eye, meaning he could see clearly at 20 ft what a normal person would expect to see at 20 ft; however, left eye had 20/200 vision, meaning he could see at 20 ft what a normal person would expect to see at 200 ft
4. Corneal abrasions appear bright green under a black light
5. Abrasion – scraping away of a layer
   ulcer–an erosion or crater, deeper than an abrasion
6. Antibiotic eye drops–to fight infection
   anesthetic eye drops–to reduce eye pain
7. To wear an eye patch; to put a lubricating ointment in his eyes if they are too dry when he wakes up in the morning; to see an ophthalmologist in 24 hours to make sure his eye is healing

Practice Exercises

Sound It Out

1. keratoplasty   2. oculomycosis   3. conjunctivitis   4. iridotomy   5. diplopia   6. glaucoma   7. hemianopia   8. astigmatism   9. blepharoptosis   10. hyperopia   11. intraocular   12. coreometry   13. cryoretinopexy   14. keratitis   15. amblyopia   16. phacolysis   17. myopia   18. cataract   19. nyctalopia   20. cycloplegia   21. nystagmus   22. phacosclerosis   23. photophobia   24. strabismus   25. hordeolum

Transcription Practice

1. Dr. Cohen decided to use cryoextraction to remove the patient's cataract rather than a phacoemulsification.
2. Mr. Blair's myopia was corrected by radial keratotomy.
3. The head injury caused a retinal detachment that required repair by laser retinal photocoagulation.

4. Because the cornea was abnormally curved, light rays were not evenly refracted, resulting in astigmatism.
5. Examination of the eye with an ophthalmoscope did not reveal any reason for Mr. Mendez's photophobia.
6. Mrs. Capers made an appointment with the optometrist because of scleritis and diplopia.
7. The baby's mother was concerned about her infant when she noticed conjunctivitis and excessive dacryorrhea.
8. Mr. Carpenter decided that it was no longer safe for him to drive after he developed nyctalopia and macular degeneration.
9. A patient's visual acuity can be evaluated using a Snellen chart.
10. A corneal abrasion occurred when sand became trapped under Karen's contact lens that was identified by using fluorescein.

Fill in the Blank

1. Diabetic retinopathy   2. Glaucoma   3. Achromatopsia   4. hordeolum   5. nystagmus
6. Myopia   7. strabismus   8. Snellen   9. Nyctalopia   10. astigmatism

Abbreviation Matching

1. E   2. I   3. A   4. G   5. C   6. J   7. B   8. F   9. H   10. D

Labeling Exercise

1. Conjunctiva **(conjunctiv/o)**   2. Pupil **(core/o, pupill/o)**   3. Cornea **(corne/o, kerat/o)**
4. Aqueous humor **(aque/o)**   5. Iris **(ir/o, irid/o)**   6. Lens **(phac/o)**   7. Vitreous body **(vitre/o)**   8. Suspensory ligament   9. Ciliary body **(cycl/o)**   10. Retina **(retin/o)**   11. Choroid **(choroid/o)**   12. Sclera **(scler/o)**   13. Macula lutea   14. Optic nerve   15. Central retinal artery and vein

Build Medical Terms

1. ophthalmology   2. ophthalmoscope   3. ophthalmoplegia   4. ophthalmic   5. keratectomy
6. keratotomy   7. keratometer   8. keratoplasty   9. retinopathy   10. retinitis
11. blepharoplasty   12. blepharoplegia   13. blepharoptosis   14. diplopia   15. amblyopia

Medical Term Analysis

1. **blephar/o**, eyelid, **-ptosis**, drooping, drooping eyelid   2. **dacry/o**, tears, **aden**, gland, **-itis**, inflammation, inflammation of a tear gland   3. **nas/o**, nose, **lacrim**, tears, **-al**, pertaining to, pertaining to the nose and tears   4. **intra-**, within, **ocul**, eye, **-ar**, pertaining to, pertaining to within the eye   5. **cry/o**, cold, **retin/o**, retina, **-pexy**, surgical fixation, surgical fixation of the retina using cold   6. **choroid**, choroid layer, **-itis**, inflammation, inflammation of choroid layer   7. **kerat/o**, cornea, **-plasty**, surgical repair, surgical repair of cornea   8. **opt/o**, vision, **-metry**, process of measuring, process of measuring vision   9. **ophthalm/o**, eye, **-scope**, instrument for viewing, instrument for viewing the eye   10. **phac/o**, lens, **-sclerosis**, hardening, hardening of the lens

Spelling

1. stye   2. correctly spelled   3. hordeolum   4. myopia   5. correctly spelled   6. correctly spelled   7. dacryolith   8. correctly spelled   9. correctly spelled   10. strabismus

Photomatch Challenge

1. dark spots in visual field, diabetic retinopathy   2. losing vision around edges, glaucoma
3. whole image is blurry, cataract   4. center of image is blurry, macular degeneration

Chapter 17

Building Otorhinolaryngology Terms

1. a. adenoidectomy; b. adenoiditis 2. a. audiology; b. audiologist; c. audiometry; d. audiometer; e. audiogram 3. a. auditory 4. a. aural 5. a. cochlear 6. a. epiglottic; b. epiglottitis 7. a. laryngeal; b. laryngitis; c. laryngoscopy; d. laryngoscope; e. laryngectomy; f. laryngoplasty; g. laryngoplegia; h. laryngospasm 8. a. myringitis; b. myringectomy; c. myringoplasty; d. myringosclerosis; e. myringotomy 9. a. nasal; b. nasogastric; c. nasopharyngeal 10. a. anosmia 11. a. otic; b. otitis; c. otalgia; d. otology; e. otologist; f. otoscopy; g. otoscope; h. otoplasty; i. otomycosis; j. otopyorrhea 12. a. pharyngeal; b. pharyngitis; c. pharyngoplasty; d. pharyngospasm; e. pharyngotomy 13. a. aphonia; b. dysphonia 14. a. rhinitis; b. rhinoplasty; c. rhinorrhea; d. rhinomycosis 15. a. sinusitis; b. pansinusitis; c. nasosinusitis or rhinosinusitis 16. a. tonsillar; b. tonsillitis; c. tonsillectomy 17. a. tracheal; b. tracheomegaly; c. tracheoplasty; d. tracheotomy; e. tracheostenosis; f. endotracheal 18. a. tympanic; b. tympanometry; c. tympanometer; d. tympanogram; e. tympanoplasty; f. tympanorrhexis; g. tympanotomy

Case Study

1. She has been feeling run-down and having headaches for about 10 years; pain is over her eyes, but sometimes it moves down and makes her upper teeth hurt; recently she became unable to detect the strong odor of cooking fish
2. Anosmia
3. B
4. Enlargement or disease of lymph nodes in neck region
5. Pan- is a prefix meaning all; infection has spread to all of paranasal sinuses
6. Temperature, blood pressure, and breathing rate are normal; pulse is high
7. Culture grows sample of infected tissue to determine whether bacteria are present; if bacteria are present, then culture can be used to identify specific type; this culture found bacteria but did not find fungus
8. Antibiotic to fight infection, corticosteroid nose spray to reduce inflammation, repeat culture to check whether treatment is working and infection is gone, stop smoking because smoke irritates sinuses, go to allergist to see whether she has allergies that could make her prone to infections

Practice Exercises

Sound It Out

1. otalgia 2. audiometer 3. diphtheria 4. pharyngospasm 5. myringosclerosis 6. dysphonia 7. adenoidectomy 8. otoplasty 9. laryngitis 10. laryngoplegia 11. laryngoscope 12. myringoplasty 13. vertigo 14. tympanogram 15. tympanometry 16. otoscopy 17. pansinusitis 18. pertussis 19. rhinitis 20. rhinorrhea 21. tinnitus 22. tonsillectomy 23. audiogram 24. tracheostenosis 25. tympanorrhexis

Transcription Practice

1. The new parents were quite concerned when their baby developed croup.
2. Meilin's deafness was due to an acoustic neuroma.
3. The DPT vaccination protects children against diphtheria and pertussis.
4. The physician ordered supplemental oxygen to be delivered by a nasal cannula.
5. His physician became concerned when Mr. Janssen developed vertigo and tinnitus.
6. Carmen's physician recommended to her parents that she have pressure-equalizing tubes because of her repeated otitis media.
7. The paramedics had to quickly determine whether the patient's condition required a tracheotomy or endotracheal intubation.

8. Ursula went to see an otorhinolaryngologist because of her repeated epistaxis.
9. For his deafness, Tariq needed a cochlear implant rather than a hearing aid.
10. After examining the external auditory canal with an otoscope, it was obvious Jackson had otitis externa.

Fill in the Blank

1. hearing, equilibrium (balance)   2. epiglottis   3. larynx   4. adenoids   5. tympanic membrane (eardrum)   6. auditory   7. nares   8. nosebleed   9. amplification device   10. malleus, incus, stapes

Abbreviation Matching

1. E   2. I   3. A   4. G   5. B   6. J   7. F   8. C   9. H   10. D

Labeling Exercise

1. Pinna   2. External auditory canal   3. Mastoid process   4. Malleus (hammer)
5. Incus (anvil)   6. Semicircular canals (equilibrium)   7. Auditory nerve   8. Cochlea (hearing) **(cochle/o)**   9. Oval window   10. Stapes (stirrup)   11. Auditory (Eustachian) tube   12. Tympanic membrane (eardrum) **(myring/o, tympan/o)**

Build Medical Terms

1. otology   2. otomycosis   3. otoplasty   4. otitis   5. otoscopy   6. pharyngospasm
7. pharyngeal   8. aphonia   9. dysphonia   10. tracheostenosis   11. tracheotomy
12. tracheomegaly   13. tympanoplasty   14. tympanometer   15. tympanorrhexis

Medical Term Analysis

1. **tympan**, tympanic membrane, **-otomy**, cutting into, cutting into tympanic membrane
2. **cochle**, cochlea, **-ar**, pertaining to, pertaining to the cochlea   3. **nas/o**, nose, **gastr**, stomach, **-ic**, pertaining to, pertaining to the nose and stomach   4. **endo-**, within, **trache**, trachea, **-al**, pertaining to, pertaining to within the trachea   5. **rhin/o**, nose, **myc**, fungus, **-osis**, abnormal condition, abnormal condition of nose fungus   6. **tonsill**, tonsil, **-ectomy**, surgical removal, surgical removal of tonsils   7. **an-**, without, **-osmia**, smell, without smell   8. **laryng/o**, larynx, **-plegia**, paralysis, paralysis of the larynx   9. **pan-**, all, **sinus**, sinuses, **-itis**, inflammation, inflammation of all the sinuses   10. **myring/o**, tympanic membrane, **-sclerosis**, hardening, hardening of the tympanic membrane

Spelling

1. spelled correctly   2. epistaxis   3. diphtheria   4. otopyorrhea   5. spelled correctly
6. spelled correctly   7. spelled correctly   8. cannula   9. spelled correctly   10. pertussis

Photomatch Challenge

1. rhinitis   2. pharyngitis   3. tonsillitis   4. sinusitis   5. epistaxis   6. laryngitis

Index

Hyaline membrane disease (HMD), 181, 184
Hydrocele, 231
Hydrocephalus, 283
Hyperopia, 327
Hyperpnea, 181
Hypersecretion, 297
Hypertension (HTN), 115, 119
Hyperventilation, 181
Hypogastric region, 45
Hypopnea, 181
Hyposecretion, 297
Hypotension, 115
Hypoventilation, 181
Hypoxia, 181
Hysteratresia, 257
Hysterosalpingography (HSG), 262

I

Ileus, 205
Ilium, 76, 196, 197, 202
Immune systems, 150. *See also* Immunology
Immunity, 152
Immunization, 158
Immunocompromised, 157
Immunodeficiency, 157
Immunoglobulins (Ig), 159
Immunologists, 150
Immunology, 149–68
    abbreviations, 159
    case study, 159–60
    combining forms, 150, 152–56
    description of, 150
    organs treated in, 151
    prefixes, 151
    suffixes, 150
    vocabulary, 156–58
Immunosuppressant, 157
Impacted fracture, 86
Impetigo, 61
Implantable cardioverter defibrillator (ICD), 115, 119
Impotence. *See* Erectile dysfunction (ED)
Incision and drainage (I&D), 63
Incus (anvil), 342, 344
Infant respiratory distress syndrome (IRDS), 181, 184
Infarct, 115
Inferior (caudal) direction, 38
Inferior vena cava, 104, 107, 108
Infertility. *See* Sterility
Inflammation, 157
Inflammatory bowel disease (IBD), 204, 207, 208
Influenza (flu), 181, 184
Inguinal region, 40
Inner ear, 344
Inner ear infection. *See* Otitis interna
Insulin, 301, 304, 305, 306
Insulin-dependent diabetes mellitus (IDDM), 304, 305, 307
Intake and output (I&O), 235
Integument. *See* Skin
Integumentary system. *See* Dermatology (Derm, derm); Skin

Intensive care unit (ICU), 119
Interatrial septum, 107
Intermittent positive pressure breathing (IPPB), 181, 184
Internal anal sphincter, 198
Internal fixation, 86, 88
Interventricular septum, 110
Intestine, 200
Intracapsular cataract extraction (ICCE), 330
Intracranial pressure (ICP), 286
Intradermal (ID), 63
Intramuscular (IM), 90
Intraocular lens (IOL), 330
Intraocular lens (IOL) implant, 327
Intraocular pressure (IOP), 330
Intrauterine device (IUD), 262
Intravascular thrombolytic therapy, 115
Intravenous (IV), 119
Intravenous pyelogram (IVP), 232, 235
Intussusception, 206
In vitro fertilization (IVF), 260, 262
Iris, 318, 319, 322
Iron-deficiency anemia, 138
Irritable bowel syndrome (IBS), 206, 208
Ischium, 76
Islets of Langerhans. *See* Pancreatic islets

J

Jaundice, 206
Jejunum, 196, 197, 202
Joints, 74, 75, 79
    cartilaginous, 75, 79
    fibrous, 75, 79
    synovial, 75, 79
Juvenile rheumatoid arthritis (JRA), 90

K

Kaposi sarcoma (KS), 156, 158, 159
Keratin, 57
Kidney, ureter, bladder (KUB), 235
Kidneys, 220, 222, 224, 226
Kneecap (patella), 76
Kyphosis, 86

L

Labia majora, 250, 252
Labia minora, 250, 252
Laceration, 61
Lacrimal bones, 80
Lacrimal canals, 320, 321
Lacrimal glands, 318, 320, 321
Lacrimal sac, 320, 321
Lactate dehydrogenase (LDH), 112, 119
Laparoscope, 262
Large intestine, 196, 199, 200
Larynx, 343
    combining form, 345
    combining form meaning, 345
    function of, 341